This book delivers a rare first-person account of international research by an African scientist. It is a book about experiments, by medical researchers facing a terrible plague, by an ambitious man in post-colonial Kenya, and by an anthropologist looking for new ways to narrate stories about African science. Davy Kiprotich Koech bravely recalled his memories of a sometimes controversial life in interviews with Denielle Elliott. Elliott's sensitive framing of Koech's testimony offers critical insight into the politics of knowledge in Africa, of power in Kenya, and of the ways that stories make selves.

Nancy J. Jacobs, Professor of History, Brown University, author of *Birders of Africa: History of a Network* (Yale 2016)

Stories attest to the profoundly relational nature of human experience and achievement. With these engaging tales from the life of one of Kenya's most prominent scientists, Denielle Elliott's book reveals the intricate web of relationship and heritage through which postcolonial citizens here and elsewhere pursue knowledge, negotiate statecraft, and navigate the promises and pitfalls of transcontinental connection.

Anand Pandian, Johns Hopkins University

Reimagining Science and Statecraft in Postcolonial Kenya

This book examines the development of medical sciences in postcolonial Kenya, through the adventures and stories of the controversial Kalenjin scientist Davy Kiprotich Koech. As a collaborative life story project, it privileges African voices and retellings, re-centring the voice of African scientists from the peripheries of storytelling about science, global health research collaborations, national politics, international geopolitical alliances, and medical research.

Focusing largely on the development of the Kenya Medical Research Institute (KEMRI) and its collaborations with the US Centers for Disease Control, the Walter Reed Project, Japan's International Cooperation Agency, the Wellcome Trust, and other international partners, Denielle Elliott and Davy Koech challenge euro-dominant representations of African science and global health in both the contemporary and historical and offer an unconventional account which aims to destabilize colonial and neo-colonial narratives about African science, scientists, and statecraft. The stories force readers to contend with a series of questions including: How do imperial effects today shape contemporary medical research and national sovereignty? In which ways do the colonial ghosts of early medical research infuse the struggles of postcolonial scientists to build national scientific projects? How were postcolonial nation-building projects tied up with the dreams and visions of African scientists? And lastly, how might we reimagine African medicine and biosciences?

The monograph will be of interest to students, educators, and scholars working in African Studies, Science and Technology Studies, Postcolonial Studies, Global Health, Cultural Anthropology, and Medical Anthropology.

Denielle Elliott is an Associate Professor in the Departments of Social Science and Anthropology at York University in Toronto, Canada with cross-appointments in the graduate programs of International Development Studies, and Science, Technology and Studies. She is a founder and co-curator of the Centre for Imaginative Ethnography, and writes on questions relating to social suffering, colonialism, morality, and the politics of medicine.

Routledge Contemporary Africa Series

The Development of African Capital Markets
A Legal and Institutional Approach
Boniface Chimpango

China, Africa and Responsible International Engagement
Yanzhuo Xu

Joke-Performance in Africa
Mode, Media and Meaning
Edited by Ignatius Chukwumah

The Media and Aid in Sub-Saharan Africa
Whose News?
Lena von Naso

Political Culture, Change, and Security Policy in Nigeria
Kalu N. Kalu

African Science Education
Gendering Indigenous Knowledge in Nigeria
Jamaine Abidogun

Power in Contemporary Zimbabwe
Edited by Erasmus Masitera and Fortune Sibanda

Unfolding Narratives of Ubuntu in Southern Africa
Edited by Julian Müller, John Eliastam and Sheila Trahar

Reimagining Science and Statecraft in Postcolonial Kenya
Stories from an African Scientist
Denielle Elliott with Davy Kiprotich Koech

Food Security for Rural Africa
Feeding the Farmers First
Terry Leahy

Reimagining Science and Statecraft in Postcolonial Kenya

Stories from an African Scientist

Denielle Elliott
with Davy Kiprotich Koech

Routledge
Taylor & Francis Group
LONDON AND NEW YORK

First published 2019
by Routledge
2 Park Square, Milton Park, Abingdon, Oxon OX14 4RN

and by Routledge
711 Third Avenue, New York, NY 10017

Routledge is an imprint of the Taylor & Francis Group, an informa business

British Library Cataloguing-in-Publication Data
A catalogue record for this book is available from the British Library

Library of Congress Cataloging-in-Publication Data
Names: Elliott, Denielle A. (Denielle Aschell), author. | Koech, D. K. (Davy Kiprotich), author.
Title: Reimagining science and statecraft in postcolonial Kenya : stories from an African scientist / Denielle Elliott with Davy Kiprotich Koech.
Other titles: Routledge contemporary Africa series.
Description: New York : Routledge, 2018. | Series: Routledge contemporary Africa series
Identifiers: LCCN 2018018226| ISBN 9781138059122 (hardback) | ISBN 9781315163840 (ebook) | ISBN 9781351672351 (mobipocket)
Subjects: LCSH: Koech, D. K. (Davy Kiprotich) | Kenya Medical Research Institute–History. | Medicine–Research–Kenya–History. | Scientists–Kenya–Biography. | Medical research personnel–Kenya–Biography.
Classification: LCC R854.K4 E45 2018 | DDC 610.92/26762–dc23
LC record available at https://lccn.loc.gov/2018018226

ISBN: 978-1-138-05912-2 (hbk)
ISBN: 978-1-315-16384-0 (ebk)

Typeset in Times New Roman
by Wearset Ltd, Boldon, Tyne and Wear

Contents

Illustrations

Figures

Preface

This project presented itself to me rather accidentally. I first heard a story about Davy Koech in 2006 in Vancouver's Downtown Eastside. During research for my doctoral studies, I sat in an urban health clinic in Vancouver, observing the clinical interactions between an HIV/AIDS specialist and his patients; in between patient visits, the AIDS doctor and I made awkward small talk. I mentioned to him that I had applied for a postdoctoral position in Kenya, to continue my research focusing on the relations between AIDS science and postcolonialism. As it turned out, the doctor had lived in Nairobi for four years researching sexually transmitted infections and HIV. In fact, Canadian medical research has a long history of research in Kenya, most notably as part of the University of Manitoba Medical Microbiology program, starting in the 1970s. As we sat there waiting for a patient to arrive he told me about the AIDS in Africa conference that he had attended in October 1990 in Kinshasa, then Zaire, now the DRC, and recounted the following story to me. In a session chaired by James Curran, the former HIV/AIDS Division Director for the US Centers for Disease Control and Prevention (CDC), Davy Koech, a senior researcher from the Kenya Medical Research Institute (KEMRI), claimed that orally administered interferon, or Kemron, was a "miracle drug" that eliminated HIV from patients entirely. According to this AIDS specialist in the Downtown Eastside, Koech stated that they had conducted a clinical trial with 200 HIV-positive patients and found that opportunistic infections had been remarkably cured. Koech's presentation was followed by a standing ovation and applause, and then a cynical comment by Curran, who suggested that if the results were true, Koech and his colleagues had just saved the world from a horrible epidemic. Immediately there were protests from the audience and someone quickly stood up and suggested that Curran was only sceptical because he thought that Africans were not capable of producing leading scientific discoveries. These counter-accusations of racism resulted in a mass exodus, with the African researchers leaving the conference.

This story often gets repeated and interpreted as a story about a "pseudo-cure" African corruption, and the inadequacy of African science. Koech was cast as a scientific fraud, trying to pass a fake clinical trial or at the very least a failed clinical trial-off for financial profit, and perhaps fame. The story stayed with me and slowly I started to investigate the Kemron controversy while I pursued research on medical science, pharmaceutical clinical trials, and transnational collaborations in Kenya. I met Koech in 2007 as I started fieldwork in Kenya for a postdoctoral project at the London School of Hygiene and Tropical Medicine. It was a brief meeting at his office in Nairobi. Eventually, a few years later, I asked Koech if he might be willing to share his stories about his life's work with me, and he agreed, though I think somewhat hesitantly. These are *his* stories and offer important insights into the creation and maintenance of scientific infrastructure in Kenya and the making of African scientists in postcolonial East Africa.

In collaboration with Koech, this project reframes a series of events, moments, and stories in his life to consider what his own personal story of scientific accomplishments and political controversies might tell us more generally about postcolonial state making and the history of medical science in East Africa (Wendland 2008). My goal then is to disrupt the ways in which African science and African scientists are imagined by examining the stories left untold, and by taking seriously contradictions and inconsistencies in the stories conveyed. I present memories, photographs, stories – all fragments – in an effort to offer an alternative rendering of history, one that challenges the typical discourses of medical science, African history, and national politics.

Koech is a central actor in medical science today as becomes clear in his stories. From the 1979 Science and Technology Act revisions that made KEMRI and all the other research institutions in Kenyan possible, to the Kericho and Kisii Hospitals, to the international collaborations with the Wellcome Trust, CDC, and the Japanese International Cooperation Agency, Koech is there, if unseen as a "public servant" as he refers to himself. But he is also a vital, if hidden, agent in national politics and state building. He was Daniel arap Moi's ally and adopted kin. He was a political strategist for him, working in Youth for KANU '92, and on his 1997 election. Koech had a significant impact on Kenya's scientific infrastructure and educational policy as he worked to secure funding for KEMRI, build a national laboratory system at the Division of Vector-Borne Diseases, created international collaborations for tropical medicine and infectious disease research, chaired the Commission into Education in Kenya, and shaped global health as we know it today. It is puzzling how he has been eclipsed in the various accounts of Kenya's history – both in politics and medical science. Except as I mentioned earlier – he is a very private and reticent man in many ways. Koech's life story is both a story of an individual scientist and a story of postcolonial infrastructure development, national politics, international relations, and African science-in-the-making. Its limitations lie in the fact that it is just one man's story, one carefully articulated, cautiously told, and deeply guarded.

As a life story project, this book is inherently and deeply a collaborative project. This project wouldn't be possible without the collaboration of Davy Kiprotich Koech and his willingness to share his stories with me over the past five years. He has been open to a critical reading of his life, one that at times must have been difficult to digest. This openness and willingness to engage in such critical work of one's self and one's work has been very courageous. I am truly thankful to him for allowing me to pursue this project and for his time and trust in sharing all the stories presented here (and the many that have been left out). He has not always agreed with my interpretation of events, or my framing of his story, but I do hope that he is happy with the final product.

There are many other people who have helped me with this project, some directly, others indirectly. I am grateful to a number of research associates whose assistance in archival research, transcription, translation, and other work made this monograph possible include Philister Madiega, Wangui Kimari, Patrick Mbullo, Kui Moko, Douglas Okelloh, and especially Victor Olago. Douglas Okelloh and Victor Olago both worked on transcribing the oral interviews into written form, and did so with precise detail. This is tiresome and time-consuming work that is also the essence of life story projects. I am indebted for their dedication and commitment to this work.

In Kenya there are many friends who over the past five years have helped me understand the larger political and scientific landscapes of Kenya and made visits to Kenya enjoyable with dinners and adventures. They include Ciru Muthiora, Nyakienda Muthiora, Moses Ndiritu, Isaac Okero, and especially Timothy Thomas. I also want to thank Stanley and Lorna Muthiora for their hospitality in Nairobi and making me feel like family.

Over the years I have had many formal and informal conversations with those working in epidemiology or medicine in East Africa who offered their time to talk to me about some of the stories recounted here, especially the Kemron clinical trial. I am grateful to Frank Plummer, Allan Ronald, James Curran, Robert Bailey, Stephen Moses, Mark Tyndall, Sam Gwer, Michael Mwaniki, and Walter Obiero Ochieng for sharing insights (sometimes very contradictory) on HIV research, the Kemron events of 1989–1990, and the history of scientific research more generally in Kenya.

Nancy Jacobs, Leslie Robertson, Noelle Mole, Priscilla Song, Elsa Fan, Kirsten Bell, Julie Cruikshank, Maurice Wallace, Anand Pandian all in very different ways have stimulated my thinking on life stories. I cannot thank Vitor Barros enough for being so gracious and generous with feedback during the writing stages of this project. His idea of "cinematic storytelling" shaped the entire organization of the book. Vitor, along with Jo-anne Roe, Deb Neill, Walter Ochieng, and Dara Culhane, all read drafts of the introductory chapter and provided crucial feedback. And yet, all errors remain my sole responsibility.

As a PhD student, my then doctoral supervisor offered a piece of advice that I now pass on to my own PhD students – sometimes you'll come across an idea, an object, some *thing* in the field that you find deeply interesting which sort of just sticks with you. When that happens, she said, don't let go of it; you may return to it one day and find it far more interesting than the thing you started out with. Koech and Kemron is very much that *thing* that I heard about in the field that I thought curious but was not a part of the research plans. And so I thank her, Stacy Leigh Pigg, for this sage advice. And I am equally indebted to Mark Tyndall who first shared the story of Davy Koech's Kemron presentation in Kinshasa with me.

I owe gratitude too to Claire Wendland and Rebecca Warne-Peters for organizing the American Anthropology Association annual conference session on "Studying Up" in 2013 where I first dared to present this material, and to Stacy Langwick, one of our discussants, for important feedback. I wasn't sure then if I was going to take on this project but they were encouraging. Without that encouragement, I doubt I would have pursued this. I would also like to thank my colleagues at York University's Tubman Institute – especially, Deb Neill, Annie Bunting, Uwa Idemudia, and Michele Johnson – where I presented a paper on the Kemron controversy on one very wintery day in 2016. Their commitment to staying on campus as a winter storm blew in and their honest yet gentle critiques are appreciated. I would also like to thank Alexandrine Boudreault-Fournier who organized an opportunity for me to present this material for the Department of Anthropology's Seminar Series at the University of Victoria. I also received important feedback from the Department of Sociology and Anthropology's graduate seminar SA840 at Simon Fraser University.

Erin Martineau, a skilled editor, helped me organize the introduction into something coherent. Claire Bell assisted with copyediting at a later stage and I appreciate her gentle approach to maintaining the voice of Koech throughout the narrative. Lina Beatriz Pinto Garcia stimulated my thinking on tropical medicine, colonialism and unstable fieldwork sites. I am also beholden to Mackie Chase who helped me work through multiple writing challenges during walks through Galiano Island's temperate rainforest and comforting meals at her home while I was on sabbatical.

Dara Culhane has been a mentor, colleague, and friend since 1999 and has, with immense generosity, shared ideas, feedback, her time, and has always pushed me to be reflective, critical, and to take seriously the stories of our interlocutors. I could never repay her for the enormous amount of intellectual generosity she has shown me. I feel so very privileged to have had a chance to learn from her and to work with her now as a colleague.

Lastly, I want to thank Leanne Hinves, the African Studies series editor at Routledge Press, whose invitation to publish this work made it all possible.

The art of storytelling/stories of science

An introduction

All stories are, in a sense, untrue.

(Michael Jackson 2013: 16)

What if the truth is not so much a secret as a public secret, as is the case with most important social knowledge, *knowing what not to know*?

(Michael Taussig 1999: 2)

The art of storytelling

This is a story of a scientist and the postcolonial state, tracing the accomplishments and controversies in the life and work of Davy Kiprotich Koech. In 1974, Koech was a 23-year-old university graduate in a recently independent Kenya, the first African to be hired at the World Health Organization's Immunology

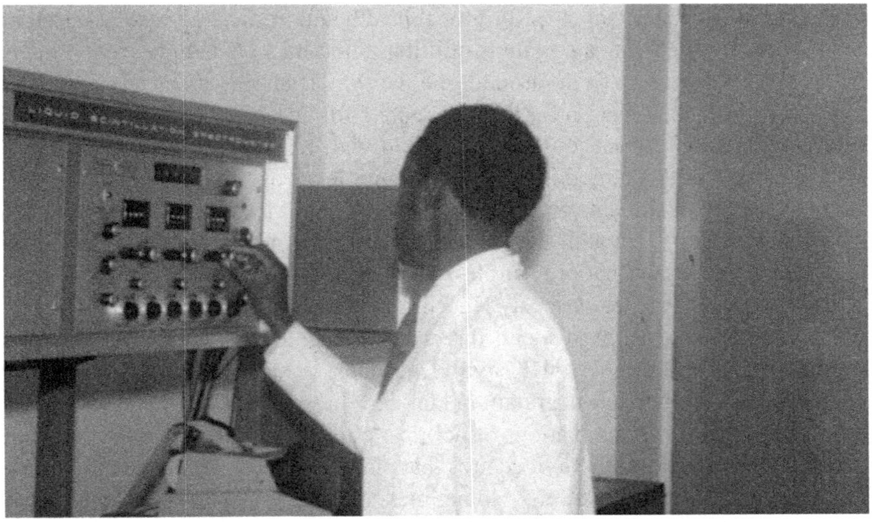

Figure 0.1 Davy Koech 1974 at the WHO Centre in Nairobi.

Research and Training Centre at the University of Nairobi and the first African researcher hired by the Wellcome Trust Research Program in Kenya (see Figure 0.1). It was an exciting time of new possibilities for Kenyans, but it was also a time of political challenges as the new nation figured out a way forward after decades of colonialism. Davy Koech grew up poor in the rural highlands near Kericho, to a father who had worked for the British as a surveyor and then colonial chief. His father saw the value in the British colonial education system and Christian ways, and he encouraged Koech from a very young age to embrace these ideals. Koech easily took to education, excelled in his studies, and managed to find his way to study science at the University of Nairobi. Later he took up graduate studies as a Fulbright-Hays scholar pursuing a Master of Science and then a PhD, while studying at schools in the United States (US), including at Harvard School of Medicine. He returned to Kenya to help shape national scientific policy and infrastructure through an industrious professional life which included holding prominent positions at the Kenya Medical Research Institute, the Division of Vector-Borne Diseases, and the University of Nairobi's School of Medicine; working as a scientist specializing in immunology and molecular medicine; and functioning as an informal political strategist and close ally to former President Daniel arap Moi. He emerged as part of a new intellectual elite in postcolonial Kenya.

In 1989–1990, a young Koech attracted the attention of global scientists, international press, and AIDS activists when he announced favourable results for a clinical trial that he and colleague Arthur Obel were conducting on a drug that became known as Kemron. Controversy emerged as rumours and erroneous stories circulated about the drug, Koech as a scientist, and the claims made about the effectiveness of the drug. This controversy stained his reputation, though he continued to work towards shaping the Kenya Medical Research Institute into one of the most important sites for global health and tropical disease research in Sub-Saharan Africa, managing multi-million-dollar budgets with nearly 60 international collaborators from around the world. Then in 2007 an American working in Atlanta, Georgia for the US Centers for Disease Control reported that funds were missing from joint accounts held with KEMRI. Koech was accused and then criminally charged in 2009 with multiple accounts of fraud, and he lost his position as the Director of KEMRI that he had held for nearly 22 years.

In this life story account, the reader hears directly from Koech, a man relatively unknown in international circles, but infamous in global HIV research. In so doing, this book takes seriously Koech's story as an African scholar, scientist, public servant, and authority with direct knowledge of statecraft and scientific infrastructure development in Kenya. This book is also an inside look at the clandestine meetings and negotiations among elite political actors, giving us a glimpse of the inner machinations of political power that were necessary to build the labs, hospitals, and research centres that many Western nations rely on today. Such complex webs of power – sometimes suspicious, sometimes unlawful – have been eclipsed in most anthropological accounts of global health or medical science in Kenya, of which there have been many.[1] Koech's stories unveil the entanglements of political violence, international geopolitics, ethnic patronage, and medical research, tracing them from his work as a student leader at Strathmore College, to his training at Duquesne and Harvard, to his involvement with the political youth group YK' 92, to the criminal charges of corruption that remain pending today in 2018.

African science studies

There are many accounts of African science and medicine, many of which are also critical of problematic discourses about Africa and Africans, but rarely do we hear directly from the scientists or medical practitioners themselves. This book addresses that gap by highlighting the intellectual projects of Africans who, in the early years of independence, worked to develop and Africanize science, medicine, and technology in their countries in innovative ways.[2] Koech's narrative makes it clear he does not see himself as a victim of racist practices or discriminatory policies in transnational science, instead he holds culpable an unfair national judicial system and the questionable practices of the Ethics and Anti-Corruption Commission (Mavhunga 2017). Koech manipulated, subverted, and at other times complied with the Kenyan state and foreign partners. He boasts proudly of his achievements in developing the national laboratory system, creating collaborative research agreements with leading global health agencies, and protecting his Kenyan employees through human resource policies meant to create equity and guarantee employment in spite of the international pressures of structural adjustment programs and aid embargos. And in spite of the controversies and rumours around Kemron, he also clearly identifies himself as a scientist who has made significant contributions to the fields of immunology, organ transplantation, HIV, and tropical medicine more generally.

Koech demanded, rightly so, that this be a project about him as African scientist, scholar, and civil servant and his role as a critical agent in creating the infrastructure necessary for medical research in Kenya. By privileging his words and his voice here, I seek to address the lack of African accounts of African science and politics (Mavhunga 2017). I hope the book will make an important contribution to the growing field of African (postcolonial) science studies, a field that takes seriously Africans as active agents who have developed and strengthened the fields of medicine, science, and technology in their own right, not as individuals who have simply imported Western science and biomedicine, or had their "capacity" developed by Western institutions, funding, and educational opportunities.[3] The book also builds on critical historical analyses of colonial and imperial science in development and nation building (Tilley 2011); German medical researchers and the development of tropical medicine in East Africa (Neill 2012); the training of African medical doctors in Malawi's medical schools (Wendland 2010); East African rumours about colonial medical personnel and the theft of blood (White 2000); and the construction of "the African" through colonial biomedical discourses (Vaughan 1991). Such work has been critical to our understanding of colonial and imperial actors, institutions, and practices in Africa, but there remains a lacuna of work that focuses on African scientists, science, medicine, and technological innovation.

The stories Koech shared with me highlight the secret deals, political manoeuvring, and bureaucratic work behind the building of this critical infrastructure. Koech witnessed and helped shape the transition from a colonial system of medicine and science, governed by the British, to a system of research governed and administered by educated Kenyans, though still largely funded and controlled by external powers. In his story, which spans more than 60 years, we see the entanglements of national ethnic politics, international policies on aid, the complicity of Western states in repressive African governance, and the global health funding apparatus. In 2012, the Kenya Medical Research Institute managed an annual budget of close to five billion KES, or US$57 million, working with partners from nearly 60 different organizations, including the Gates Foundation, Pfizer Pharmaceuticals, PATH, the Global Alliance Against TB, the WHO, and the US Embassy. The work of the Wellcome Trust, the US CDC, and university partners like Liverpool, Oxford, Manitoba, Chicago, Texas, Duke, and so many more, could not have been done without the extensive medical and scientific infrastructure that exists in Kenya. Though often discussed in the context of "global" health, these collaborations are also situated within national scientific projects that involve African scientists, politicians, and workers, all of whom make these larger global health projects possible. As Nancy Rose Hunt reminds her readers, "Global health operations in Africa today … are the new present in relation to which most of us now write; and this fact alone has implications for how we conceptualize and cast our historical work" (Hunt 2013: 11). Koech's stories help us understand the politics of such a landscape.

Drawing on documents that Koech provided, as well as more than 100 hours of interviews with the man himself, archival research, and other interviews, the book delves deeply into the context of Koech's life story, encompassing Kenyan's political independence, national politics, his academic and career aspirations, and the deeply personal tragedies that affected him and his family. While his story is largely one about science and postcolonial state projects, it is also a book about the tensions and antagonisms in collecting and curating life stories. I present photographs, newspaper articles, documents, narrated memories, and stories – all fragments – here in an effort to offer an alternate rendering of history, one that challenges the typical discourses of medical science, African history, and Kenyan politics. I do not wish to suggest that Koech's account is a more "accurate" or "authentic" history of medical science or statecraft in postcolonial Kenya, but rather I present it simply as an alternative African account that might problematize Western accounts of Kemron and Koech given by folks like Peter Piot (2012),[4] scholars writing about East African politics or African science, and of course the AIDS doctor from Vancouver, Canada who first conveyed the story to me (as conveyed in the preface) (Yoshimizu 2015). Following the lead of anthropologist Michael Jackson, my main goal here as an anthropologist is to neither try nor exonerate Koech but to explore "the ways in which people struggle against disadvantages of their circumstances and recover from the adversities of their histories" (2013b: 21). Jackson explains further: "Knowing why things happen, or judging people for the errors of their ways, is thus less important than trying to understand how, in the face of hardship, human beings still find life worth living, and endure" (ibid.), or as Koech poignantly reflects at one point, decide to give up. I want readers to see his life stories of struggle and triumph within larger networks of power, privilege, and political histories which speak to a larger set of questions that scholars are asking about the effects of colonialism, the politics of aid and development, and contemporary geopolitics. My approach is to prioritize the social and political aspects of Koech's life as a way to offer deeper insight into the controversies, and the quotidian work of building and sustaining scientific infrastructure. The value of his personal story, in part, is not that it declares his innocence or exposes his guilt, but that it is representational of a larger collective of scientists, civil servants, and policy makers in postcolonial Africa (Jackson 2013b).

Koech offers untold stories that are a critical piece of Kenya's history. In his telling of his life's work, Koech indirectly raises, and sometimes addresses, a number of questions: How were postcolonial nation-building projects tied up with the dreams and aspirations of African scientists? How do imperial effects continue to shape contemporary medical research and national sovereignty? How did the colonial ghosts of early medical research and politics haunt the struggles of postcolonial scientists trying to build national scientific projects? What do accusations of corruption and fraud tell us about colonial imaginaries and racial logics in contemporary scientific collaborations?

The truth?

When I first made the decision to work on this project after hearing the Kemron story, many colleagues in Kenya, whom I had come to know through my work on medical research and clinical trials, discouraged me, insisting Koech would never tell me "the truth". And during our many hours of interviews, Koech insisted repeatedly that he was telling me "the truth" and he would provide documents to "prove" his account was truthful. My approach here is to think of all stories as partial always unfolding and evolving (Clifford 1986). I am not only thinking in terms of Koech's stories, but all those that circulate in Kenya and in global health circles about him, including anthropological, other scholarly, and scientific stories. They are all partial stories, reflective of a brief moment, as too are Koech's.

Michael Jackson suggests that all histories and stories are "in a sense, untrue" (2013a: 16). As a point of departure, this project takes a particular cautious approach to "the truth", highlighting instead the "vexed and unstable contrasts between truth and untruth" (Jackson 2013b: 45). Koech's stories reveal the ways in which the act of storytelling allows narrators to "rework reality in order to make it bearable" (Jackson 2013b: 36). I started to think about the stories here – those from Koech but also all those other stories told by people who think they know what happened, or think they know Koech, including some anthropologists, historians, and political scientists writing about Kenya – as *intractable*. Slippery, fractured, contradictory, sometimes debatable. In a sense then, there are parallel projects within this book: Koech is telling a story about Kenyan politics, his life's work as a scientist and state actor, and his role in establishing Kenya as a preferred site for both bioscientific research and population health programs (especially for maternal health and against HIV and malaria). But the book is also a methodological reflection on epistemologies of memory, storytelling, and ethnographic accountability. Influenced by the work of Ruth Behar, this life story offers "a double telling", with both Koech and I narrators and readers, though in very different ways (1990: 224). Some may doubt Koech's account of history, and accuse him of distortion, exaggeration, or evasion. Like all stories, his are partial, fragmented, and incomplete. And some may read them as simply biographical, a man attempting to (re)write his own history, to redeem his reputation in science and politics, to leave a legacy. But his stories are also stories of science-in-the-making and the work of building infrastructure among the ruins left behind by the British after Kenya's independence in 1963.

Behar (1990) prefers the designation of "life story" over "life history" for the way in which story underscores the "fictions" or the "colour" that a narrator adds in their telling of their life, the exaggerations and edits. The process of remembering has the effect of blurring fact and fiction, truth and falsehoods. Writing life stories forces us to think about how we remember our past. Psychologists like Daniel Schacter (2013) suggest that memories are biased because of our emotions and that they are fundamentally "constructive processes", and thus by nature remembering includes forgetting, confabulation, and distortion. Memory, Portelli also explains, is "an on going process of elaboration and re\construction of meaning" (2005: 5). This reality, along with understanding that storytelling is a way for humans to make order of a disordered world (Behar 1990), may lead some to an epistemological scepticism for life story projects.

Filmmaker Tim Burton addresses the problems in storytelling in his film *Big Fish* (2003), which speaks directly to how humans use storytelling to make sense of our lives and how we rearrange the events in our lives to make ourselves sometimes seem like "big fish" or the "big man". It is a story of son, William Bloom, who returns home to see his dying father Edward, who has spent his life telling tall tales to his son. William is desperate to make sense of the truth amidst all the stories and colourful characters and crazy adventures his father has told him. It is only at his father's death that William realizes that the stories *are* his father. Though at times rearranged, at other times exaggerated, the stories are true; they're just better versions of his life. As with Davy Koech, telling stories of great exploits and pursuits all the while leaves the man somewhat unknown. Edward is never portrayed as someone being dishonest or deceitful, and at his funeral all the wild characters of his stories show up to pay their respects. William eventually realizes the gift his father has given him, adopting the storytelling practice as he says good-bye to his father at his deathbed. In this framing of stories, misremembering is equally important in a radical retelling. But rather than proving the falsity of such memories, I consider exaggerations and misunderstandings as another part of the story. Even erroneous, fragmented stories give critical insight into the politics of science and nation building; they also reveal experiences hiding in the shadows.

Speaking for others

> Even the best ethnographic texts – serious, true fictions – are systems, or economies, of truth.
>
> (James Clifford 1986: 7)

"There is no one you can trust," said Koech to me, in response to my question that he must trust Caleb Atemi, a Kenyan biographer, with whom he had partnered to write his biography. His lament reminded me that anthropological fieldwork and the monographs we produce demand a profound level of confidence from our interlocutors and rely on the relationships we form in the field. From the beginning of this project I realized I was asking a fair amount of Koech. He had gone from being Moi's close ally and friend, leading the country's medical research institution, and holding many other key roles, to a man whose home was searched and properties seized, who was arrested in public and lost his job, and who was then shunned by friends and colleagues. I was asking him to trust me with his stories even though I was a stranger. Writing and editing another's stories is an enormous responsibility, and anthropologists have crafted an entire discipline based on this practice. We collect stories and then retell them for larger audiences, hoping they convey more than just fragments of one person's life. But there are multitudes of ways to share such stories. As a student in the 1990s, I found the poetic stories and songs of the Bedouin women in Lila Abu-Lughod's (2008[1993]) work, the Athapaskan and Tlingit elders of Julie Cruikshank's (1991) research, and the story of Esperanza, the Mexican peddler of Ruth Behar's (2014[1994]) research compelling for their intimacy and honesty, and for the carefulness of the anthropologists' prose. They offered a different type of anthropology – one that did not assume the role of the anthropologist was to "interpret" the lives of others. Their work, along with many others since, showed that many of our interlocutors and research participants are critical theorists of their own lives and the larger contexts in which they live and work.[5] Of life stories, a genre of ethnographic writing, Behar (1990) explains that it offers novel and creative ways to think about the relationship between theory and stories. I like the life story format for the subtle way in which theory is conveyed, rather than spelling out positions and debates in capital letters, or inaccurately imposing interpretations of the stories. Or, in Hannah Arendt's words, "narration reveals the meaning without committing the error of defining it" (Arendt 1979: 169, cited in Cavarero 1997: 3).[6]

There are multiple sorts of storytelling going on here. There are the stories people tell about Koech, KEMRI, and Kemron, and all the stories about politics, corruption, and the everyday work of science both within and without Kenya.

Then there are the stories that Koech has shared with me over a span of five years. And lastly there are the stories that I am retelling or creating, sometimes re-purposing, as I make sense of all these other stories. Jackson (2013a) sees storytelling as a strategy, used to account for that which is often lost in conventional social histories or biographies: the accidental, blurred, and imagined, and that which disturbs, disrupts, and distracts. His approach to storytelling and memory helps to destabilize histories that privilege particular regimes of truth, especially those of Western scientific thought. Stories can transform both the storyteller and the audience (or listener and reader); they can create a space for agency and help us recover "a sense of ourselves as actors and agents in the face of experiences that make us feel insignificant, unrecognized or powerless" (Jackson 2013b: 17). I sense this is an important part of the project for Koech, a "restorative praxis" in telling his stories (Jackson 2013b: 23). As one can see from the different chapter lengths, there were particular issues that Koech spent a great amount of time discussing. He retold certain stories – of 2007 when he was forced to leave his position at KEMRI and the 2009 arrest – over and over again even though I had audio-recordings of the stories. The minor details sometimes changed in those stories over the five years we worked together but the overall surprise and frustration that he voiced never faded.

Storytelling can transform a superficial caricature (a "fraudulent scientist") into a complicated, paradoxical person with an impassioned and entangled life; it can humanize scientists who have been flattened by sound bites and newspaper headlines (Fassin 2008). I hope in Koech's stories readers will see not only the political agent for Moi but also the grieving father, the Christian who feels abandoned by his community of faith, the young scientist trying to make it in a competitive global world, and that his life was shaped by the larger landscape that he was trying to navigate. Jackson argues, "human action always involves more than a singular subject; it occurs within fields of *inter*action", with states, with collaborators from other nations and transnational agencies, with political actors and other allies within Kenya (2013b: 18). Jackson draws on the theoretical insights of Hannah Arendt, as does the other scholar who is helping me make sense of the genre and method of life story, Adriana Cavarero. What I like about Cavarero is that she theorizes life stories and narration as a form of political action and she emphasizes its relationality (Cavarero 1997: xxiii). She explains, "Exposed, relational and contextual, the Arendtian self leaves behind a life story that is constitutively interwoven with many other stories" (1997: 124). That is true of all the stories Koech tells. We can only understand the stories of Koech in relation to the larger politics of the nation, the story of Moi, and myself as his interlocutor. Stories emerge in a multitude of relational contexts and "within webs of interlocution" (Lucas 2017: n.p.). As well, his actions and the decisions he makes are also relational. That is, they emerge out of real and imagined conversations and debates with others, guided by certain moral judgments, moral imperatives, social opportunities, and political necessity. Jackson reminds us that,

> Because our lives unfold in the indeterminate or potential space between ourselves and others, our original intentions are often confounded and our assumed identities eclipsed, leading us to do things we did not think we had it in us to do, and obliging us to constantly rethink the very notion of who we are.
>
> (2013a: 18)[7]

Yet, the stories circulating about Koech, or Kemron, or KEMRI, or even the nation itself, tend to eclipse the relational character of lives and stories. This is especially apparent when contrasted with the stories Koech recounts about Kemron, the *Saba Saba* demonstrations of 1990, and the interference by the Permanent Secretary of internal security, which all illustrate how relational the Kemron events were.

I offer this introduction as a sort of road map for readers who may not have detailed knowledge of Kenyan politics or who may not be familiar with the academic debates about the use of life stories. The introduction works as an "act of mediation" on the life story (Behar 1990: 224); the stories are Koech's, the argument is mine (Tomaselli 2003), and this introduction situates the two. The danger of such an introduction is that it may seem to undermine Koech's telling of his life story, replacing his African voice with just another non-African, academic telling. This is not my intention. Koech's stories are compelling, revealing, and critical in their own right. Some readers may wish to skip the introduction and go straight to Chapter 1.

A scientific biography

Koech has plans to write a biography and we often talked about the difference between this project and what his biography might look like. In our many discussions I continually framed this as a "scholarly life story project", the sort of project that is common for anthropologists (as discussed). Yet, I also envision this as a sort of scientific biography, one that, in the tradition of science and technology studies, highlights the desires, dreams, and failures of an African scientist trying to negotiate multiple, overlapping fields of power: kin relations and responsibilities, a personal wish to be a respected national and international scientist, political alliances to Moi and Moi's family, and a desire to build a world-class system of scientific research that would benefit his fellow East African citizens, all the while attempting to achieve his own professional aspirations. In contrast with more mainstream biographies like that by Andrew Morton (1998) or Caleb Atemi (Musyoka and Atemi 2016), scientific biographies situate the life's work of a scientist in relation to their field and the concepts they developed (see those of Barbara McClintock (Keller 1983), Stephen Hawking (Mialet 2012), and Warren McCulloch (Abraham 2016)). They are not so much biographies of individuals as they are biographies of epistemologies and of new scientific fields, as well as accounts of the entanglements of politics, culture, economics, and science (Nye 2006; Porter 2006).

But this is not the usual scientific biography. Though the book is imperfect in that it is "like all scientific biographies, just a snapshot taken from a particular vantage point in a much larger historical vista of ever-changing science and lives within it" (Richards 2006: 303), it unveils critical stories, including a very different version of the Kemron drug trial and insights into Koech's private relationship with Moi. As a boy, Koech often had to sleep in barns, he went hungry during his elementary and middle school years, was impoverished at college and university, who then became an elite, Harvard-educated scientist with extraordinary access and power. One of the things I find most compelling is how key political actors – including the head of Internal Security for Kenya Hezekiah Oyugi, US Ambassador Smith Hempstone, Texan veterinary scientist Joseph Cummins, or African American religious leaders and physicians – are imbricated in Koech's narrative of medicine and science in Kenya.

Yet if readers are expecting the inner workings of everyday science in Kenya's laboratories, like those in the tradition of Latour and Woolgar (1979), they will be disappointed. Koech spoke rarely about actual scientific practice, even though he has a PhD in Medical Pathology and Immunology and has authored or co-authored many scientific papers. One exception is presented in Chapter 9 where he reflects on the scientific research he participated in at Akademgorodok, in the former USSR. And then in Chapter 10, where he describes in detail his work in developing tissue-typing, which transformed live kidney transplants in Kenya. Though the book does not focus on the technicalities of science in his labs, they do tell us a great deal about the politics of science. Koech's stories give us a sense of the challenges African scholars and scientists have faced in being seen as intellectuals and preeminent scientists, and of the exclusionary practices that exist in so-called global health or transnational science (Mavhunga 2017). Koech was the first African employee of the WHO Immunology Research and Training Centre and first African scientist employed by the Wellcome Trust in Kenya. He and Moi both spoke about the strength and capacity of Africans to do their own scientific research and to develop world-class interventions. Koech's career and the building of KEMRI occurred at a time when many nations were focusing on the Africanization of science, medicine, and education, and when Kenya was developing national policy on the Kenyanization of medicine and science.

An inconvenient interlocutor

I admit here, with some embarrassment, that Koech was not the interlocutor that I expected. The collaborative research process we undertook forced me to reflect critically on a variety of assumptions: those I inherit from the disciplines that I work within (cultural anthropology, African Studies, and science and technology studies), those that are shaped by my own politics, and those that come with being a foreigner doing research in a country that is not my own. As I recounted in the preface, I first heard about Koech when a colleague told me a story about the Kinshasa HIV/AIDS conference in 1990 that he had attended. At that conference Western scientists accused Koech of being a scientific fraud, leading to a divisive meeting between African and Western scientists. In 2007 more stories surfaced about him when he was forced to step aside as CEO of KEMRI after an employee from the United States Centers for Disease Control and Prevention accused him of misappropriating funds from their shared accounts. In both cases, Koech was being challenged and accused of being corrupt and unethical by Westerners. I thought such experiences would lead him to be critical of Western interventions, the legacy of colonial scientific projects, and the inherent discrimination and racism of contemporary global politics. I was wrong for the most part. Certainly, he did not offer the anti-colonial critiques I expected, nor did he rally against a neo-imperialist American agenda.

I came to this project through ethnographic research on the tensions inherent in transnational clinical trials being conducted in western Kenya by Americans, Canadians, and Europeans. I found these clinical trials to be problematic given the labour inequities inherent in such collaborations, racist practices in everyday work contexts, and the unintended consequences of such trials that further marginalize the very communities they aim to help (Elliott 2016). I imagined that Koech would also be critical of Kenya's and KEMRI's ties with the West, and of the reliance on funding from the Americans and British. Instead, he spoke about these collaborations with pride, and had only kind things to say of most of his counterparts at the American Embassy, the CDC, the Walter Reed Project, and the Wellcome Trust.

Koech refused to portray himself as a victim of colonial or neo-colonial projects, or as a passive agent in them. Rather, his stories of politics, negotiating aid, and setting up Kenyan's national system of medical research cast him as an active actor, manipulating international ambassadors, shifting the terrain of aid from foreign donors, and refusing to admit defeat. It is a narrative of triumph in the face of a lifetime of adversity. This is a life of strategic calculation, adopting Western projects when they benefited, and resisting or undermining when they did not. Koech speaks highly of his American comrades at the CDC even though he lost his job as a result of their accusations, and even though the criminal court case that could exonerate him has been stalled in the Kenyan judiciary since 2009. When others have suggested that the collaborative agreements between KEMRI and organizations like the Wellcome Trust that he set up sacrifice Kenyan workers for British foreign agendas, he defends these practices as being in place to protect Kenyan workers from inequitable salaries. He has fond memories of Kipng'eno Arap Ng'eny who his family proudly educated. Ng'eny was the first student at his father's school in Soliat, a man known in Kenya for being one of Moi's appointees, who was accused of mishandling funds, and then charged by the Kenya Anti-Corruption Commission in 2001 (Hornsby 2012). Koech recounts the brilliance of Carey Francis, the British mathematician who was known for believing Africans shouldn't receive advanced education and Kenyan independence had been rushed (Kareithi 2013). Koech also boasted proudly that he was known as the "Paramount" at the Meriada Garden's café, where we often met; the British, under colonial law, designated local African leaders as “paramount chiefs”.

Grace Musila reminds us that the postcolonial struggle for independence was not necessarily anti-colonial or anti-Western, but often it was “a case of being anti-colonial personnel but pro-colonial ideals and principles” (2015: 51). This is evident too in Koech’s narrative as he sometimes questions colonial authority, structures, and practices, and at other times embraces Western systems and agents. He lauds the British education system in Kenya, and at the same time challenges the myth of African inferiority, demanding he be recognized for “beating them” in their own schools. Recounting stories of his father’s concern for order, timeliness, and self-discipline, Koech shows how his father’s life and his own character have been shaped by British colonial values. His stories remind us that many contemporary African scientists and policy makers were born under colonial rule, went to schools run and taught by colonial actors, and grew up in a country where they were second-class citizens to white settlers. Colonialism as a structure and its historical racism, discrimination, and violence still clearly cast a shadow on the scenes of politics and medical science in Kenya.

Koech’s stories draw attention to the artificiality of such colonial/postcolonial binaries. Never does he speak of his or of Kenya’s history within these temporal (or political) designations. While they are not useful to how Koech orders his past, this is not to say that colonialism and colonial actors are not critical to his story: they very much shape the man he is today. More than 60 years later he recounted the shame he felt for being left-handed when colonial missionaries taught that it was sinful, and how as a young man he was chased by a white hotelier from Kericho’s Tea Hotel (a hotel he now owns majority shares in). I concur with Branch and Cheeseman that contemporary Kenya “presents an example of the manner in which the capacity and knowledge structures of government developed during colonial rule continue to shape the post-colonial state” (2006: 14). A careful reading of Koech’s stories makes visible the innocuous ways that British colonial values, practices, and knowledge continue to inform scientific infrastructure, education, and transnational collaborations in Kenya.

Koech is absent from scholarly histories of politics in Kenya. What can we make of his erasure or absence from political histories and histories of medical science in Kenya?[8] He explains that he worked to be an invisible actor behind Moi, declining political appointments in favour of working as a “public servant” in state science, and avoiding public outings or travel with Moi despite invitations to attend. But given his account of his influence on national leadership races (not only with Moi, but Mwai Kibaki and Jaramogi Oginga Odinga as well), his relationships with foreign ambassadors and international funding agencies (like helping convince the US to lift the aid embargo in the 1990s), and his connections among Kenya’s political elite, the absence of his name in histories of Kenyan politics is puzzling. Koech helped create a transnational scientific assemblage that has attracted thousands of researchers, millions of dollars in funding, and countless research projects from dozens of nations, demonstrating that the Kenya Medical Research Institute is a preferred site for public health, clinical, and epidemiological research. It is equally curious to see that his name is absent from studies of medical science in Kenya, given that he was an instrumental player in getting the Science and Technology Act amendment passed, which made all scientific research institutes in Kenya possible; his work advocating for funding from Moi to build the Kenya Medical Research Institute; and his leadership role there, not to mention his work with the World Health Organization, the Division of Vector-Borne Diseases, and the medical school at the University of Nairobi. How can we understand this absence? How can we make sense of these many acts of scholarship that erase such an agent of change and scientific development? Given the penchant for informal news, gossip, and rumour in Kenya, it seems doubtful that his omission and invisibility from scholarly accounts can be attributed to him "working behind the scenes" or his elusive character. After all, as I have noted elsewhere, many of the stories Koech told me were public knowledge, stories I had heard many times before (Elliott 2014). I suspect many readers will agree with me after reading his stories and wonder – how have these stories not been told yet? For they are fascinating, detailed, and genuine.

Given the many conversations I have had about Koech and his work – with Kenyan citizens and researchers, with global health scientists, and with anthropologists and historians who have provided feedback after reading drafts or hearing presentations – I have concluded that it is his role as an inconvenient interlocutor, an actor tainted by scandals and controversies and a relationship with Moi, that has made his story too embarrassing, too uncomfortable for us to tell. The messiness and contradictions of his stories, his connections to Moi and the violent regime of the Kenya African National Union (KANU), his alliances with Western agencies and actors, and Koech's effort to remain a hidden figure, made the story of his contributions to Kenyan science and statecraft too difficult to tell. Further, his story highlights that many international actors and states were complicit in the institutional arrangements that demanded, or made possible, Koech's acts.

Stories of science

On states and infrastructure

The everyday bureaucratic and scientific infrastructure of global health and transnational science is often overlooked, almost invisible. In stark contrast, Koech's life story centres the work of the KEMRI and the Kenyan state, as well as his work supporting these national projects, and thereby contributes a valuable perspective to our understanding of global health and tropical medicine research. One might get the impression from organizations working in Kenya and other newly developing nations that these countries lack the scientific infrastructure or "capacity" required for transnational science, that they require Western interventions to support, build, fund, mentor, and develop its citizens and its institutions. And though outside funding has certainly contributed to Kenya's scientific infrastructure (for instance, the impressive laboratory at the Kisian field station was strengthened with resources by the CDC or the facilities at the Kilifi research site), and offered Kenyan citizens new possibilities for training and work, such claims erase the histories of people like Koech and his many colleagues in politics, medicine, and science who worked to develop these institutions and collaborations, and the networks and alliances required for infrastructure. As Simone explains, "infrastructure configures specific engagement and circuits of exchange and attention", circuits negotiated largely by Koech in the realm of medical science (2012: n.p.). One of the reasons that KEMRI has such a large budget – nearly US$57 million – is because it has been a preferred site for research. Given the way the US government works, US researchers and institutions looking to do global health or tropical medicine research need to find collaborating nations with existing infrastructure. In Kisumu, Kenya, where I worked before starting this project, it was a common joke that the Lumumba research site buildings had been built with Canadian plywood. The Lumumba site was the location of the male circumcision trials, conducted by the University of Nairobi, University of Illinois-Chicago, and the University of Manitoba, among other interventions and studies. Historically, US funding could not be used for buildings or infrastructure development (exceptions include renovations), but Canadian funding could be, so US funds went to salaries, equipment, and other allowable expenses, and the Canadian funds were used to build structures. Such US aid and development policies therefore limit locations where US-funded research can be done; as Koech explained, "creative" negotiations around such policies are necessary. Koech's stories help us understand how these funding mechanisms work, and what sorts of symbolic and material exchanges are required as he negotiates international foreign aid regulations. His stories highlight the possibilities and the limitations of scientific infrastructure, the role of the Japanese, and the entanglements with geopolitical developments like the end of the Thatcher/Reagan era. As such, his stories also contribute to a reimagining of Kenyan science, state building, and the histories of medical institutions like KEMRI, the Division of Vector-Borne Diseases, and the Kericho and Kisii District Hospitals (Hunt 2013).

Whether it is land acquisitions, communication technology, laboratory construction, security systems, vehicles, licensing, or clinics and office buildings, many forms of infrastructure are necessary for contemporary scientific research. These have been oddly "invisible infrastructures" (De Boeck 2012) in anthropologies of medical science and global health research (exceptions include Umlauf and Park 2017), but Koech's stories of how he navigated global politics, foreign ambassadors, national politicians, and administrative hurdles bring infrastructures to the forefront again. He details the quotidian administrative, bureaucratic, and political choreography required to make it all happen, and the statecraft behind national scientific institutions and projects, and the transnational collaborations with other states and organizations (Gupta 1995, 2012). Koech negotiates land purchases for new building sites as Germany loses interest in Africa when the Cold War thaws, secures funding from Margaret Thatcher's government to build his lab, makes back-door deals with the US Army to set up satellite communication, develops creative ways to ensure he would not have to lay off any KEMRI workers under structural adjustment policies imposed by the International Monetary Fund (IMF).[9] In Chapter 15 he describes the process of working with the Japanese members to facilitate the construction of KEMRI buildings in Nairobi that would meet the regulatory codes regarding seismic provisions in Japan. The heavy reliance on funding from Global North donors reveals how fragile the Kenyan scientific research assemblage is: less than 10 per cent of the KEMRI budget is provided by the Kenyan state, not enough to cover basic wages for its 3,000-plus employees. Revealing for what it tells us about the everyday workings of bureaucracy and the complex relations mediated by state actors in the contemporary African state (Larkin 2013; Gupta 2012, 1995),[10] Koech's story is an important contribution to ethnographies of the state and infrastructure.[11]

Daniel arap Moi

Koech's story reveals a very close relationship with former President Daniel arap Moi, one that forces us to seriously consider the entanglements of ethnicity, national politics, and science-in-the-making. Though Koech did not have political aspirations and turned down appointments offered by Moi, he worked closely with Moi and other political leaders behind the scenes to build medical and scientific research infrastructure, work that involved him in national and international politics and statecraft. We can't understand the story of KEMRI, global health research, or the Kemron drug trials without apprehending Moi's role in Koech's life.[12] This relationship highlights the complex ways that state power shaped not only an individual scientist's work but also the development of scientific institutions and policies that made Kenya one of the most desirable nations for global health, pharmaceutical, and infectious disease research in Africa. This is, for me, one of the interesting paradoxes about Koech's life story. We see that his relationship with Moi, something many people find questionable, even distasteful, is also what helped build the system of medical research that many countries have come to rely on. The uncomfortable reality is that while Moi was detaining people without arrest during the *Saba Saba* demonstrations in 1990, his government also had long-standing collaborative agreements with the US, the United Kingdom, Japan, and many other nations (Brown 2001). Canadian researchers working in Nairobi in the late 1980s, who witnessed the spectacle of the Kemron launch, reported that they felt they had to carefully self-censor any critiques they might have of Moi or his government. As James Kariuki writes of Moi's reign, Kenya was at that time "a country in which the government [was] afraid of its citizens, and the citizens afraid of its government" (1996: 70). This apparently was also true of foreigners working within Kenya, fearful they would be detained or forced to leave. It wasn't as if those working for the CDC, the Wellcome Trust, the US Army, or the University of Manitoba in Kenya did not understand the sort of state they had collaborated with. They benefited from the practices and policies that Koech, Moi, and his ministers, enacted at KEMRI and the University of Nairobi's Faculty of Medicine.

The accusations, the controversies, the suspicious rumours that have surrounded Koech's life's work and that surround the institution he largely built highlight not only Koech's complicity in the Moi regime (assisting him being re-elected on two occasions) but also the complicity of so many others. Stephen Brown has written at length about how Western nations and actors supported Moi and his re-election, and contends their rationale to doing so was to avert a breakdown in the economic and political order, "even if this meant legitimizing and prolonging the regime's authoritarian rule" (2001: 726). Samwel Ong'wen Okuro (2009) describes the way in which the IMF and World Bank structural adjustment programs imposed on Kenya resulted in weakened medical and educational systems and Moi's forced compliance with the demands of international donors during the 1990s. Koech's stories help us understand that the actions of Kenyan state institutions do not occur within a national vacuum, but are shaped by international organizations and geopolitics.

Moi started his career as a teacher but quickly rose to power once he made the decision to go into a life of politics (Lynch 2008).[13] In 1955, Moi was elected as a Legislative Council member for the Rift Valley, and just a few years later he made a fateful trip to visit Jomo Kenyatta, who was imprisoned by the colonial state. Though he had been discouraged from going by the colonial elite, he insisted and thus was the first African politician allowed to visit Kenyatta (Morton 1998). In 1963, Kenya became independent under Kenyatta's leadership, and in 1964, Moi was appointed Minister for Home Affairs in Kenyatta's new Cabinet. In 1966 when Kenyatta revised the constitution so there were eight Vice-Presidents, one for each province and one for Nairobi, Moi was elected the KANU Vice-President for Rift Valley. And then, later that year, after Joseph Murumbi resigned as national Vice-President, Kenyatta chose Moi to replace him. Moi had been loyal to Kenyatta, and he represented and guaranteed the vote of the Rift Valley Kalenjins. According to a number of historical sources, Moi's position was precarious during those years, with plots to kill him, especially as Kenyatta grew old and his health started to fail (see Kariuki 1996; Hornsby 2012). These sources also claim that Kenyatta's "family" (largely elite Kikuyu allies in government) did not want Moi to be in a position to become the next President and so Moi was constantly being undermined (Kariuki 1996: Hornsby 2012; Lynch 2008). But on 22 August 1978, when Kenyatta died, Moi was quickly sworn in as the new President, for a 90-day period until a new election could be held.[14] On 10 October 1978, he was elected (as sole candidate), then sworn in at Uhuru Park in Nairobi on 14 October 1978, and he remained President of the Republic of Kenya until 2002 when he stood down. Moi was Kenya's longest-serving President and, many argue, the most repressive and controlling, famous for the Nyayo House torture chambers (Adar and Munyae 2001; Kagwanja 2003).[15]

As is quite well known, ethnicity plays a major role in Kenyan politics and this was equally true under Moi. Historian Charles Hornsby notes that between 1978 and 1981 there was a gradual "de-Kikuyuization of the administration", as Moi dismissed relatives of Kenyatta (the first President) in senior parastatal positions and replaced them with Kalenjin members (Hornsby 2013). Although Moi had promised to rid Kenya's politics of corruption, it only worsened under his leadership. Hornsby explains, "State resources were increasingly diverted into the parasitic sector, the off-book sectors of the economy in which insiders extracted resources from the state for private benefit via bribery, abuses of procurement and perks of office" (Hornsby 2013: 369). Growing corruption, increased police violence and human rights violations, and an increasingly suspicious state characterized Kenya's political landscape in the 1980s.

During this entire reign, from his time as Vice-President until today (as this goes to press Moi is retired, rarely seen in public, and 94 years old), Koech has maintained a relationship with Moi. He recounts early meetings with Moi as Vice-President and the deepening of that relationship over the years as Koech came to see Moi as a father figure. While most who think they know the story of Koech, KEMRI, and Kemron believe that Koech benefited from the patronage of Moi, a re-reading of the story shows Moi may have also been Koech's downfall. The relationship and the rumours tarnished his reputation and by all accounts destroyed any prospects for the drug Kemron. When Moi was no longer in a position of power, the political elite discarded Koech.

One of the uses of storytelling is the way in which it forces us to move away from the polarized descriptions of individuals: corrupt/clean, ethical/unethical, honest/deceitful, oppressor/victim, colonizer/colonized. Koech's story helps complicate our understanding of Moi just as much as it complicates Koech's own self-portrait. Most accounts of Moi's presidency have focused on the repressive regime, the political torture within Nyayo House, and the paranoia of both the government and its citizens during that era. However, our understanding of Moi is incomplete if we don't listen to Koech's stories of how Moi helped build scientific and medical infrastructure, improve health care, strengthen the education system, and of the friendship that he offered Koech. However uneasy people may feel about the relationship between Moi and Koech, or Moi's practices, their collaborations built KEMRI, developed a national laboratory system, and helped create world-class facilities for global health research used by many Western institutions and scholars, including medical anthropologists.

Koech's narrative also speaks to the historical and on-going weight of ethnicity in Kenya's statecraft and national politics, and the consequences for his own life as a Kipsigis/Kalenjin scientist. Although the ethnic designation "Kalenjin" is perhaps one of the more contested, because it represents a political affiliation as opposed to a typical ethnic category (for instance, based on a shared language), it does link Koech and Moi if only in an ethnic imaginary (Lynch 2011). During our interviews, Koech was careful to note that he was not a relative of Moi, noting that he was a Kipsigis, an ethnic sub-group of Kalenjin, and Moi a Tugen (from the Baringo Lake area). Culturally and linguistically related, these ethnic sub-groups are brought together under the political umbrella Kalenjin, a relatively new ethnic construct in Kenya (Lynch 2011). Moi was well known for appointing Kalenjins in senior government positions starting in 1979, but especially after an attempted coup d'état in 1982, and again in 1990 after the assassination of Robert Ouko when he replaced Kikuyu members with Kalenjins and other allies, regardless of member's local affiliations (Cohen and Odhiambo 2004; Hornsby 2012). Within a relatively short period of time, Moi created a generation of educated Kalenjins, like Koech (who was granted funding to study in the US when Moi was Vice-President), through his control and influence over the Ministry of Education, the universities, public exams and school placements, the Teachers Service Commission, government scholarships, and health services, which now constitute a significant proportion of Kenya's elite (Lynch 2008).[16]

Charges of corruption

Koech's stories raise many questions about the entanglements between political corruption, international aid, accountability of public resources, and global health research. Advancing from my earlier framing of lives and stories as relational, shaped by relationships with peoples, ideas, and structures (such as class, race, gender, nation), I want to suggest that we understand corruption within medical science and global health similarly as "not merely selfish and private but profoundly social, shaped by larger sociocultural notions of power, privilege, and responsibility" (Hasty 2005: 271). After serving as Director of KEMRI for

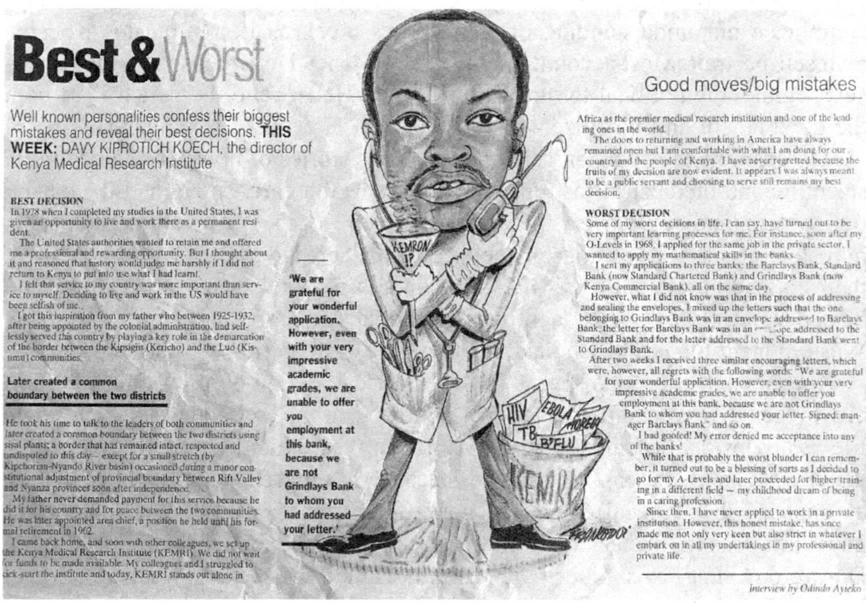

Best & Worst

Good moves/big mistakes

Well known personalities confess their biggest mistakes and reveal their best decisions. **THIS WEEK:** DAVY KIPROTICH KOECH, the director of Kenya Medical Research Institute

BEST DECISION

In 1978 when I completed my studies in the United States, I was given an opportunity to live and work there as a permanent resident.

The United States authorities wanted to retain me and offered me a professional and rewarding opportunity. But I thought about it and reasoned that history would judge me harshly if I did not return to Kenya to put into use what I had learnt.

I felt that service to my country was more important than service to myself. Deciding to live and work in the US would have been selfish of me.

I got this inspiration from my father who between 1925-1932, after being appointed by the colonial administration, had selflessly served this country by playing a key role in the demarcation of the border between the Kipsigis (Kericho) and the Luo (Kisumu) communities.

Later created a common boundary between the two districts

He took his time to talk to the leaders of both communities and later created a common boundary between the two districts using sisal plants; a border that has remained intact, respected and undisputed to this day— except for a small stretch (by Kipchorian-Nyando River basin) occasioned during a minor constitutional adjustment of provincial boundary between Rift Valley and Nyanza provinces soon after independence.

My father never demanded payment for this service because he did it for his country and for peace between the two communities. He was later appointed area chief, a position he held until his formal retirement in 1962.

I came back home, and soon with other colleagues, we set up the Kenya Medical Research Institute (KEMRI). We did not wait for funds to be made available. My colleagues and I struggled to kick-start the institute and today, KEMRI stands out alone in Africa as the premier medical research institution and one of the leading ones in the world.

The doors to returning and working in America have always remained open but I am comfortable with what I am doing for our country and the people of Kenya. I have never regretted because the fruits of my decision are now evident. It appears I was always meant to be a public servant and choosing to serve still remains my best decision.

'We are grateful for your wonderful application. However, even with your very impressive academic grades, we are unable to offer you employment at this bank, because we are not Grindlays Bank to whom you had addressed your letter.'

WORST DECISION

Some of my worst decisions in life, I can say, have turned out to be very important learning processes for me. For instance, soon after my O-Levels in 1968, I applied for the same job in the private sector. I wanted to apply my mathematical skills in the banks.

I sent my applications to three banks: the Barclays Bank, Standard Bank (now Standard Chartered Bank) and Grindlays Bank (now Kenya Commercial Bank), all on the same day.

However, what I did not know was that in the process of addressing and sealing the envelopes, I mixed up the letters such that the one belonging to Grindlays Bank was in an envelope addressed to Barclays Bank, the letter for Barclays Bank was in an envelope addressed to the Standard Bank and for the letter addressed to the Standard Bank went to Grindlays Bank.

After two weeks I received three similar encouraging letters, which were, however, all regrets with the following words: "We are grateful for your wonderful application. However, even with your very impressive academic grades, we are unable to offer you employment at this bank, because we are not Grindlays Bank to whom you had addressed your letter. Signed: manager Barclays Bank" and so on.

I had goofed! My error denied me acceptance into any of the banks!

While that is probably the worst blunder I can remember, it turned out to be a blessing of sorts as I decided to go for my A-Levels and later proceeded for higher training in a different field — my childhood dream of being in a caring profession.

Since then, I have never applied to work in a private institution. However, this honest mistake, has since made me not only very keen but also strict in whatever I embark on in all my undertakings in my professional and private life.

Interview by Odindo Ayieko

Figure 0.2 Davy Koech caricature.

over 20 years, Koech was forced to step aside in 2007 because of allegations from the CDC that he had misappropriated funds from their accounts; specifically, he was accused of embezzling near 19 million KES, a charge he finds laughable, pointing out that if he was going to steal money from a three to five billion KES budget, he'd be smart enough to take more than "a mere 19 million shillings". He maintains that all charges of corruption are false.

Did he benefit from his relations with Moi in ways that many would find unethical? He doesn't say. Maybe, maybe not, but certainly no more or no less than the Kenyan system of patronage has typically sanctioned (Musila 2015; Shilaho 2017). Arthur Obel, Koech's early collaborator on the Kemron drug trials, retained his academic and political appointments after two claims of pseudo-cures for HIV/AIDS. *Lancet* reporter Rebecca Dodd (1996) wrote that the fact that he seemed untouched by such false claims suggested "friends in high places". Though constitutional reforms in 2010 made attempts at correcting the culture of impunity that has existed in Kenya since colonial law, Koech still raises concerns about the legitimacy of the anti-corruption bodies and the judiciary itself.[17] His letter to the Attorney General points out the faults and failures in the case against him and certainly questions the legitimacy of the Ethics and Anti-Corruption Commission (EACC) (and its predecessor the Kenya Anti-Corruption Commission).

The influence that Moi and his family had in Kenya over the courts, police, and political offices, and how this altered outcomes of trials and investigations, has been well documented (Moore 1998; Lynch 2008; Hornsby 2012).[18] We can assume, at the very least, that the loss of Koech's position as CEO and his arrest at the hands of the Ethics and Anti-Corruption Commission in 2007–2009 would never have happened under Moi's leadership or protection. Daniel Branch explains that in Kenya, "the government's control over the police, judiciary, and electoral system ensured that there was no possibility of punishment for major crimes, even if they attracted considerable attention in the press", which created a "culture of impunity" (2011: 21). Koech's outrage and frustration that he was charged, which he often voiced during our meetings, is understandable given this history of impunity. He refused to ask other politicians for help because, he explained, doing so would be a costly endeavour, requiring payments to officials. At other times he explained that he believed in the court system; they would come to see that he hadn't taken any money.

Koech has operated within a national system characterized by economic insecurities and political anxieties, so his opportunistic strategies might be generously understood as skilful manipulation of political relations to the advantage of the national projects he supported, but also to his benefit. His stories point to systems of patronage maintained by elites, benefitting certain individuals or ethnic groups (Song 2017; Hornsby 2012; Shilaho 2017). One of the questions guiding this book is – How do we make sense of these two entangled lives: an elite, political strategist and close ally for a repressive leader and a national scientist dedicated to building a system meant to save lives? These uncomfortable paradoxes are critical to our understanding of how national political projects and individual lives of scientists and bureaucrats are co-constitutive.

Koech's story is one of a well-connected man, with important political acquaintances. He met with Hillary Clinton and Barack Obama, among others, and had unrestricted access to Moi. For some time, Koech's Twitter account featured a photograph of him and Barack Obama shaking hands (see Figure 0.3). Family photographs taken at his eldest son's funeral in 2002 show Raila Odinga and Daniel arap Moi both in attendance. An older photograph taken on the grounds of KEMRI in Nairobi during a special event shows Koech walking side-by-side with Moi, leading an impressive parade of elite Kenyan men. Walking *behind* Koech is Mwai Kibaki, who was elected the third President of Kenya in 2002 (see Figure 0.4). Koech acknowledges he worked as a political strategist for Moi, suggesting tactics that helped get Moi elected, working to arrange secret meetings with Jaramogi Oginga Odinga and Raila Odinga, setting up other secret meetings with the Japanese and American ambassadors, and working with the political youth group YK' 92.

These admissions have raised serious questions about Koech's complicity in the violence enacted by Moi's government. Though he speaks openly about helping Moi win re-election (and with some amount of pride), he never speaks of the well-documented accounts of torture, violence, and disappearances under Moi's rule. Some readers will wonder if I questioned him about these. I did not, because I feared that posing such questions would risk the relationship I had built with him, and risk the project. Others have asked how I navigated the ethics of such collaboration, given these close ties to a violent political regime.[19]

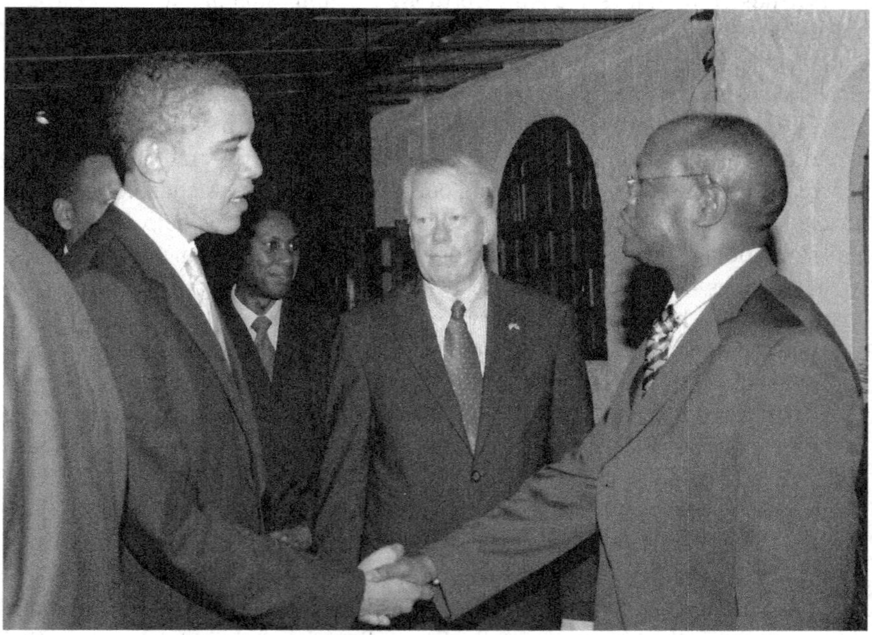

Figure 0.3 Davy Koech and Barack Obama.

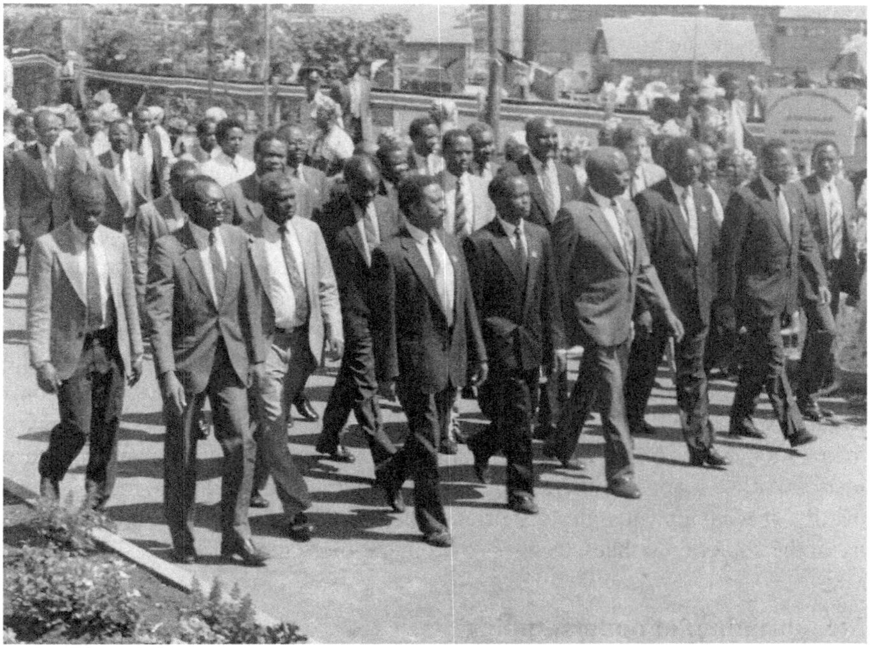

Figure 0.4 Daniel arap Moi and Koech at the Kenya Medical Research Institute.

Michael Taussig asks, "what if the truth is not so much a secret as a public secret, as is the case with most important social knowledge, *knowing what not to know*?" (1999: 2). This is true not only for many of our interlocutors, but often for us anthropologists too.[20] From the beginning of this project people asked me of Koech, "Do you believe him? Do you like him?" During our interviews Koech was always a kind, soft-spoken, gentle person. We sometimes would have to interrupt interviews to pick up and deliver one of his kids from one location to another. He was clearly a dedicated and doting father. As far as I know, Koech has never been accused of being directly involved in the violent acts that Moi's regime became known for, but the relationship with Moi haunts his narrative, this narrative, and leaves many questions unanswered. As scholars we have to question what value this sort of work has for public scholarship or anthropology, and what it means for us to engage in ethically murky collaborations with people who do (or might have done) bad things, whether directly or indirectly through their complicity and silence. For me it was important to understand Koech as one actor in a larger, complex political and social system that was governed by a distinct, if ever shifting, set of rules, a system that enabled African and non-Africans alike, as Western states engaged in, profited from, and influenced the political system and the development of scientific infrastructure.

Koech's tale is a cautious one. These stories also help us understand that those who we suspect of being involved or complicit in violence may also be victims. Given the history of disappeared and murdered bodies, and especially in light of the International Criminal Court charges levied after the 2007–2008 post-election violence, it is not surprising that he is unwilling to openly point a finger for the endless delays in the case. He only blames the original complainant in the 2007 allegations, who has since died, and the Americans working for the CDC who did not follow what he sees as legitimate channels of authority. We might understand his vague answers to my questions and his convoluted stories as being products of fear. In Chapter 27, when Koech reflects on his night in detention, he remembers that guards warned him that people go missing from the jail. In response, a family member slept outside the police station in a car all night, ensuring that if Koech were taken from the station in the middle of the night to be "disappeared", at least they would have a witness. However uncomfortable we are with Koech as a man – with the accusations, the controversies, the relationships, and the underlying violence that haunts his narrative – his story insists that we recognize the complexity of an individual's life's work, the complexity of Kenya's entangled histories of politics and science, and the complexity of the sometimes-shady business of contemporary global health.

Memorandum of understanding

Koech and I first sat down to meet and discuss this project in 2013 but I had begun thinking about the possibilities of this project in 2007, starting by tracing the rumours of the Kemron case, which involved a 1989 drug trial using oral interferon in the treatment of HIV, and trying to reach Koech who had seemingly disappeared from public life after he was forced to leave KEMRI. I approached Koech with the idea of this project, imagining that it would give him an opportunity to make sense of the controversies that have followed him. We agreed that in the beginning we would meet to talk but these original conversations would not be recorded. I sensed he wanted to get to know me, to see what kind of person I was, and if indeed I might be an ally, sensitive to the particular story he wanted to tell about himself. I returned to Kenya to formally start the interview process with Koech in June 2015 after securing a small grant to conduct the research. For our first appointment in 2015, he requested we meet at Meriada Gardens around noon, a restaurant owned by Luo friends on Muthangari Gardens, just off Gitanga Road. He began the interview, the way many Kenyans start their life story, which is with their birth. Over the next three years I would return during my research leave in the summer months to continue the interviews, and to conduct archival research when possible.

Before Koech and I started the formal interviews, I drafted a memorandum of understanding that outlined how this collaborative process would work. Not legally binding, such documents set out principles that guide ethical and moral practice between the anthropologist and the interlocutor, and acknowledge the value and necessity of the interlocutor's time, stories, and knowledge in the project, contributions which are often ignored or eclipsed in the formal production of academic texts. They are also attempts to level the traditionally unequal relations between the anthropologist and her participants in the field, giving power and control to participants over their stories and the way they might like their stories told.

As part of this memorandum of understanding, I committed to Koech that I would, before submitting anything for publication or presenting material publicly, send him drafts to review. I welcomed his suggestions and edits regarding factual errors in the narrative. He did not have veto rights on publications, but when we disagreed on points of analysis, I offered a number of strategies that might move us toward a resolution. For the most part, in earlier papers and presentations this proceeded relatively straightforwardly. His edits focused on factual errors (an incorrect date, a misinterpretation of a conversation). For this book, a monograph based on his narratives, he was offered an opportunity to review and make suggested edits on all 29 narrative chapters, and the introduction.[21] I also invited him to write an epilogue and be listed as collaborator. During the first phase of editing, Koech's requested changes were either factual (to correct dates or names that he might have forgotten or mixed up during the interview or in which were recorded incorrectly during transcription) or to remove material he had provided during the interview but felt was inappropriate to share with a wider audience. All such latter instances were in the context of larger political events or international relations that might be considered politically charged. It was my feeling that he came, over five years of interviews, to tell me very private, somewhat confidential stories, forgetting that these narratives were being recorded and would be transcribed for publication. Or perhaps, with reflection, when seeing them in text form, the idea of sharing some of these more politically contentious stories was a bit too unnerving. Though I felt that this process of deleting these parts of the narratives did a disservice to the larger story I respected his decision. After all, he still lives and works in Kenya and many of the people related to this story are alive and well. He lives with the possibilities of repercussions from these stories, which I escape. I don't have to worry about the Kenyan political elite or American officials blocking me from further work in Kenya or global health, court cases being further stalled, or running into colleagues at the grocery store or at Meriada where many meet for drinks. Nor do I need to worry about actual physical harm, "disappearing", which continues to be used as a tactic of silencing those who go against the state.[22] These are real possibilities for Koech. They may pose a certain risk for me when I travel to Kenya but that is a privilege I have: a choice to travel to Kenya or not.

For the most part, the following stories are drawn from transcribed interviews. Koech was provided copies of all transcriptions and audio-recordings. As editor and curator of Koech's life story, these are his words, albeit edited for clarity, flow, and detail. I did the first round of editing and then I returned to him for further clarification and to ensure the edits accurately reflected what he had wanted to say. When the process of editing transcripts started, Koech asked that the narratives be edited to form a coherent, linear story from beginning to end, with no repetitions; he wanted them to be reworked into a written history rather than a life story based on oral interviews. But I wanted the reader to be able to "hear" Koech when they read the scenes of each chapter, and so I have edited them in the form of a "direct monologue", as if he is speaking directly to the reader. Koech has a unique pattern of speech that I tried to retain and an ever-so-slight stammer. Though I have edited the pauses and disruptions in speech, I have worked to preserve other idiosyncratic speech patterns in order to maintain his voice and his style of narration as much as possible. For instance, I have kept his manner of affirming the last sentence spoken with "yes", an interjected statement that asserts that what he has said is a matter of fact. I included most of these.

We discussed the tradition of anonymizing actors in ethnographic texts but we both agreed that it would be difficult to tell the story in the way Koech wanted and for readers not to know who the characters were. It would be difficult to anonymize presidents, ambassadors, and ministers unless we created a fictional nation in which this took place, but then it would no longer be Koech's story. So in this sense, we adopt the strategies of science and technology studies in scientific biographies, treating Koech's story as an important historical document. On a few occasions, I decided to edit material that I thought was problematic. These pertained usually to the characterizations of different ethnic groups in Kenya. Given the extremely volatile and sensitive political landscape following the 2017 (and 2007) elections, I felt it important that the stories did not contribute to ethnic generalizations.

Koech also skilfully narrated and edited a story that he wanted to tell. While memoranda of understanding are meant to rectify the historical imbalances in the research encounter, they do not account for different sorts of power imbalances present in encounters among those of us who study highly educated, powerful men like Davy Koech. Even in his fallen state, he is very much a part of the political elite in Kenya, with an on-going close family relationship to Moi. When I started this project, Kenyan colleagues urged me to reconsider, suggesting the project could put me in danger because of Koech's close relationship to the Moi family. I rarely felt like the power imbalances were in my favour during this project, except at the very end when the monograph was being edited and the introduction written.[23] He chose if we would meet, when we would meet and where, what he was willing to share, and what he refused to discuss. He simply ignored my dozens and dozens of requests for additional materials (documents, archival materials, and so on), or made excuses why he could not, and then he would share materials that I did not request or find useful. Those were documents that supported or duplicated the stories he told me. Sometimes such documents were almost verbatim stories but in text form, such as his letter to the Attorney General that carefully recounts the errors in the judicial and bureaucratic process and how he was unfairly accused, but he refused to give me the actual charge sheet from the Kenyan police.

I am doubtful that there is any such thing as a "neutral biography" or life story but this one is particularly political and perhaps contentious given the wide range of actors who are entangled within it (Robertson and the Kwagu'l Gix̱sa̱m

Clan 2012). And it is far from impartial in its telling. Koech has a clear, specific narrative that he wanted to tell and when it wavered, he made efforts to amend it during writing, editing, and in the final production. During interviews he often refused to answer questions by simply ignoring my queries, changing the topic, or promising to discuss at a later date. But those later dates never arrived. I often found myself frustrated by his refusals to discuss certain questions. At other times, I was surprised by how much he did tell me. He is a skilful narrator and controlled the agenda of this project. His stories were meant to deflect those of critics that suggested he was fraudulent in scientific practice or administration. He framed his life's work as one of public service, guided by a moral imperative to advance science and aid Kenyan citizens, to a state that has forgotten and deserted him.

In Chapters 1 through 6, Koech reflects on his father's life, growing up in the Kericho highlands, his schooling, and trials and challenges that he suggests shaped his character. Chapter 7 is a brief reflection on an encounter in the 1960s at the Tea Hotel in Kericho with a white hotelier, another life-changing moment. In Chapters 8 through 11 he details his experiences in training to become a scientist, including his research in the US, his work with the WHO, his time in Siberia, and his contribution to developing the Science and Technology Amendment Act which transformed the shape of scientific research in Kenya. He discusses his relationship with Moi and his involvement in national politics in Chapters 12 and 13. Chapters 14 through 19 detail his work as the Director for the Kenya Medical Research Institute as he set up and negotiated complex bureaucratic cooperative agreements with a range of states and agencies conducting global health and tropical medicine research in Kenya. The story of the Kemron trial and the repercussions of are accounted for in Chapters 20 to 22. Chapter 23, another brief interlude, speaks to his eldest son's death. Chapter 24 sets up the complex fiscal arrangements between KEMRI and other nation states which leads to the accusations of corruption, his arrest and loss of job, all discussed in Chapters 24 through 27. In Chapter 28 he discusses his work as a businessman, including companies for dredging the channel off Mombasa. And then the book concludes with the influence of the Christian faith on his life in Chapter 29. Koech concludes with an epilogue that reflects on his life's work but also on the collaboration between he and I in producing this book.

Cinematic storytelling

One of the challenges I faced as Koech's interlocutor on this project was how to present these stories. He recounted them in fragments, moving from past to present and back again, over a period of five years. Constructing a linear narrative seemed inauthentic given his practice of storytelling. Therefore, the following chapters are 29 vignettes, each one with a purpose, telling a story within the larger life story. I adopt a form referred to as "cinematic storytelling", each chapter is a scene, conveying both the quotidian of Koech's life and the larger networks of power that shape his work and the social worlds in which he is embedded.[24] I understand scenes to be "set within the fabric of everyday life but also function as an imagined alternative to the ordinary, work-a-day world".[25] I find them useful for thinking through Koech's struggles, aspirations, and achievements because they offer a creative way to imagine "utopian moments", allowing "otherwise ignored or disappeared communities and subjects to find a home" (Woo, Rennie, and Poyntz 2015: 288). The ordering and progression of scenes guide how we see and understand problems, events, and institutional relations. These chapters then act "as spaces of assembly engaged in pulling together the varieties of cultural phenomena": the geopolitical alliances, national politics, kin obligations, and scientific dreams of Koech (Straw 2015: 477).

A scene, as defined by Woo and colleagues, "is a starting point and not an ending point for investigation" (2015: 288). Many scenes are followed by an "intermission" – a newspaper article, photograph, document, an obituary – meant to help further contextualize Koech's stories (written or added by Denielle Elliott).[26] These intermissions also sometimes offer alternative perspectives. For instance, in the intermission after Chapter 12, where Koech reminisces about his friendship with Moi, I offer information from the Human Rights Commission's report on Moi's legacy of violence. Many chapters mention various actors who weave in and out of Koech's stories and the intermissions help explain who those people were and what is known about them. While the chapters do have a sort of gradual linear movement through time starting with Koech's father in the 1920s and 1930s when Koech was a young boy, I have avoided the typical life history temporal logic. Instead the book presents stories, antagonisms, and political moments that emerge from Koech's narrative.

The scenes presented here vary in length, in depth, and in intensity. The length of each scene largely reflects Koech's preoccupation with the story being told in it, or his reluctance to tell certain other stories that I pushed for. For instance, Chapter 7 about the Tea Hotel, although a very short story told after the audio recorder was off, is a poignant reflection on the history of segregation and racism in colonial Kenya as Koech is chased out of the hotel by a *mzungu* [/white person/]. Just two pages in length, some may wonder why it was included. In contrast, the story of the Kemron clinical trial and subsequent controversies take up considerable space, as do the stories of Koech losing his job with KEMRI. But I hope that as readers move along from scene to scene, arriving at the climax of Koech's life – the criminal charges levied against him by Kenya's Ethics and Anti-Corruption Commission – they will begin to sense the complex entanglements of science, politics, and international aid, and see how Koech presents his life story as a series of unfolding events, leading to a state of uncertainty.

Notes

1 For instance, see Booth 2004; Geissler 2011; Elliott 2014; Graboyes 2015; and Hutchinson 2017.

2 For instance, see the work of Verran 2001; Mavhunga 2017; Peterson 2014; and Geissler 2011.

3 The field of African science studies includes many outstanding works, all of which cannot be discussed, but those that have influenced my thinking on Kemron, Koech's story, and the development of a national scientific project in Kenya include the following: Hecht 2012; Tousignant 2013; Carney 1996; Redfield 2002; Jacobs 2006; Bonneuil 2000; Pollock 2014; Neill 2009; Osseo-Assare 2008; Fullwiley 2011; Lachenal 2017; and de Laet and Mol 2000.

4 Like other accounts of Kemron (see Krotz 2012 and Nattrass 2013), Piot writes critically of Koech in his memoir-style account, suggesting that Koech had not conducted a legitimate clinical trial and made false claims about the effectiveness of Kemron. As part of this project, I wrote to Piot to request an interview, since he dismissed Kemron as a "quack remedy" in his memoir (2012: 298). In response I received this email from his administrative assistant, "Can you let her know I really don't have anything to contribute. Thanks,peter. [*sic*]"

5 There is a rich history within anthropology of the life story genre and those who have preferred to share the stories of their research participants or key interlocutors in their own words. Some other exemplars include Chernoff 2003; Jackson 2004; Robertson and Culhane 2005; Robertson and the Kwagu'l Gix̱sa̱m Clan 2012; Menchú 2010; Shostak 2014; and Pandian and Mariappan 2014.

6 Yet, as I point out in endnote 12 below, there are moments in this book when I felt some elucidation of the approach that I have adopted for making sense of complex lives and the art of storytelling for both anthropologists and our interlocutors. I realize this may seem counter to what I have proposed, and it may very well be. It feels a tension in the difference between a typical biography and a scholarly life story project, the latter which aims to situate the life within larger contemporary methodological or theoretical questions.

7 For more on the uses of thinking about relationality or intersubjectivity in ethnography of lives, see Jackson 1998.

8 For instance, Koech is not mentioned in Hornsby's (2012) detailed and lengthy history of Kenya; Branch's 2011 book on Kenyan politics since 1963; Lynch's (2011) study of Kalenjin politics; Branch, Cheeseman, and Gardner's (2010) collection; or Murunga and Nasong'o's (2007) edited collection on Kenyan politics.

9 On the challenges and failures of structural adjustment programs in Kenya, see Murunga 2007.

10 For more detailed considerations of infrastructure, especially in Africa, see Von Schnitzler 2013; Larkin 2008; Mains 2012; Edwards 2003; Droney 2014; Geissler and Tousignant 2016; and Star 1999.

11 See Branch and Cheeseman 2006 for a detailed discussion of bureaucracy and the Kenyan state.

12 On this account, Koech disagreed with me. In response to the introduction he wrote to me by email,

> You have put much emphasis and weight on my relationship with Moi to the extent that the reader may interpret that my lifeline support was from Moi. It is true that Moi had soft spot on me, mainly because I never at any time went to him for favours or take false reports to him in order to seek favours. Not at all. He was a friend because of that … I completed all my studies during Kenyatta presidency, before Moi was President. I used my friendship with Moi for the best of the country. I have been my own person. My friendship with Moi was only an added advantage.

This response forced me to reflect on the challenge we face when scholars and their interlocutors have differing interpretations of the stories presented, or when we attach different meanings to particular events. In spite of his insistence that his story is his and his alone, my approach (as I explain in the introduction) is to understand lives as being shaped by ethical and moral interactions with others, always being produced in relation to the lives around us, and our social contexts that limit or open up possibilities.

13 For detailed accounts of Daniel arap Moi see Gabrielle Lynch's (2008, 2012) work and Andrew Morton's 1998 biography of Moi. Although the latter has been dismissed by many academics as inherently biased, it provides useful information and insights, as it started out as an authorized biography by Moi.

14 There are excellent discussions of the political intrigue and manoeuvering during this era in Kenya surrounding Kenyatta, Moi, and the leadership of Kenya. See for instance, Hornsby 2012, Morton 1998, Lynch 2008, and Kariuki 1996.

15 See Hornsby's (2012) detailed history of Kenyan politics for a comprehensive and deep description of Kenyan politics, including under Moi. wa Thiong'o (2011), Anderson (2005), and Elkins (2005) have written now classic books on Kenyan's political history under colonialism.

16 As Shilaho (2018) argues, Moi's actions were not dissimilar to those of Jomo Kenyatta, Mwai Kibaki, or Uhuru Kenyatta. They all engaged in the same sort of elite patronage where they used their political power and reach to their own benefit, or to the benefit of elite supporters. According to Shilaho, Moi was unique in the way he responded to resistance to his patronage: by firing Cabinet members and state violence.

17 In May and June 2018, as this manuscript was being prepared for publication, Kenyan news sources were reporting daily on new corruption scandals within state agencies and parastatals. Kenya's Chief Prosecutor Noordin Haji pursued charges against a range of (approximately 50) senior officials in a number of corruption related offenses particularly with the National Youth Service and Kenya Power. Given the lengthy and endless delays with Koech's case, it's difficult to imagine how the Kenyan courts will handle these new charges.

18 Also see Michela Wrong's account of Kenyan corruption and the West's complicity in such practices and networks (2009).

19 A number of anthropologists have taken on projects with groups or individuals whose lives have been characterized by immoral, illegal, or violence actions. Sidre Bangstad (2017) recently raised the issue of what it means to do ethnographic fieldwork among "people we don't (necessarily) like" and suggests our current moment of neo-fascist groups, alt-right movements, and clearly immoral and violent political leaders offers an opportunity for new anthropological inquiry. Vincent Crapazano's (1986) *The Whites of South Africa* remains a classic as a critical reflection on Whites during South Africa's brutal apartheid regime. Alexander Hinton's (2016) story of Duch and his trial for torturer with the Khmer Rouge in Cambodia and James Waldram's (2012) study of a treatment program for sexual offenders in one of Canada's prisons both examine the lives of those who have engaged in violent acts, or been complicit in systems of oppression, racism, or abuse, and force us to face the perplexing complexities of humans.

20 And the reason that many anthropologists and writers find more freedom in writing fictional accounts (see discussions on this dilemma in Gordimer 1989; Gibb 2006; Hecht 2007).

21 Since I wrote the preface, introduction, and intermissions, and the arguments made in the introduction are solely mine, I do not write as "we" in these introductory chapters.

22 Such practices in the Kenyan context have been written about by many Kenyan and non-Kenyans especially in light of the International Criminal Court cases against Uhuru Kenyatta and William Ruto in the 2007 national elections (see Lynch 2015) but also in the most recent 2017 elections when the Electoral Commissions Chairman, Chris Msando, was allegedly tortured and killed just prior to the August vote (Burke 2017).

23 Tomaselli (2003) has written a lovely paper on power dynamics in fieldwork that speaks to how scholars can try to neutralize unequal relations between researched and researcher.

24 I owe special thanks to Vitor Barros for introducing me to the idea of cinematic storytelling.
25 On scene studies see the following: Blum 2001; Straw 2001, 2015; Woo, Rennie, and Polnytz 2015; and Yoshimizu 2015.
26 I drew inspiration from Kim Fortun's *Advocacy After Bhopal* (2001) and Martha Lampland and Susan Leigh Star's *Standards and Their Stories* (2009) and their use of photographs, letters and other documents as intermissions.

1 Daudi

To the best of my knowledge, or at least I was told that, I was born on Tuesday the 21st of August 1951. Do you know during that time there was no recording of dates? It was in the afternoon because my middle name is Kiprotich. Yes, that means it was between three p.m. and four p.m. It might be necessary for you to know how the Kipsigis nomenclature works. Yes, the middle name represents time of day so at least the time of birth is always remembered. If it was a little earlier in the day, it could have been Kibet. Or if it was in the morning I would be Kipng'eno, or Kipng'etich, but Kiprotich that means "when the cows are coming back home". Goats usually come later in the day. Cows come home a little early because there is the milking process. And so my name means I was born when the cows returned to be milked.

Davy was not my first name. Actually I was David. Yes, actually not even David, but I was first Daudi. Yes, we had different names and then eventually I converted the name to be more sophisticated. I decided to call myself Davy. That was there about 1966. This is not unusual. You know in this country people call themselves various names. It is only when they end up having to get a formal identification that they actually settle on something. Davy Kiprotich arap Koech is my full name but then there are also other descriptive names. I am also named after my grandfather. So I am Arap Seng'eret. You see, in between those, there are other names. As I was telling you, you have so many names but at some point you must settle on something. So as is known on record, I am Davy Kiprotich Koech. I dropped the name Arap.

But I was not born Koech. I was born as Daudi Kiprotich but this changed when I had gone through the Kalenjin rite of passage for boys. I acquired my father's middle name, Kipkoech, after the rite of passage in 1962. Among the Kipsigis, those are my people, the males go through the rites of passage from the ages of ten to 14 years of age. I was one of the youngest to go through the rite of passage because my father was pushing me to go early. In fact, I had to go through the rite of passage before I was even ready. Yes, that one was now in 1962.

My father was always pushing me to start things early. I started the school at the age of four. I was too young. I had to be taken to school because I could not manage to walk from home to Soliat alone, which was close to 4 km away. So I

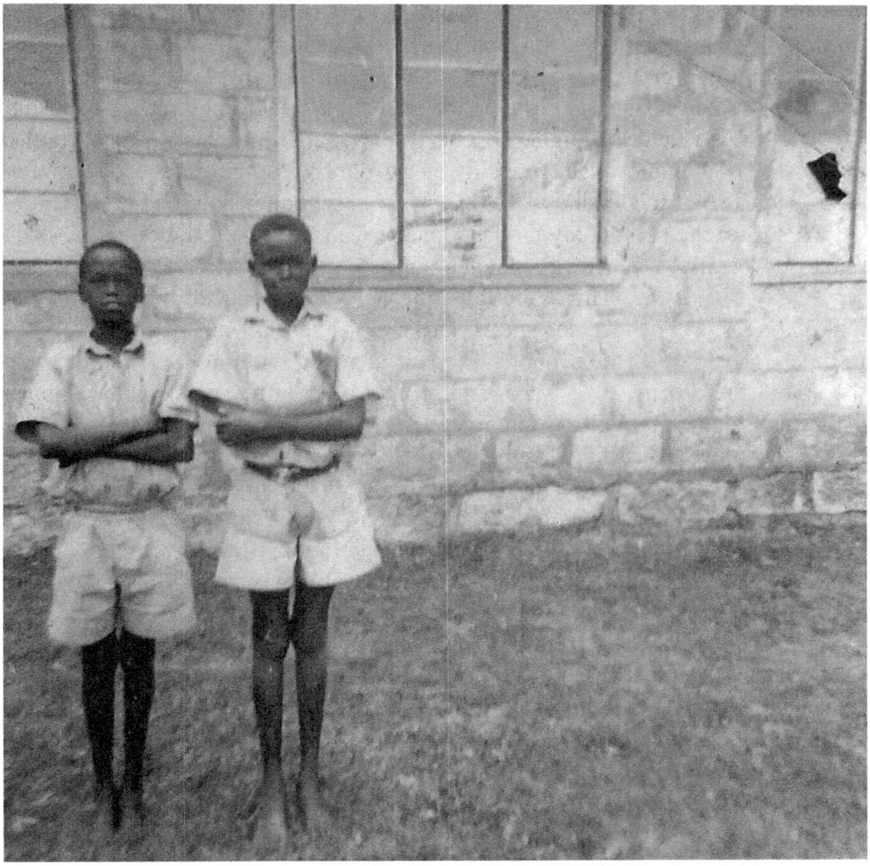

Figure 1.1 Davy Koech [left] with a classmate in primary school, 1960. [The first photograph in his life. He is nine years old.]

was taken halfway to school and then from there I would make the rest of the distance on my own. In the evening I used to run back home and an incident happened which is very difficult to forget. I had just been bought a pair of long khaki shorts as part of my school uniform, towards the end of 1955. I went to class one for only one term and then I was promoted to class two in 1956. I was living at Motero village back then. So, at the age of five, before I was due to even go to nursery school, I was promoted to class two at Soliat Primary School.

"Soliat", like the name sounds, is named after a grass. It is a tall grass, which you see in the grasslands. You may have seen in the grasslands that some animals will hide under the grass and so the school was named after this particular type of pasture. This grass grew everywhere at that time because we did not have the problem of today with overgrazing. And so, I was at school, and at ten, maybe 11, in the morning I picked one of the stalks of grass and started to chew on it. You know, the way kids do. Yes, I was exactly five years old and I chewed it but instead of being reprimanded by my teacher, he said, "please don't do that". When I continued, he took me by the hand and he was about to cane me when all hell broke loose! I immediately went straight toward the teacher's index finger, and bit it, leaving a permanent scar. In fact, the finger was disfigured! It was no longer straight. Of course, I was then beaten and so I decided that I was not going to wear those silly pair of shorts that they had made us wear. And I left them at school and walked away from school, heading home.

When I reached home, my mother was there and she then said to me, "*Kiprotich …*" Actually, when we pronounce our names, the Ki remains silent, so she would say, "*Protich.*" This is because the Ki was introduced by *wazungus* to make it more pronounceable. She says to me, "Where is your pair of shorts?" I told her, "They are at the school." She was annoyed with me. So eventually, at the end of the day my elder sister and brother brought my pair of shorts home. This event made a real change in my life because I had bitten the headmaster's finger and actually that finger remained disfigured for the rest of his life. I think he passed on recently. When my father returned home, I was not disciplined but he was cross at me and he said, "I understand you. You get very angry very easily." I had not yet learned to control my emotions. I was still very young anyway. So at the end of the day my sister brought my pair of shorts home and in the village I was the only one, besides my brother, who had a pair of shorts. Others did not have any. So it was privilege. Yes, it was a privilege to own a pair of shorts back then because people had very little.

I come from the Kipsigis sub-tribe. The Kipsigis is the predominant tribe among the Kalenjin-speaking people, about 58 per cent of all the Kalenjins. Both my father and mother were Kalenjin. I have many siblings from two mothers. Christine is the eldest, followed by Elizabeth then Elijah, Paul, me then Musa, Florence, Sarah, Rachel, John, Jane and Solomon. We have middle names that may be difficult to explain here. Elijah is Kiprono, and Paul is Kipkoros. Do you remember I told you about my brother Kipkoros? I follow him. Then my younger brother, Musa, follows me. They have all gone to their own houses and they are married. In fact, I realized recently I have so many nieces and nephews and I don't know all of them so very soon now I will have them come now to my house for a family gathering.

My father passed on in 1988 at the age of 92 years. I believe my father passed on because of shock. My father died, I think I would say organ failure, because he was okay until one day when he was going home he met some guy on the road, that winding road walking home. He met a certain person from home who says, "Hi *mzee*, how are you?" My father replies, "It's okay … yes yes yes." And then the fellow asks, "How was the funeral?" My father said, "Which funeral?" "Your sister?" And so this is how he came to know that his sister had passed on. His sister Opot Tolony was staying very far from our home where most of the relatives were, in the Waldai area. You see that is where she was married and that's where she was staying but she and my father were very close. So he didn't know that she had passed on. Actually I cannot understand. So he started feeling unwell as a result of the shock from the news that she had passed and then he started having multiple organ failure, and then six weeks later on he passed.

He was a strong man and healthy throughout his life. He never went to hospital even a single day. No, not even for a single day he had never been to hospital. When we realized that the kidneys weren't working because he could not pass urine, and we knew there was a problem, we took him to the hospital. The kidneys were partially working and he had a lot of uric acid in the blood and urea … and then the kidneys failed. Yes, this all happened within six weeks. And so he passed on at the age of 92 and this was in 1988.

My mother passed on in 2004 when she was 86 years old. She was slightly diabetic but she didn't pass on because of complications of diabetics. She woke up from her bed to go to the bathroom and then she slipped, and broke her hip. She came to stay at my house in Kericho to recover, but she had a clot, an embolism in her lungs, and died.

2 Colonial administration

By the time my father, Samuel Kipkoech arap Mitei, dropped out of school because of distance, he knew how to read and how to write. I think that gave him an advantage and it is why he was selected to be a border guard under the colonial administration. I think during the First World War he was able to see what other people were doing, he was exposed to new things, even though he was just a cattle rustler. You see, he was too young to join the First World War. So during that particular time he was asked to go and collect cattle. These young men were the ones looking for cows and so on to bring them to a certain locality where they could be collected and then processed for meat to feed the

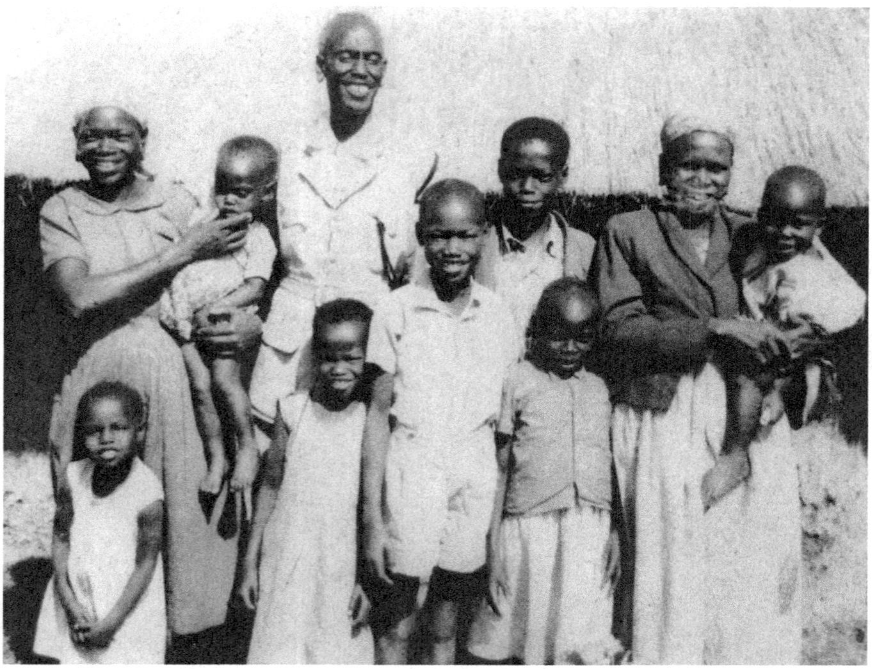

Figure 2.1 Koech's family, with father in uniform.

soldiers. That used to happen during the First World War, and the Second World War the same thing occurred. People, like my father, used to collect cattle from farms, then they are taken to be slaughtered, and then the meat is transported to feed the soldiers in the war. So although my father during the First World War was too young to go to war, he was not too young to be sent as an errand boy. So he was sent to go and collect the cattle and then push them back to a particular place, the *Boma*. This is what we call the place in Kiswahili. *Boma* means a corral. Yes, where all the cattle are held and then from there they are taken to be slaughtered and then the meat transported. Yes, the meat could go to various parts of the world. So that was the role of my father during the First World War.

Yes, at the beginning of the First World War he was just about 16 or 17 years old, because he was born in 1896, and at that time they thought this slightly too young. They could not be trained to handle guns or something like that. Then in 1925, after the war, the colonial government was now doing the boundary demarcation of the Colony and Protectorate of Kenya. The colonial government identified my father to participate in the demarcation of boundaries, the area largely between the Kipsigis and the Luo. So my father was doing the boundary between Kisumu and Kericho district from a place called Chemase, on top of Kisumu up in the hill, all the way up to Sondu. So every two steps they put a sisal, another sisal, another sisal, and my father was negotiating with another person, *Mzee* Oliech, who was identified among the Luo community to participate in the boundary demarcation. They had to agree on the boundary. So they did this between 1925 and 1932. My father worked almost for free, on a pro bono basis, between 1925 until 1932.

And those boundaries have never changed until even today.[1] There has never been any border dispute until today, except one minor change made by a constitutional amendment in 1964, which allowed the Luo to follow the Nyando River further to the east where the headwaters are. So instead of the boundaries going straight from one point, it starts beyond the river and then makes a small peninsular, and then back again. That was the only constitutional amendment of the provinces, which was done by Jaramogi Oginga Odinga when he was the Vice-President and the Minister for Home Affairs.

My father became a border guard before he married my mother. And then he was a chief. My mother was involved in church activities. She was a lay pastor, which meant there was some restriction within the village. Because of my father's discipline with public administration and my mother's role in the church, we were not involved in some of those cultural activities that could be seen as destructive by the colonialists.

Soon after the border work my father was appointed as a Chief under the colonial administration. His main role was purely administrative matters, like settling conflicts within his area of jurisdiction, and they were involved in collecting taxes. We used to have what we call a hut tax, I think it was one shilling.[2] For every hut that you see, the British collected a tax on it. In fact, until recently they used to have this hut tax. As Chief, he was involved in making sure that people lived in harmony, people cultivated their farms. The Chief was everything in the society. He was like the CEO of a village and in charge of the government, what we called "On His Majesty Service" (OHMS) until 1952 under King George. OHMS was even written on the vehicles, either On His Majesty Service or On Her Majesty Service, something like that.

The chiefs of those days were fairly powerful. But my father did not need to exercise that authority because of the kind of people he was dealing with. They were just fellows from home, cattle thieves, and so he had to return the cattle which had been stolen from the Luos to Kipsigis or vice versa. Sometimes it was people who were drunk and disorderly, even managing them, and things like that. Basically he was responsible for keeping order. Order in any system and making sure government regulations were obeyed. If it was time for planting, he must ensure there was planting. So from 1932 all the way until just one year before independence in 1962 when he retired from the public service. Yes he worked for about 37 years for the public service. He got his pension, which was 1080 KES at that time, for all those years of service. I remember he was very angry when he retired. He was given his pension and his pension was 1080 KES total. Can you imagine – 1080 KES for having worked in the government for 37 years from, 1925 until 1962?!

I remember him talking about independence. He said, "You know what? I am happy we are getting independence." He retired in 1961, one year before independence. Having worked for so many years for the colonial state, he believed the transition to independence would turn out well. He felt deeply about it because he was part of the group that was organizing, on a diplomatic front, to bring independence to Kenya, telling people not to resort to arms. Telling people not to engage in violence. He believed to do it correctly, to succeed from the British, there should not be any bloodshed. So he was part of that group, the prime movers demanding settlement by peace and not killing each other. Yes. He didn't want violence because he said, "It will stiffen the heart of these imperialists." It would stiffen their hearts so it was good to approach it with some level of wisdom and caution.

He was one of the greatest influences in my life. For example, in regards to planning. I would see him often because at home in the village he had his own house, the main house, because he wanted to wake up in the morning to go to work but he didn't want to disturb anyone in the family. So he had, we call it *singiroino* [/a gazebo/], like a small building outside. In most homes, most of our rural homes, they have one, it is an outside building. A small outside building where you could meet with friends, you could meet with people, and so on like a gazebo or a banda. Yes. So he used to stay there and I used to sleep with him. He didn't want to wake up any of his wives when he was ready to go to work and did not want to disturb anyone. So in the evening, I would watch him – before he sleeps he would fetch his clothes for the morning, and he made sure everything was ready, setting them by the bedside. Of course we are dealing with little huts. The whole room could be a couple metres at most, but he would organize it. And he would say to me:

"Listen, see what I am doing? What am I doing?"
"You have prepared your clothes, father."
"Am I wearing them now?"
I say, "No. You are wearing them in the morning."
"Precisely. What else have you seen?"
"I have seen you have organized your *sufuria* [/pan/] there for tea."

He used to love tea, and a small cup with some milk. Then he would prepare the fire to be lit in the morning. You know the three-legged stones for cooking? Yes, and he would say to me,

> What you are going to do tomorrow, plan it today. What you are going to do next week, plan it this week. What you are going to do next year, plan it this year. What you are going to do the next decade, plan it this decade. So he said, son, plan. Plan. Plan. You will not succeed by waking up in the morning you don't even know what is where. Before you go to bed you must know what you are going to wear tomorrow.

Although there was no wardrobe to select from so that you cannot get confused as to what to wear! You wear the same thing every day. This lesson is ingrained in me until today. It is not possible for me to sleep without knowing what I will wear tomorrow. It is part of me. It has become a habit. Yes. It doesn't matter whether I come home very late, or drunk, and so on. No. No. I must always know how am I going to wake up, what am I going to wear, and I always prepare what I am going to do. Every day of my life it had been like that, even if I have nothing to wear, I decide I am going to wear the same. During that time I think the British instilled some level of discipline in him, yes, about keeping time and being prepared.

So my father had a very big influence on me, especially in terms of planning and patience. He used to talk to me, telling me stories when I was younger that before he joined the government, during the First World War he was one of the youths who were used to drive the cattle for food for the soldiers. I have told you about that. Yes, I am usually consistent because that is the truth. Yes. I will not tell you something else today and then I tell you something the following day. So that was around 1914. He was almost the age of Jomo Kenyatta, our first President. I think they were born at around the same time. What Kenyatta was doing, my father was doing the same, and they were about the same age. During that particular time, in between the periods of war, and there was no government work to do he would wake up early, using oxen to plough people's farms. You see, during that era, my father was one of the leaders who introduced maize to our country. You see maize was not our staple food and the British introduced it when my father was in the provincial administration. In fact, people were being encouraged to put in maize as a staple food as a very good source of carbohydrates by the British.

But there was a problem. People would boil it the previous day before they planted it but, of course, the moment you boil it, you have killed the germ. It will not germinate and grow. So they would go and plant but nothing would grow, until my father had to go with the grain to plant the day of planting. So there was a lot of resistance to some of those things the British introduced, not because it was necessarily bad, but it was a way of rebelling against the British. There was a lot of rebellion, though often it was silent. If the British introduced it, we said we don't need it. But the people who could see a little further ahead into the future could say, "No, let us try." It was an exotic thing and we were not used to it, but now we have used it and as a way of making money in Kenya but we didn't need it earlier on. We now have a very large industry built up around maize.

It was during this work with the British that he also had exposure to education. He had little formal education but it was when he was already old. He was not a young man in school. When he was already big he was trying to read and write and so on, but after that he joined the administration. My father then became increasingly interested in education and schools and so he created a new school, which is now a major school in our home.

Notes

1 For more information on the history of boundary demarcation in Kenya under colonial rule, see Ogot 1963 and Hornsby 2012.

2 The 1901 Hut Tax Regulation imposed by the British demanded a payment of one rupee, payable in kind or through service (Waris 2007).

3 Soliat Primary School

My father had a passion for education as a result of two things: one, at that time he was working for the colonial administration, as I have said. He wanted to impress upon them that he liked school and they were impressed because he had actually gone to school. If I showed you where he lived and where he attended school, you would be amazed at the distance. He went to school for only three years because it was too far, it was about 40 km one way. You see, because it was near impossible for anyone to travel those distances by foot. Yes, so he only finished about three classes.

My father established a lower primary school in 1949 in Soliat. So he created an opportunity for people from the village to go to school, otherwise people would not have had the opportunity. It was not a missionary school; it was just a public school open to all. When my father created the school he didn't have his own children to go there yet. At that time I had not been born. My eldest sister was already too big. Yes, so my father went round the village areas and he found a boy who was taking care of goats, and he pulled him from there.

So the first person to go to my father's school eventually became a minister in the Kenyan government. It was 1949 and he was the first student to be enrolled in the school. My father said to us, "Take him as your eldest brother", because without him that school would have not been created. Without him we would have not gone to school. And without my father he would have not gone to school. You see because there was no local school, the boy was just taking care of the cattle and goats. When my father found him, he was wearing just a sheet; we call it a *leso*, and taking care of goats. But my father said to him, "You are the one going to start this school. You are young enough, you are intelligent enough. You must." He didn't have any clothes. My father said, "Come the way you are. I want you to be the pioneer student in the school." But the boy's father himself was not really interested in education. He was not. He was very busy doing other things. He was involved in this and that but it was long ago. The father didn't have any idea about schooling but my father recognized the potential of Kipng'eno Arap Ng'eny, as a pioneer student. So, he said, "I am taking you as one of my children and it is me who will educate you." And that is precisely what my father did. So my father educated him until he completed and went on to other schools.

Yes then he went to intermediate school elsewhere, close to Kabianga, because we had some relatives there so my father handed him over to his kin so that he could continue his studies.

He was called Kipng'eno Arap Ng'eny. Yes, from there he went to study in India, then after India, he went to Russia. He studied civil engineering and then in 1966 he was appointed as the Director of water services for the Republic of Kenya. Yes, so it was the pride of home that once he agreed to go school, it opened up ways for us as well, so then my sister managed to go to school (not the first one who was already married). And then the rest of us followed, and we managed to go to school as well, but we could only attend this school for four years and then we had to change schools. From there it was a struggle due to the distance we had to travel. But my elder brothers and also my sister continued at upper schools, and then from they went for training after finishing their "O" Levels.

Kipng'eno Arap Ng'eny passed on recently, in July 2014, but he was still a very important person. He was the Minister of Water Development. He was in charge of the Kenya Posts and Telecommunications Corporation in this country. He was a Member of Parliament for Ainamoi.

He created Kenya Industrial Estates. He was loved in Kenya for the work he did. He passed on last year due to an extended illness.

When my father retired from the public service, because he had reached the retirement age as set out at that particular time, he continued to be passionate about education.

Intermission

Kipng'eno Arap Ng'eny, Koech's father's first student, became a rather infamous figure in Kenyan politics. Though, like Koech, he came from humble beginnings, he went on to be the long-term Managing Director of the Kenya Posts and Telecommunications Corporation (KPTC) (now defunct), an appointment made by Daniel arap Moi in one of Kenya's key state institutions. Many Kenyans adored him, in part because he was known for over employing many Kenyans at KPTC. Reports suggest that he left the institution with over 85 billion KES of debt and far too many employees, a debt and over-staffing that are said to continue to plague subsequent Kenyan state institutions that replaced KPTC (Telkom Kenya and Posta). Telkom Kenya was forced to lay off 15,000 employees in what was considered a very expensive process. The International Monetary Fund and the World Bank reportedly pressured Moi for many years to get rid of Ng'eny, due to the mismanagement of funds. Some accounts suggest that one of the conditions set as part of the agreement that the IMF lift the aid embargo to Kenya was that Ng'eny be removed from his position (Gathii 2009). He left KPTC in retirement in 1993 (aid started flowing again in November of that year) but then was appointed to lead the Kerio Valley Development Authority. He later joined politics as the Member of Parliament for Ainamoi, and then became the Water Development Minister during Moi's government. A Kenyan friend told me that Ng'eny and Moi eventually had a disagreement, resulting in

Ng'eny falling out of favour so much so that when he became ill and wanted to travel to the West for treatment, Moi's government forbid him from leaving the country.

Ng'eny was eventually charged in 2000 with corruption (for fraudulent practices involving 186 million KES) by the Kenyan Anti-Corruption Commission (KACA), those charges were dropped and then in 2001 the Kenyan High Court forbid the Attorney General's office from bringing any more charges against Ng'eny due to a nine-year delay between the original accusations and the charges (Gathii 2009, Hornsby 2012).[1] Ng'eny was also sued for defaulting on bank loans upwards to 100 million KES (Hornsby 2012). KACA was eventually declared "unconstitutional" by the Kenyan judiciary because the powers for prosecuting corruption were based solely with the Attorney General. According to Gathii, "The rise of an anticorruption authority in the context of an authoritarian and corrupt government was met with judicial disapproval. The entire government was corrupt" (2011: 3). The revised 2010 Constitution allowed for the creation of the new Ethics and Anti-Corruption Commission (EACC), which charged Koech (and colleagues at KEMRI) in 2009. There are resonances of Ng'eny's case in Koech's criminal cases as he details in Chapters 25–27.

Note

1 For a detailed review of anti-corruption legislation in Kenya, see Gathii 2011. And see Gathii's detailed discussion on the barriers preventing national anti-corruption agendas (2009).

4 Growing up during independence

In life we may not remember every bit of what has happened in the past but there are major events that get implanted in one's memory, yes. The very nice events may be the things that you can remember when you were very young. For others the memories may be if you were very hungry, there was no food, because that also gets ingrained into your being. Some major challenges in life are the ones that we remember and the great successes. Not the in between, whether you slept or woke up, the fact is because we do them daily, we won't remember them.

So my life dates back to more than 62 or 63 years now. My memory of the past may be about 63 years to 62 years and during that time, when I was young, there was difficulty accessing some of the essential facilities, like school, because that is the time when our nation was fighting for independence. During that particular period we were experiencing a period of colonial influence. The rules, the do's and the don'ts, of those days were largely either from our parents or from the colonial administration. We were taught at that time that being left-handed, for example, was sinful. We were told that it was not godly, and so we were taught we must self-correct ourselves to use our right hand only. I was born left-handed and so later on when I was about to go to school, I was told that I must learn to write using my right hand and the reason for that was that left-handedness was un-godly. It was against God's teachings but I don't know what sort of teachings they were talking about. That is what frustrated us a little bit. And I became a little rebellious in response. When one of the American missionaries visited us I noticed that he was left-handed. He was working and writing using his left hand and I already taught myself to use the right hand. I was confused – here is this missionary and he is supposed to give us the good word and the good word is that you should technically be a right-handed person yet he is writing with his left? Yes. So that is what disappointed me but eventually I wrote a book with the American missionary, Rev. Gerald W. Fish. He passed on in 2005. These are the kinds of things that influenced my thinking, the paradoxes of colonial rule, my formative years as I matured.

So, you are starting to see that I have come through a lot of challenges. From Soliat Primary School, I proceeded to Sitotwet Intermediate School in 1960, some 20 km from home. Yes, besides bearing the yoke (story follows below), there were more challenges. That incident was immediately followed by periods of hunger because I was walking for 20 km from home to school at the age of nine. It is like walking the distance from here in Lavington to the airport, even slightly past the airport. Sometimes I would go to local homes and stay there, but in some of these homes they converted me to be a slave boy. Then I would go looking for other homes but they would not accept me. There were two homes, though, that gave me some of the greatest comfort. Yet, that comfort was really not what you would imagine. In these homes, I would stay where the maize is stored. I would sleep on top of the grains and then a boy in the house would come with a bowl of mashed potatoes in the night for me to eat. And I would eat this very quickly; he was stealing from himself to feed me, as he was sharing his portion with me. Yes, I was so hungry that I would eat very fast. He could bring me some of the water he was drinking as well. But some nights there would be no food and I would go to sleep hungry. Then in the morning I would go to the open grass, because in the maize store it is full of a lot of dust, and I would try to wash the dust off by using the grass in the pasture. I would wash my legs using the grass and then use soap as a lotion, but come 11 a.m. it is all cracked!

At school, if we were thirsty we drank water from the school tank which was storm water collected from the roof, the run off. Unfortunately, that roof had been covered with algae for four years and this is where our water came from. And would you believe the roofing was made of asbestos roofing? But thank God I never came down with mesothelioma as a result of the asbestos materials. Yes. So these are some of the challenges that I was balancing because it was not possible to travel the 20 km on a daily basis. I would be so tired that I could not manage to

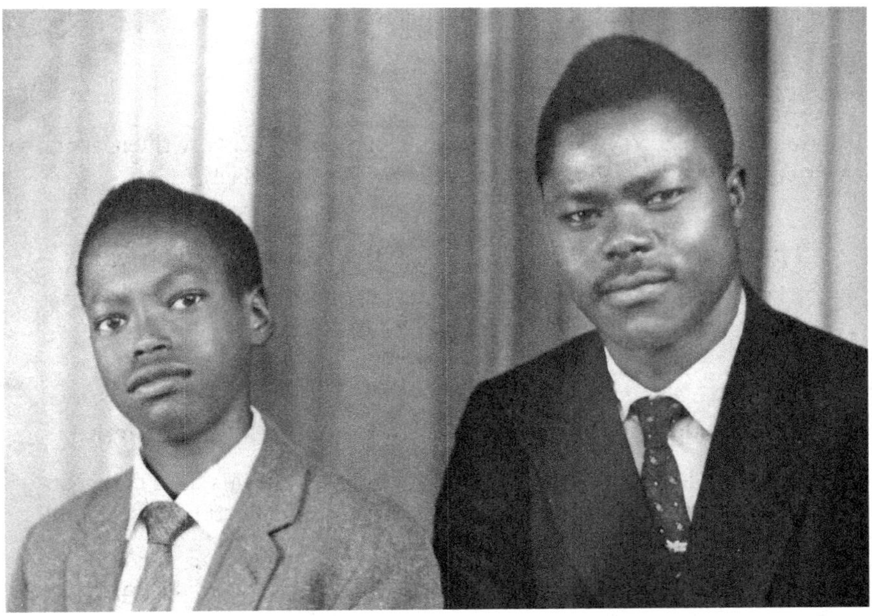

Figure 4.1 Davy Koech [left] in a studio photo with classmate Timothy Siele, 1964.

wake up. I would arrive in the morning, and then it is late when you go home. My father would be waiting for me, and it might be raining. I only had one pair of clothes, which we used to wash over the weekend so when it was raining we had to put it by the fireplace for it to drip water but there was so much smoke.

Then people in the village used to mock my father, saying he had taken his children to school including with this little one. In the village where I was, the people who were working for us were actually those kids who never went to school but my father used to encourage me. He would say to me, "At least you are going to school! You have a uniform and you have home clothes so at least you have two pairs to change. These kids don't have a change of clothes. At least you have two handkerchiefs!" He would offer these encouraging remarks. He told me that I would learn how to read and write, you know, how to communicate and to learn English. I think these experiences and his lessons ingrained in me some kind of stamina and determination in the presence of all adversaries, so that even leaving KEMRI and going to court is nothing. I have had a lot of experience with challenges when I was young. But when I attended secondary school I didn't have any major challenges because we were boarders so we were all equal before the eyes of the headmaster and I was made a dormitory and a school prefect so I had some level of authority then.

I went to this other school called Cheribo where I spent one year in 1964. To get to this school we had to cross a big river, Chekoson River. In the morning on our way to school, we would come to the river, undress, tie our clothes around a stone and then throw them across the river and then swim across. When you go there you drip dry and then you put on your clothes and then you go to school. I mean it was challenging but funny now to look back.

Intermission

The following excerpt is from Davy Kiprotich Koech's written narrative "A Price to Pay and the Penalty for Success" (Koech, no date).

The Birth of a Prince and the Challenge of the Yoke Bearer

East African Standard

Monday, February 22nd, 1960

Second Lead Story: Commonwealth Celebrates Royal Birth

Commonwealth celebrations marking the birth of Queen's third child continued throughout the weekend and messages of congratulations are still pouring into Buckingham Palace.

Congratulations from Kenya and Nairobi were cabled by Acting Governor Mr Coutts and the Mayor of Nairobi Ald. Mrs. Needham Clark in wishing the young prince long life and happiness.

On behalf of the people of Nairobi, the mayor expressed the hope that the future will hold health, happiness and peace for the Royal family.

In common with other Commonwealth capitals and the entire British Empire, a 21-gun salute was fired at Government House Nairobi on Saturday by men of the 11th K.A.R.

The ceremony was watched by Mr Coutts, Lady Renison and the G.O.C, East African Command Maj. Gen. N.P.H. Tapp.

Kenyan schoolchildren have been granted a special holiday today.

Special prayers of thanksgiving for the Queen and the new prince were offered yesterday in cathedrals and parish churches throughout the Commonwealth.

The prince

Prince Andrew

(Later became The Duke of York, Earl of Inverness and Baron Killyleagh.)

Profile

The Duke of York was born on 19 February 1960 at Buckingham Palace, the second son and the third child of The Queen and The Duke of Edinburgh.

He was the first child to be born to a reigning monarch for 103 years.

Named Andrew Albert Christian Edward, he was known as Prince Andrew until his marriage, when he was created The Duke of York, Earl of Inverness and Baron Killyleagh.

(… and there ends the story)

The yoke bearer

Davy Kiprotich Koech

(A malnourished village boy who later became a consummate corporate executive and an international scholar who has been tried and time-tested for over three decades. Prof. Koech is the Chief Executive, *Centre for Clinical and Molecular Sciences*; Professor of Immunology & Molecular Medicine; and Distinguished Professor, Australian-Asian Institute of Civil Leadership.

On the morning of 22nd February 1960, he carried a yoke for 20 km as his school handicraft, but had to return the entire distance of 20 km because he hadn't known that there was no school in the entire British Empire and Commonwealth in celebration of the birth of the prince!)

Cruelty and medical negligence propelled him into the health profession. A malnourished village boy grew up from the ashes of poverty into a respectable Professor of Immunology and Molecular Medicine in several universities.

... and the story begins

From a malnourished village boy to fame

The journey to school was always a nightmare. His tiny feet would be sore by the time he reached the grass thatched structure. Malnutrition conspired with hunger to give his thin frame a painful gait. Villagers laughed at him as he laboured up the rocky and dusty pathway. His head, they joked, was bigger than his anatomy. Boys laughed at him. Girls teased him: "Monitor Lizard" they called him.

The yoke and the birth of a prince

Koech laboured on. At an early age, Davy Kiprotich Koech learned to ignore jeering detractors. But he never ignored one incident which occurred on Monday morning, 22 February 1960. After walking almost the entire 20 km to school with a cart/ox yoke for presentation as handicraft, he was stopped by one old man who told him that there was no school that day. Reason? *Ati* the radio said that Queen Elizabeth II gave birth to a prince the previous Friday and a public holiday had been declared for today, Monday, in the entire British Empire and Commonwealth to celebrate the birth of the prince! (Born Prince Andrew, and later became The Duke of York, Earl of Inverness and Baron Killyleagh.) His annoyance was not on the holiday, which he would have loved; but on the thought and the agony of having to carry the yoke, more than half his weight, back home, but this time for the entire distance without the assistance of his father who was not aware of the change of schedule!

5 Hospitalization

When I was nine years old, turning ten, on the night of Wednesday 9th May 1961 in the course of the evening there was an important event in my life. I was far from home and, you see, it was the rainy season so it was difficult for me to travel all the way home and then back to school. Yes. I could be rained on for five hours walking home on the road, and then sleep for just two hours. That is not even enough time for my clothes to dry. And then I would have to return to school the following morning in the rain again, so it was extremely difficult and my father had arranged for me to stay in a home near the school when it was raining. So it was one of those days when I was looking for a place to sleep. I was walking from where I was getting some food to eat to another place where I could manage to get accommodation for the night. It was during that night that I was now trying to jump across a trench, one that had been dug for the water to flow away from the house, and I slipped and fell and broke my leg. That is what happened.

Yes. When I fell down I knew something was wrong with my leg. I couldn't move my right leg. Whenever I tried to move, the leg would bend the other direction. I knew the right femur bone must have broken. In fact, the bone was pricking into the skin, into the flesh, inside. It was not an open fracture so they didn't know what was going on and so they sent somebody to look for my elder brother Paul who was staying somewhere else. Then he came and we looked for another *mzee* [/elder/], a family friend, Jacob Birir Araap Cherinyit, who was the only one with a pick-up truck in the village. But, from where I broke my leg to where that person was staying, was several kilometres away so they went looking for him, told him that this child has broken his leg, so please assist us in taking him to the hospital. And he came on the following day, 10th May.

I was taken to Kericho District Hospital, reaching the hospital at around midday the following day, 11th May. I was crying and at the hospital they said, "This one is going to be a broken leg." I was taken to one of the wards waiting for an X-ray. But, back then, the X-ray machine was in another place, it was not within the Kericho Hospital, it was at the Central Hospital, a private hospital belonging to Brooke Bond Liebig, a large tea growing company in Kericho. I had to travel about 3 km to get the X-ray but there was no vehicle from the hospital so we had to wait until Friday when there was transportation. So then I was taken to this other hospital and by then, in fact, my leg really was swollen, and we were to do the X-ray. The X-ray results would not be ready until the following Wednesday. So I was taken back to the hospital, waiting there for the X-ray results. There was nothing they could do until the X-ray came so I just waited. When the X-ray came, they confirmed it was a broken femur, it was split, and for this they said, "You have to be taken to the theatre for surgery." I don't know what is so unique about Wednesday but there used to be only one doctor who was based in Nakuru, and he would go round to the various district hospitals in the whole of Rift Valley. From Nakuru he would go to Kericho, then to Kapsabet, to Kajiado, and so on.

So when the X-ray appeared on Wednesday the doctor said in order to align the bone, they would have to put it in traction. It was not possible to put on a plaster. The doctor would be available for surgery only the following Wednesday. The question of pain management ... that technology was not available in my home district hospital, yet it could have been available elsewhere. It may have been discovered in 1900 but it had not reached our place. It may have been routine in other areas of the country or the world but not in our district hospital. So the doctor said he would return for surgery the next Wednesday.

I was still in a lot of pain and so I waited for that Wednesday. That is the time I was given some anaesthesia, it could have been halothane, or anything in those days. I was put to sleep and then they aligned the leg preparing it for traction. Then from there they put a pin in, just below my knee to support it. You see at that time it used to be put on what is called traction, with a pulley and a weight. So that is precisely what happened with my injury. I was forced to stay in that particular position, with my leg up in traction, and then after about three weeks, I told them – "Listen this traction, the pain, not on the leg, but where the pulley was put, it is too much to bear." I said, "It is unbearable. There is something wrong despite the fact that I do not know what you did." Yes. There was something definitely wrong. I told them: "I feel the pain in the leg below the knee, but where it was fractured was only slight pain."

But where they had put the pin in was really hurting, and I complained until they said, "Fine, if this is the case let us call the doctor again." They waited for another Wednesday when he would return. The whole of the hospital administration looked at it and they agreed that given the amount of pain that I was experiencing, that there may be a problem. So they removed the traction and then disconnected the pin from the weight and they opened it up, where the pin had been put, and then they realized that instead of putting the pin through the bone they had put it on top, and it was tearing the flesh. When they tried to remove the pin, it came with the flesh, tearing and rotting. So now they started concentrating on where the problem was but they didn't know what to do. They decided to put a plaster on the lower part of the leg, and then create a new pin at the end of the plaster. It was plaster of Paris and then they create a hook to attach for the traction, to the weight.

This was complete and I was put back into traction but after a few days I started crying again. I again complained to them and said, "It is bad!" Then they realized that they had not allowed for any ventilation, the plaster even covered my toes, they were not exposed. Then the clinical officer who was doing this plaster was a drunk. He could come to the hospital totally drunk! So again they asked themselves – "What can we do? We have to now remove the cast." So they removed the cast. When they removed the cast, one month had passed. Now I am going into the second month complaining still, not because of the pain in the fracture, but because of the pain in the lower part of the leg. There was a problem and they realized that they made a mistake so they said the only thing that they could do is to remove the cast. When they removed the cast, the lower part of the leg was becoming gangrenous. They now bandaged the lower leg. Then when it was bandaged, they created another hook for traction. And then they said, "What we need to do now is to put the hook at the end of it." Then they reduced the weight to ten pounds. All this time I was lying in bed, unable to move. There was no movement at all. You see the back of my head was even getting bare, and very soon I suffered from bed sores.

I stayed there for another one or two weeks, and then I told them again, "There is a problem." "What problem is it?" I said, "The pain is unbearable!" The skin is being pulled! So these fellows at the hospital said this boy has become very naughty, complaining, what do we do? What we are going to do is go do another X-ray? No, they didn't and instead they said, "He has become a problem so the only thing we are going to do is to amputate the leg." Not where it was broken, but down in the lower leg where they created the problem. They said, "Let us wait a little bit and observe it." Then one day while I was still lying with a bandage on the leg, suddenly the skin gave way, it fell off with the plaster. There was blood, and the clinical officers could see that my skin was going all the way down to the floor. The skin was now peeling off! You see, all this time they never bothered about the actual broken bone. They were sorting out the mess they had created. They said, "No, we now don't think the leg is going to heal. We are going to amputate." So they made a recommendation that my lower leg should be amputated. So the doctor who could perform this only came to the Kericho Distract hospital one Wednesday in a month. So now we had to wait again.

Yes and then they said, "Now let's decide where to amputate the leg. Either we amputate the leg from the actual fracture point, or the place where he has been complaining." Of course, you know that was outright medical negligence. The option I was left with was to turn to God and make a covenant with Him. I asked him to save my leg from being amputated. In return, I would go into the caring profession.

The hospital staff said about me, "This one has got a problem." But on the day the doctor was supposed to come, he didn't turn up. I don't know what but something held him up. The hospital staff were disappointed, but inside me, I was happy that my prayer had paid off. So, these other guys stayed and then said, "What we need to do is to dress the part of the leg and allow it to heal and when he heals we discharge the guy." And that is precisely what happened. So it was a covenant I made maybe about 2nd July 1961 that I made that covenant with God. So since the doctor didn't come and cut the leg they started to dress it until it became okay and then they discharged me. I had spent three months lying in one position.

6 Student life and education reforms

When I finished my "O" Levels, before I went to Strathmore College in Nairobi to study for my "A" Levels, something had happened. I joined Kericho High School in 1965. When I was at Kericho High School I was very good in mathematics. There was no arithmetic problem I could not solve. Yes. We used to have a textbook written by a person called C.V. (Clement Vavasor) Durrell titled *Certificate Mathematics* and there was one time when we were doing the usual daily tests and working our way through the book. The teachers had an answer book, which they used for grading. So I remember one sum that I was marked wrong on because the answer book gave a different answer.

I was marked wrong but I knew it was correct. I went to my math teacher and I told him, "Sir, I think I am right." The math teacher said, "According to the answer book, you are wrong. The answer is this …" But I told him, "No, the answer book must be wrong on this one." So it became an issue, because I would not relent, until they got in touch with one of Kenya's greatest teachers of mathematics of the time, which everyone remembers till today – Carey Francis. Yes, Carey Francis. If you ask anyone about Mr Francis anywhere in this republic, you will hear that he was one of the greatest mathematicians of all times. He taught mathematics at Maseno High School and Alliance High School, and then eventually he went to Pumwani High School where he taught mathematics until he passed on. In fact, he was buried at Alliance. Yes, the remains were interred at Alliance. We called him the father of mathematics in this country. So my own mathematics teacher had to call him because we were using the same textbook in the entire secondary school system in this country. At that time our textbooks were provided free, which was beautiful. We were not being forced to go and buy books as they are today. You just paid the usual amount of money for the fees, and then you are given exercise books for English, mathematics, literature and whatever else you were studying. My mathematics teacher at Kericho High School was a *mzungu* [/white person/] called Mr Wilson, an American, so we had to call Pumwani School to ask Carey Francis because I argued with the teacher. I said, "Let us look for the Mathematician of our times!" I was only in Form 2.

So the two men talked and then my teacher looked for me and said, "Koech, you are right." I was vindicated. So there was no problem that I could not solve.

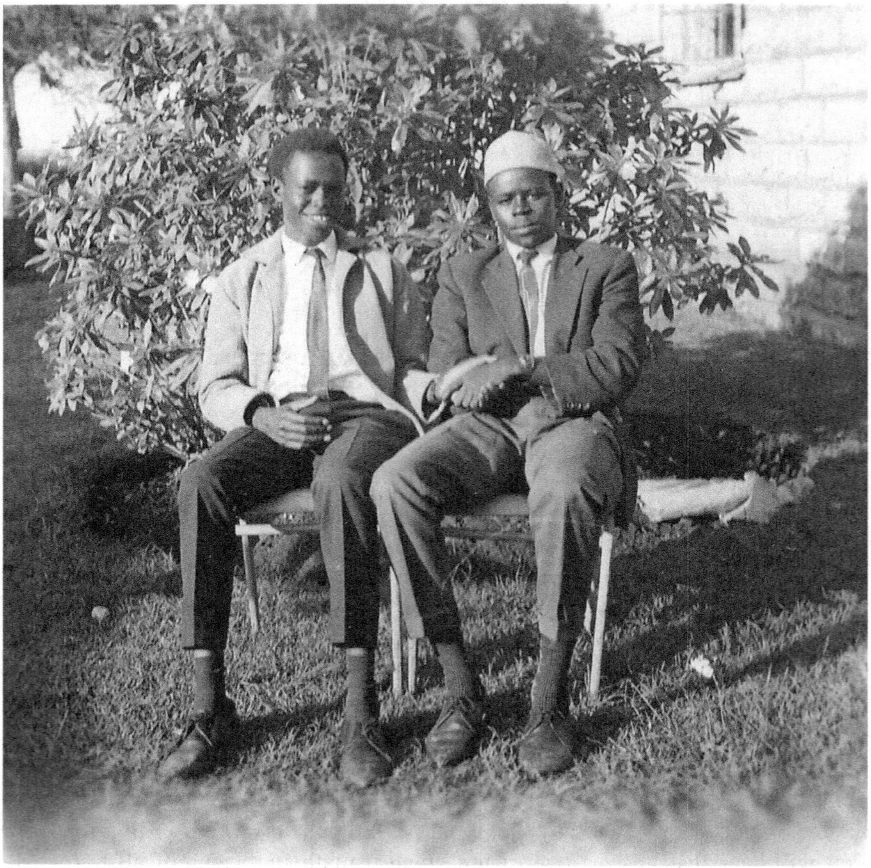

Figure 6.1 Koech with classmate, 1968.

Yes. So we stopped making reference to Carey Francis and I took over. Yes, but at times they called me Durell. We used his book, the *Certificate Mathematics*, in our secondary schools up to the mid-1970s. Yes, I did very well in high school and I demonstrated a lot of originality, and after that I went to Strathmore College in Nairobi. That is where I studied for my "A" Level course in 1969. That is the period I fell in love with *this* neighbourhood (Lavington) because I attended Strathmore for two years. When I was at university I participated in student politics. Back then we were all in student politics at the university. I was at one time the minster for foreign affairs for the university and the current Senator James Orengo was my President.

Strathmore, just down the road here, was an institution, I would say, for the representative of Kenya because despite being a private faith-based school, it was deliberately non-denominational, and all communities of Kenya were reflected in the study body at Strathmore. It was Kenya's first multi-racial school. From Kericho, though, I was the only one in my class attending at that time. But there were also students, some friends of mine, from Kisumu, from Mombasa, so many different locations. The administrators wanted a balance in representation. It was also a school of accountancy, and of arts and sciences. You did not need to come from one of these large families, or prominent homes. No. You just came because of whom you were.

During the holidays at Strathmore, I would go straight home. I had my first cousin who was working as an accountant in Kericho. I would go and stay with him on and off during the holidays. There was one time when I had finished secondary school and a company called Brooke Bond employed me in Kericho within the tea industry. There are two major corporations of tea in Kenya: one was called Brooke Bond, which is now part of Unilever, and the other one called James Finlay. Those are the two largest tea firms in this country but of course there are other smaller ones like George Williamson and Sasini plus, and then the small-scale tea growers under the giant umbrella Kenya Tea Development Association (KTDA). When you fly over Kericho there is nothing else except fields of tea. One day I joined the US ambassador to Kenya when flying from Nairobi to Kisumu preparing for Obama's visit when Obama was still a senator. So we were flying very low using an American plane, which was around temporarily. I even saw my house in Kericho from the plane. It was lovely. But usually, because of Mau Forest, there are a lot of clouds and air turbulence, which forces the planes to fly at a higher altitude. But there is a way planes manoeuvre the route to Kisumu and then you can see thousands of acres, to the farthest the eye can see, nothing else except tea interspersed with some other bushes or forests. For instance, forests of Eucalyptus trees are planted as a source of local firewood for the factories and for the houses of tea managers. Yes. On one occasion, I was employed in their own laboratory where they were doing research, extracting a malaria drug called Chincona, which is a source of quinine. They were trying to see whether the synthetic version was better than the natural version, or something like that, and I was there doing the technical work. But eventually I left because I was only being paid 231 KES per month.

When we were at Strathmore College we were together as a community even though we came from different areas. However, in areas of government we could see something different happening. I was in Nairobi attending Strathmore College the same year that Tom Mboya was assassinated in town. He also lived in Lavington just by the shopping centre. Yes, that is where his house was. So at that particular time Jomo Kenyatta had taken over the country's leadership. He had been President of Kenya for about six years. We saw the divisions in government: Jaramogi had decided to part ways with Kenyatta. Now we started to realize that you can go and join the government depending on who is in charge and then you secure a very big or important position. You get large tracts of land even without working for it. As long as you know how to make use of it. So that is what caused some kind of concern to us students but because, at that particular time, Kenyatta was an authoritarian, together with his own henchmen, people could only complain in murmurs. They could not complain openly. There was no open democracy. There was no open criticism of the government.

The character of my college principal, Professor David Sperling, had an influence on me as a student during my time at Strathmore. He is of American origin. He is a Harvard and Yale graduate and a member of the Opus Dei. I never became a member of Opus Dei because the lifestyle requires a total makeover! He is still around to this day. He was at one time at the University of Nairobi but he is currently a research professor at Strathmore University. He never forced us to do anything and he gave us a little bit of freedom, responsibility and self-discipline, and there weren't even uniforms except the college blazer. You could wear anything so long as it was presentable, which was very good for me because I could not afford to buy any uniform then. I had only two pairs of trousers, one grey and one black, for the entire two years that I studied there. You could see through the grey one because the fabric was so thin, it was worn-out. And I often went hungry at Strathmore.

Soon after that I joined the student government at the University of Nairobi and so we could see exactly what was at play. At that time, Moi was the Minister for Home Affairs and he was in charge of the police and security. It is only thereabout 1975 when another famous politician, a Kikuyu called Josiah Mwangi Kariuki, was murdered and then his body dumped in Ngong Hills somewhere, eventually discovered by some Maasai herders. The students from the University of Nairobi demonstrated in protest in the streets of Nairobi, and the government broke it up with riot police! Then the government closed the university.

Moi had been misled, he had been told by his security officers that Kariuki had gone to Zambia. He wept in Parliament, saying that he was misled. Moi disclosed to everyone that he was deceived. But Kenyatta wouldn't sack Moi. Because Kenyatta knew that if he touched this guy, the country would go up in flames. He knew Moi's community had influence through the Kalenjin land. The consequence of that was too great for Kenyatta's regime. And that Jaramogi had been proscribed, his party was proscribed; many people were killed and injured during Kenyatta's visit to Kisumu. So Kenyatta thought very seriously and said no. What he did instead was to transfer the entire police department to the Office of the President so Moi was no longer in charge. But it was in the Office of the President for only four or five years then Moi became President. Then he said, "No, it was brought over to me" and it has stayed there until today. The rest is well documented in several documents.

As university students we were concerned about the rights of the students but also involved in national politics, not just local but African affairs generally. We were fighting for the freedom of Zimbabwe with demonstrations in the streets. We were fighting for our own rights. We were also fighting for greater say in government, fighting for extra funding for the students. I was in the student government as the Minister for Foreign Affairs and an editor-in-chief for the students' magazine, *Platform*. At one time we had a riot at the university and it was closed for several weeks, quite a number of months actually, and then the government dismissed some students. The students' magazine was proscribed! But we were fighting for other things as well. Our fights were not too violent but with purpose, unlike what the students do at the moment. James Orengo was our student president during my time and I was his special advisor so I was involved in all sorts of politics. Importantly, the students that were there at that time were not only Kenyan students but they included foreign students largely from other African countries at large. That is not commonly being practiced at the moment in our public universities.

I was also a student representative in the faculty of science. I had been admitted in the faculty of medicine, but could not join it due to some logistical issues, so instead I went into science. So when I was in the faculty of science I fought for curriculum changes. Let me explain. At that time students were at the university either for three years, four years or five years depending on the degree course a particular student was pursuing. At the end of any particular degree programme, and as per tradition, each student sat three examination papers on each subject: Paper number one was to test the learner on material learned as from the first year of entering the university, basically recall. Paper number two was to test the learner on the material learned during the year current year of study. While paper number three was devoted to practicals in science-based subjects and projects in other subjects. Any previous terminal or end-year examinations were not considered during the grading for the award of the final degree.

Personally, I felt it was unfair to be graded on the basis of a few hours' performance at the end of the degree course without consideration of performance during the previous years. When I was a student representative in the faculty of science, I went to address the entire senate of the university in 1972. You see the Internet was not available then. It was 12 years before the Internet came to Kenya. I had not studied outside the country, nor did I have any knowledge of what was going on in other countries. I knew at that particular time that the British were very traditional and we were following their system. So I advocated for this change until it was approved at the end of 1972, but it did not take effect until around 1975 when it started from the faculty of science. That I think was my first contribution in the area of education. This is fairly routine at the moment. Some public universities call it the Unit System while most private universities call it credit system or something similar. They mean the same thing. It is about credit accumulation.

It was as a result of my female student colleague, the details of which remain personal. I was so passionate about it. I moved from student politics, which was fighting in the streets, to academic advocacy in the college. I remember what my father once told me: "When you want change you are more likely to be recognized when you go about it in a diplomatic manner." He said, "You see, you don't need to shout if you have to do something." So I adopted this peaceful way to advocate changes in the education curriculum and the way in which the examination system would be accumulated. Yes. So it started in the faculty of science, and then spread to the rest of the faculties. I am proud of this work that I was able to communicate to the institution and to the senate and make important changes to education. This direction was strengthened when I was a member and later the Chairman of the Commission for University Education, then the Commission for Higher Education in 1984 until 2003; and when I chaired the Commission of Inquiry into the Education of Kenya, between 1998 and 1999.

Intermission

EDWARD CAREY FRANCIS

L. A. PARS

Carey Francis was born at Hampstead on September 13th, 1897, and died at Nairobi on July 27th, 1966. He was educated at William Ellis School, Hampstead, where he showed extraordinary promise both at work and at games; he was Head of the school, and captain of football, cricket, tennis, and athletics. He served in the First World War, holding a commission in the H.A.C., and being mentioned in despatches. He came through the war unscathed, and after the war he took up the scholarship to which he had already been elected at Trinity College, Cambridge. In his undergraduate days he maintained the same high standards, both academic and athletic, that he had shown at school. It was generally believed that he headed the list in the Mathematical Tripos of 1921, though of course the title of Senior Wrangler had long ago been abolished.

His mathematical interests were mainly in the field of analysis, and he was much influenced by three Trinity mathematicians, Hardy, Littlewood and Pollard. In 1923 he was awarded a Rayleigh Prize for a substantial essay on the Denjoy–Stieltjes Integral, and two papers " On differentiation with respect to a function " and on " The Lebesque–Stieltjes Integral " appeared in the Proceedings of the Cambridge Philosophical Society in November 1925. He was a Fellow of Peterhouse, and Director of Studies in Mathematics, from 1922 to 1928, and during the last four years of this period he also held the office of Senior Bursar. He was a brilliant and immensely popular lecturer. He was one of the original University Lecturers when the Faculty System was established in Cambridge under the new Statutes of 1926, and he also served as Secretary of the Faculty Board of Mathematics.

But his great promises as a mathematician was not fulfilled, not because of any lack of ability, but because there were other things that counted higher in his scale of values. His heart had always been in the Mission field, and his friends were not surprised when, in 1928, he left Cambridge and went to Kenya as a lay teaching missionary under the Church Missionary Society. He first taught at Maseno, in Nyanza, and it was here that his pupils gave him the name of " Achuma "—the man of steel. But Maseno was only the training-ground for his real life-work, which was the Headmastership of the Alliance High School in Kikuyu. This position he held from 1940 to 1962. It was here that his most important work for African education was done, and here that his immense reputation as an inspiring leader and teacher was built up. Under his guidance the school attained an almost mystical prestige, and to be a pupil of Carey Francis at Alliance was a highly valued and a much-coveted distinction. More than half of the members of Kenya's present cabinet are old boys of this school.

His last years were a little clouded by unhappiness about political developments in Kenya; he was convinced that independence had come much too early, that the country was not yet ready for self-government. Nevertheless he set out, with characteristic courage, to make the transition work as smoothly as possible. When he died the House of Representatives stood in silence in his memory—an honour usually reserved for its own members and for Heads of State. He was buried in the grounds of Alliance, the institution to which he had devoted so many years of his life, and in which the influence of his lovable and impressive personality will never die.

Jesus College,
Cambridge.

[J. London Math. Soc., 43 (1968), 368]

Figure 6.2 Obituary for Carey Francis.

7 Kericho Tea Hotel

Davy Koech told me this story after we had finished an interview and the audio recorder had been turned off. I asked him if he would retell it for me since I had made only rough notes after the fact. He wrote this to me by email in 2017.

As for the Tea Hotel, in Kericho, one evening in 1969, my cousin Josiah Chepkwony, who was working at the then Brooke Bond Kenya Ltd as an accountant, took me to the Tea Hotel for a drink. The hotel was the property of Brooke Bond, the single largest tea grower in Kenya. At around 7.30pm, the lights went off and darkness engulfed the hotel. Upon realizing that there was power in the neighbourhood, I personally took the initiative to establish whether the problem was restricted to the hotel as opposed to being a general problem. I found out that the main fuse controlling power to the hotel had blown off. I did a makeshift rewiring and restored the power. I met the hotel manager upon exiting the distribution box along the path to his office. He asked me who I was and what in the world I was doing on the corridor to his office. I tried explaining to him that it is me who was fixing the power. He didn't listen and assumed I was trying to steal. He instructed me to leave the hotel immediately and never to come back to the hotel for the rest of my life. My cousin was furious when he heard and wanted to start a fight but was restrained by the hotel patrons.

Sometime in the nineties, while travelling the UK and in the company of a senior colleague, we met the same fellow working on a lawn-mower cutting grass in Sainsbury area. My colleague recognized him immediately and I was introduced to him as the new principal owner of the hotel and the one he chased out of the hotel in 1969. He stared at me and quietly responded – "I am sorry." We bid each other bye and proceeded with our mission.

My fieldnotes from the first time he told me the story, read as follows.

Fieldnotes, dated 12 July 2015.

I met with Davy Koech at around noon, staying with him until 5 pm at Meriada Gardens. A solid interview but after the audio was turned off, and we had a beer, he told me this story about being a young man, sometime in between high school and college, when he returned home to visit Kericho and was staying in Kericho town with a cousin. I can't recall all the details now but the gist of it was – he must have been staying in some small room in the hotel with his friend, and there was no power in part of the hotel, so he took it upon himself to find the fuses and make the fix. Which he did – but after or during, he was caught by a *mzungu* [/white/] manager or owner who berated him, told him to immediately leave the hotel and that he was to never return. He said of course that it had been a deeply humiliating experience and that he was hurt that this foreigner would ban him from a hotel that was deeply associated with his rural home.

He now owns majority shares in the hotel. And I had noticed recently in the news that there is an investigation into his majority shares. The other 40% of shares are owned by a local company, Yasangwan Holdings, made up of many (300 plus) local tea farmers including, he explained, people like his mother, uncles, and cousins. It came up in conversation today because the day before a fellow, William, who is the manager of this company (the 40%), had come to Nairobi to show Koech some letter. I got the distinct feeling that there was tension between the two. Neither seemed sincerely happy to see the other but I could not follow the conversation since they spoke in their vernacular. The news article in the *Standard* said Koech and his company Sololo Investments were being sued. The current Director of Yasangwan, Henry Belosi, wanted to know how Koech had come to own such large shares, which he had apparently purchased in 1991 from the Kenyan Tourist Development Corporation. The case was eventually dismissed by the courts.

8 On becoming a scientist

I finished my Bachelor of Science exams at the University of Nairobi in 1974. Two days later I went to a medical laboratory at Kenyatta National Hospital. I went to the Director of the lab, Dr Itotia, and requested to work there. He asked if I had graduated. Yes, I told him. "What were you studying?" I told him and then he wrote a small note, a handwritten note, and because he was a pathologist the hand note was just terrible actually! He sent me to the University of Nairobi where there was a new unit being created called the WHO Immunology Research and Training Centre, in the Department of Pathology. It was being managed by the World Health Organization.

I went there and when I arrived I met Professor Vaclav Houba. He read the note from Dr. Itotia and then called me into his office. He asked me one question. This question was almost the same question that I had been asked in my final exams the previous week. He said, "How do you measure protein?" One single question. I thought about it and the most obvious thing that you can do is use the optical method, but then I remembered a very old technique called the Kjeldahl method which was more complicated than the optical density technique, which was a lot easier and so on. Yes. So he told me come back for the letter in the afternoon and so I went across the road. I didn't have any money and so I ate *githeri* [/mixture of corn and beans boiled together/] and returned later in the day. I got the letter of appointment to work at the University of Nairobi in collaboration with the Wellcome Trust Research Laboratories because Professor Houba was affiliated with both institutions.

I was the first African employee of the WHO Immunology Research and Training Centre. I was employed as a research officer trainee. And at the Wellcome Trust I was also the first Kenyan to be employed at the scientific level. We were working then with the University of Liverpool's School of Tropical Medicine, the London School of Hygiene and Tropical Medicine, and Oxford University. You see, Oxford didn't have a School of Tropical Medicine so we worked in molecular medicine, which is a type of laboratory medicine. Professor Houba was in charge of immunology within the medical school and he was an employee with the WHO. We were researching schistosomiasis, filariasis, malaria, and leishmaniasis. So those were the areas I did my first work and then my first scientific publication was in 1976. We were trying to map out the cellular mechanisms of individuals affected by schistosomiasis, examining the immunity of baboons we had raised, which were within the Wellcome Trust. The Wellcome Trust was also within the National Public Health Laboratories at the Kenyatta National Hospital Complex. From there we went into human clinical trials. That is where I was first exposed to human clinical trials for schistosomiasis studies. I even trained as a trial monitor during that time.

In May, about one month into my research there, we had some fellows from Case Western Reserve University coming to do research on schistosomiasis, along with researchers from the Harvard Medical School, and others from the Liverpool School of Tropical Medicine and Cambridge University. The encounter I had with these highly rated researchers was the beginning of a long journey for the next 40 years in science, medicine and technology. Within the University of Nairobi Medical School there was a department of microbiology that was dealing mainly with the biology of parasitic and viral diseases. It was part of the Department of Pathology at the medical school. I was one of the founding members of the laboratory at its beginning in 1974 at the University of Nairobi with WHO consultant Professor Houba. Yes, I think she was Czech or Slovakian, one of those countries in Eastern Europe, but a WHO employee. So we were together in the laboratory and concentrating on immunology which was a new unit of the Department of Pathology.

At the University of Nairobi we established a nascent department in 1974 and then soon after that we received some support from another new institution. At that time it was the International Laboratory for Research on Animal Diseases, called ILRAD, which is at the moment called ILRI, and this was an international research unit based in Kenya's Kabete area. They didn't have a permanent location but it was being financed by various institutions and governments like the World Bank, the US government, the Canadian government, the Swiss government, and I think the UK was involved, and a few other international aid agencies which contributed funds to do research on animal diseases. You see, basically most of the diseases that affect livestock, like sleeping sickness, theileria and a few other animal diseases, are actually very close to what we were seeing in human diseases. ILRAD were researching animal diseases, although we had another institution, which belonged to the government dealing with those particular subjects, but the scientific strength of those and the facilities were not sufficient. ILRAD expanded its mandate and eventually changed its name from ILRAD to the International Institute of Livestock Research Institute, or ILRI. These researchers were using my laboratory when I went away to the US for graduate studies because they were still establishing their own lab.

Then in 1976 I won a Fulbright-Hays Scholarship to study in the US. I had received a different scholarship to go to Montreal for some further medical training at McGill University in Canada.

I was going to McGill but in the process the President's (Kenyatta's) PA (personal assistant) who happened to be a very powerful man at that time blocked me from pursuing the studies in Montreal. You know, Vice-President Moi had met us as university students and said he had a scholarship and he asked for me to come see him. When I reached Jogoo House, I was not allowed to see him. Then two weeks later I received a phone call saying that I had gotten a Fulbright-Hays Scholarship to go study in the US instead. I was a Fulbright-Hays fellow for two years.

And so I went to the US to study a combined master's degree in clinical medicine and clinical pharmacology. Yes, this was at Duquesne University and the University of Pittsburgh Medical School. As part of this master's program, I was also attached to a research program with my professor at the University of Pittsburgh Medical School who was a neurosurgeon, Professor Robert Selker. In fact, I think he passed on in November 2010. It was the time when we described the mechanism of apoptosis also described as programmed cell death in brain tumours.

Although it was a two-year master's program, I completed all requirements within 12 months. At which time I moved to Harvard Medical School where I started my doctoral program. This was the end of 1977. There I pursued doctoral studies in pathology and I was granted a PhD in clinical pathology specializing in immunology from the University of Nairobi where I had transferred a couple of years after starting. In my master's I had dealt largely with drug-to-drug interaction but when I entered the PhD program I said I am done with drugs. Let me go now to pathology. Yes. When I was doing my master's degree I realized that there was a lot of work to do with the pathogenesis of disease.

Yes, I was also exploring the pathology mechanisms that are happening even in our local diseases. You know what sort of effect do, say, these diseases have?

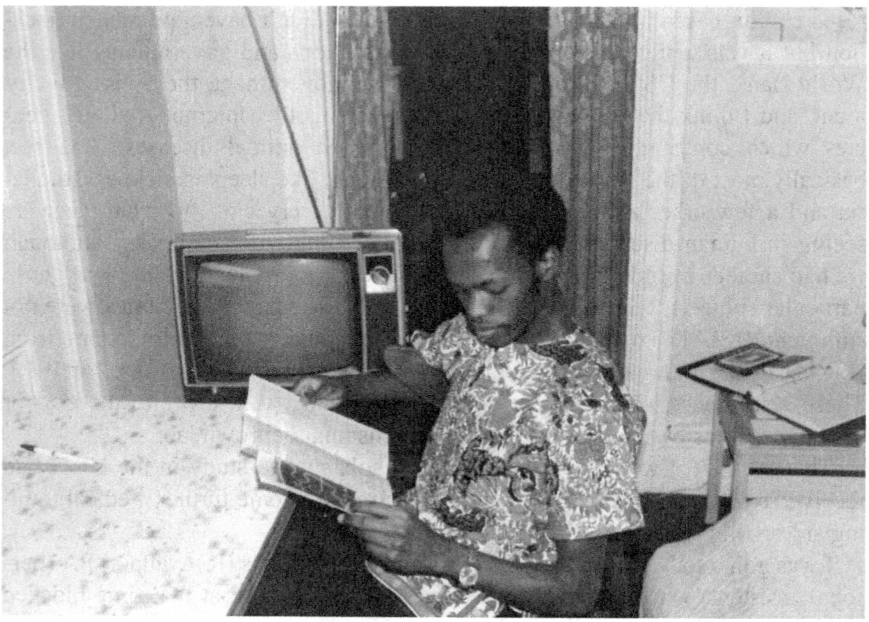

Figure 8.1 In his room while at Harvard University Medical School, 1978.

Like, for example, if you measure the blood count. If you measure the blood count, say yours – you come from a temperate country and you are not exposed to parasitic infections all the time, but one critical issue is that there is another person who is exposed to these infections. When you look at the blood profiles and immunoglobin profiles, plasma profiles, etcetera, despite the fact that the two are clinically normal individuals, they are totally different. Yet, you are treated the same by laboratory and clinical standards. So, we now raised a concern that the standards that we have been using in laboratory work, are derived from Caucasian (white) populations in the Northern Hemisphere and they may not apply to those living in the South or Africa.

So, what we are trying to do now, one of the projects I am involved with, is to set up about 156 centres in this region to do local biometric and biological test standards. May I tell you – according to international standards if you look at the blood pressure of people here in Kenya, everyone is hypertensive! You encounter a significant percentage of presumably clinically normal people who are considered hypertensive according to these international guidelines and so they end up getting treated because of that. Yet, they are perfectly normal individuals. What is the reason of having a blood pressure of 140 over 90 as the maximum limit? What is it? We will send you to the cardiologist, you will be treated with anti-hypertensives, but it may be that you are not at the same risk of stroke as someone from the Northern Hemisphere. These local variations needed to be investigated. So those are some of the things we want to correct for.

But my main areas of interest were on three main diseases: schistosomiasis, leishmaniasis, and malaria. Most of my more than 200 publications were on those three diseases. And then, this is thereabout 1984, that is the time when we started hearing rumours about HIV/AIDS and I had the first contact with a person living with AIDS in Nairobi, together with my friend, called Professor Arthur Obel. And then we went on to work on HIV and we published our first publication on Kemron together.

I went back to the US where I now did my postdoctoral work. We started a course called the Biology of Parasitism in the Marine Biological Laboratory at the Woods Hole Oceanographic Institute which is known primarily for research on ocean life and marine animals and so on.

9 Siberia

In 1981 I was sent by the World Health Organization to do some work in the Soviet Union. I went to an institution in the Novosibirsk hub, half way between Leningrad and Vladivostok. I used to hear about this place in my geography lessons when I was in school and sometimes on the radio. There used to be a radio program that we would listen to. The program would begin with the sound of the train, representing the train to Vladivostok, which is on the east end of the then Soviet Union to Leningrad through Moskva [/Moscow/]. Yes. So somewhere in between is a place called Novosibirsk. From Novosibirsk you travel inland to another institute, I was at the Institute of Cytology and Genetics. Yes, of the Soviet Union. It was in Siberia. I tell you it was exciting. I was there for probably very close to three months.

I was studying genetics of disease and disease manifestation … and there were quite a number of things that we were doing. It is a place called Akademgorodok.[1] Which means academic city in Russian.[2] Yes, so this academic city had about 22 institutes then. Yes, there is nothing else there except science. This was 1981 and the Cold War was at its highest. Actually, I will tell you the effect of the Cold War on the development of the Kenya Medical Research Institute (KEMRI) later.[3]

So this is where I went to stay. This is actually the place where the Soviet Government banished scientists. They developed it in 1956 and then they said, "Here you can do your science." One of the criteria for being there was that you see you must speak and understand English, and then of course you must be good in all the other sciences to be associated with one of these 22 institutions. Yes. That is the place where people were working on proton (particle) accelerators. It is the centre where they did trials on the proton accelerator in one of the physics institutes. Yes. I was working on the genetics of human disease, anything in human diseases, including parasitic infections, viral infections. And most of the things that we know at the moment about genetics and DNA were not known at that time. The discovery of genomes came later, and all these other things came in, and so we were part of those to develop this new knowledge about genome expression. For instance, there was a non-healing ulcer we were working on. So we wanted to find out exactly the pathologic mechanisms that were taking place in this ulcer. You see, you cannot explain the aetiology of an open wound if the cause of it is not parasitic. If it is not this, then is it genetic? And so we had to find out if these cancers indeed could be treated and, if so, eventually what forms of therapy would work.

It was interesting work but the situation, because of the Cold War, it was exciting in the sense that when you are with friends, the KGB is spying on you. At that time, KGB activity was at its highest. Yes. There was something very interesting – we could meet with a person like you, maybe an acquaintance. Yes, and then will ask you one question. Like, "By the way, are you married?" That's all they would ask. If you say yes or no that is enough. Somebody else out of the blue would catch you unaware and ask, "By the way, do you have children?" And this information is entered into their databank so by the time you are through, they knew either you are married or not, whether you have children or not, what are their ages, and so on. But these questions were not asked on the same day. Out of the blue, without asking anything else, on different days, random questions. It was odd. I realized the effect of the Cold War where everyone was being treated with a lot of suspicion. Yes, that was at the height of the Cold War. There was a lot of suspicion and I had first-hand experience. I had taken my camera, taken many photographs, back then of course we had film not digital cameras, and when I returned home, all my film was blank. Yes, so they gathered a lot of information on the individual. In fact, it was an extremely interesting time because it was also a period that the Soviet Union government did not allow food products to leave one republic to another one. You see their states were called republics, yes, so when I was there I was permanently eating potatoes and animal parts. I don't know whether it was beef or what and then they are giving you vodka. It is a very interesting mindset or ideology that whatever you produce in that republic is what you eat; you must have some special permissions to transport it to the next republic.

The Russians would ask me if I was from Angola because it was one of the very close allies of the Soviet Union. I told them, "I don't even know where Angola is!" It is too far from where I come from. Fortunately, I had a friend from Cameroon, from the University of Yaoundé, Vincent Titanji, who became a good friend of mine and family friend who was also studying there. Even after we left, we stayed friends and we have visited each other's family. We are editors of the *African Journal of Health Sciences* which I started soon after I became the Chief Executive of KEMRI. Yes. He had studied in the Soviet Union himself and he spoke fluent Russian.

You will know that Kenya has historical ties to Russia. You see the reason for that is because of two Luo politicians in this country from Nyanza, Jaramogi Oginga Odinga and Tom Mboya, the latter who was assassinated. Tom Mboya was one of those persons who organized the airlifts to America, including Obama's father, Obama Senior. He was airlifted by Tom Mboya in 1959 and 1960. While Raila Oginga Odinga he had his own airlift arrangements with the Soviet Union. That is why most of the people you find in Nyanza have travelled to the Soviet Union for education. That actually caused a major rift between (Jomo) Kenyatta and Jaramogi Oginga Odinga at that time because of the differences in ideology. Kenyatta was considered neutral during these days of fighting for independence and justice in Kenya. Kenyatta also went to the Soviet Union but he only went briefly, instead he lived in the UK.

But I went to Russia, which was actually the USSR at that time, when I was an adult. I was not a part of the airlifts since I was not going for education. I had already completed my postdoctoral studies in 1981. I went there on a specific research mission where we were studying some newer techniques in immunogenetics. The choice of that place was made largely by the World Health Organization since I was travelling there under their sponsorship so I was not a solitary individual trying to find my way through the Soviet Union, I thank God. That was 1981.

Notes

1 For a detailed account of Akademgorodok see Josephson 1997 and Ninetto 2001. Like the Kenya Medical Research Institute, the scientists at Akademgorodok were largely state scientists.

2 In Russian, the name is Академгородóк, a combination of академия (*akademiya*, or academy) and город (*gorod*, or city).

3 Also see the paper by Khapoya and Agyeman-Duah (1985) on the effects of the Cold War on East African politics and Anderson and Rolandsen (2014) on how the Cold War superseded colonialism in East Africa.

10 HLA tissue-typing and kidney transplants in Kenya

In 1984 I was appointed the Director of the Biomedical Sciences Research Centre at KEMRI (Kenya Medical Research Institute). As a professional researcher what I did first was to find out how best I could participate in the development of new technology for ease of diagnosis and management of diseases, based on my training in immunology, pathology and pharmacology. Yes. At that time, I realized that even simple testing for individuals who needed organ transplants was being done in other countries. The tissue and blood samples were being sent to the UK, to Germany, or South Africa where the analysis would be done to identify possible donors and recipients, depending on who was the most appropriate individual genetically. I realized there were some issues with this process. One, there was a lot of cost involved in shipping these samples to Europe or South Africa. Two, it was taking too much time, putting patients at risk. And then lastly, three, patients were forced to wait for organs. I said myself, "Why do we do this?" And then I asked myself, "Did you go to school?" I said yes. "Do you know this subject?" I said yes. "Can we identify the problem?" I said yes.

So the then Director of Medical Services, Dr Wilfred Koinange, asked one of my colleagues who was administratively my boss if it was possible to do these tests in Kenya. This person responded that we would not be in the position to develop this technology in Kenya for at least another seven years. Yes. So then I was asked and I said, "Okay, give me the authority and the money and I will be able to provide this in two months." I knew where to procure the materials, I knew what to do, and I knew the technology required, and so on. I had a few technical staff, one of them who is now a professor in the university because I was very good in developing staff (capacity). They said, "Sir, why can't we try this particular method?" I could listen, so I would say, yes, let us try that ... I had extremely competent technical staff members who were capable of doing this sort of work so we went ahead. Yes. After I agreed, they (the Government of Kenya) asked me how much money this would require. Within 12 hours I gave them the figure – roughly 2.5 million KES. At that time, in 1984, that was a lot of money for us to do this.

At that time, I had now entered into a new laboratory where I had procured new equipment so we were well positioned to take on such a project. You see, in fact my laboratory was not in the original list of laboratories funded by the Japanese. So, sadly, I had an almost near empty laboratory. I had no laboratory equipment to do the work. What should I do? Fortunately I had a way of getting some money. Margaret Thatcher's government, which was in power in the UK then, funded the laboratory. In less than a year it was fully funded and operational. It was a grant-in-aid to the Kenyan government that I had made an application for through the National Treasury. Somehow I received the money so I furnished the laboratory. The Japanese had not funded it because they believed that it was too technical and specialized a subject because we were focused on basic research, not service provision. So, I applied for a grant when Moi University in Eldoret was applying for funding for their library, aptly called the Margaret Thatcher Library. Her government funded it and then she actually made a trip to Kenya and visited the university in 1988. It is through the same funding process that I managed to filter in my request.

I had a window of opportunity because I happened to have been involved with the education sector, which I will be able to tell you more about later on. Yes. So out of that work I knew there was some funding and part of it was from Margaret Thatcher's government. So I filtered it through the treasury. So, in fact, my funding was even faster to come through because the library was infrastructural development, they were putting up the buildings, and so on. It was expensive to put up a library. Yes, so when they brought my request, it was very quick. Within three months I had furnished my laboratory. Yes. And I was the first government official to get a PC (personal computer) in Kenya and that was 1984. Microsoft had not been developed and so I had a Commodore 64.

So my colleague was saying it was going to take us seven years to develop this technology but I said, "Give me the money and I will produce it." I will perfect this technique within two months.

So eventually after about two or three weeks of work, I went back to the Director of Medical Services and I said where is the money? They said, "We are still looking for it." And so he said to me, "Do you have any money? Can you please use that money and we shall refund you?" So, out of my grant for the laboratory I had the resources to assist. I had the equipment, the materials, the technical staff, and within seven weeks I had perfected the technique. And within one week after that we were able to do tissue-typing for kidney transplants. So it is through me that we had the very first successful kidney transplant from a living donor in Kenya.

Yes, and then we continued perfecting that technique until I created a computer program that we still use today. You know, in any given individual there could be as many as 100 different types of genes that are critical in terms of particular gene loci, which are responsible for transplant antigens. They are responsible for the safe upkeep of foreign bodies or a foreign organ. Yes. So we had mapped those out and then we realized at the time there were as many as probably 100 to 150, but less than 200, different antigens so, utilizing what other institutions and laboratories had done, we were able to bring this battery of antigens. Those specific antigens that are responsible for graft rejection, we normally call it graft rejection. Yes. So they were the markers. So we went through our populations and we were able to identify markers for graft rejection.

But out of those more than 150 different gene expressions responsible for graft rejection or uptake, you may not have all of those. You may be having 40, you see, you may be having 20. So it is up to that but people have different genotypes. Yes. So to begin with I had to screen most of our local population for the spread and frequency of particular genotypes and then I realized that it is now possible to map these specific antigens. Because you could try to do actual manual comparison but it was tedious. Most of these genes are dominant, there is nothing which is recessive. If you have too many which are opposing antigens the organ won't take. Yes, but you could not achieve 100 per cent. Even in twins you may not have 100 per cent. You know, even fingerprints in twins are different. So a fingerprint is a very powerful identification tool because fingerprints are different from one individual to the other one, even in identical twins. Each time we were doing the analysis, each time we were doing this and then I knew the spectrum of all the possible gene antigens that are responsible for graft rejection or uptake. So I have to computerize them and then eventually I had a computer package so I could just plot those particular genes into the computer. When we were beginning, these computers were new so we struggled. There was no ready-made computer package, which you can purchase and then do a little bit of modification. It is easier at the moment of course.

We had to start from scratch creating the program, so I pursued another friend of mine to assist me in creating a program for that. Yes. So eventually I was able to perfect the system where we could match a patient, what we normally call the recipient, with the possible donor. We feed the required information into the program and then there is a print out, together with my name and signature at the top. Yes. Various laboratories in Kenya said, "Unless we receive Koech's signature we are not going to pursue because we don't believe you." It was all printed out even for me and so the only thing I had to do is to sign and say okay the most appropriate person out this group to donate is so and so but there was also what we called a pass mark. It would indicate for instance, the percentage of compatibility. Maybe it is a 70 per cent compatibility match. I have only given you the laboratory results, then you as the surgeon decide, they go ahead to check other clinical conditions of the individuals, because some of the possible recipients may be having a genetic disease which at the end of it might prevent them from getting a transplant organ. In fact, we had a family where they had a genetic trait for developing some kind of a tumour, so we knew this person was going to come down with a tumour at some point so why deny another person an opportunity to live because we are giving this kidney to someone who cannot survive due to other complications? We said, "No, that one we cannot give despite the fact that he is compatible with this one.'" So, we would have to look for alternatives and we had to also counsel him and other donors and recipients. Say people who are single girls who are not married yet, we have to counsel them because there is a possibility that future husbands could reject the girls, saying – "You are not total." You have lost a kidney. You have only one kidney so you are not a total being. So there are some of those issues involving stigma that we want patients to be aware of, so there is a counselling session that accompanied procedures, offered by counsellors. Yes. So that is how it happened. So we were able within two months to utilize the money, which I had from my grant; we were able to create this new system, and make it available in this country. The test takes only two days. It is very quick. You donate blood, today we do the assessment, in the afternoon we are feeding it to the computer, and tomorrow morning, I am signing off. This was way before the Human Genome Project had started.

The problem was that you cannot use ABO compatibility[1] in order to do a transplant. It is not possible. If you are donating blood there is no problem. Doing ABO compatibility for blood donation – that is not an issue because you are dealing with blood, you are not dealing with tissue, the transplanting of tissue. We have had transplantations, which were based on ABO compatibility, but what we want to avoid there is haemolysis. We did not want blood to become haemolysed because of incompatibility or even a reaction in the body. People have even died out of adverse reaction because of ABO incompatibility. The body kind of sees it as a foreign substance. Yes, so to begin with we had to do ABO compatibility tests which is routine. Then, number two, is when we now do HLA compatibility. HLA refers to Human Leucocyte Antigens tissue testing. Then later on DNA testing came in so I edited the program to account for this. We made the technique available to most of the laboratories.

In 1984 we were only doing kidney transplants because the most critical organ that needed transplanting here was the kidney. Yes. Things like liver and lung were remote. These were very remote and it was purely academic if you wanted to do it. But we did not encounter too many clinical cases that required lung transplants or liver transplants. Although the liver is possible to do, the liver is also capable of growing itself, unless the total liver is bad, but if you only remove the bad part of the liver, it can grow and repair itself. It is one of the organs that can actually re-grow. Just like the tail of a lizard.

I think this was an important development for Kenya because we were now able to increase the speed and the rate with which transplants were being done in this country. We reduced the amount of time people were spending in hospitals doing dialysis. It was a very expensive exercise and extremely exhausting. Just sitting by the dialysis machine, about two or three times a week, and then having the blood go through, and each time patients are waiting two to three hours just lying down, wearing you out psychologically too. Those are the kind of things that affected me as an individual and that I was concerned about as a scientist. In fact, fortunately the Chairman of the KEMRI Board of Management by that time was a nephrologist, and still is a nephrologist. Yes. He did his master's degree on kidney diseases. So I am happy today when I look at what we accomplished. You reduce the time of waiting, you reduce the stress of going through dialysis while waiting for an organ, you reduce the cost of travelling too because at that time some people would travel out of the country for transplants. I am not a surgeon myself. I support them through laboratory work, even up to today. So they were able now to sharpen their skills.

You know we must weigh the decision for organ donors – who should donate the kidney vis-à-vis the chance of rejection, so one has to make a judicial, a very careful decision. Because you do not want to give a kidney to somebody and then it is rejected and this person has lost their life. That was my critical view. By the time I sign off on the donor, I know clearly in myself that this candidate should not reject the organ so long as the correct drugs are given to maintain this patient's health. That is required for the next several years. That is what I did and not a single time did any of the people I recommend, ever, ever reject and the graft continued to hold for a long time, even several years. At times I said, "No, let us not take chances." You see at times relatives could come and say, "Koech, listen, I would have wished that so and so donates the kidney. Please let it be." I said, "Here there is no bribing. You don't bribe for organs!" And it is science, you cannot say "so and so gets it instead of so and so" because someone asks you to. I said you cannot and I cannot make a mistake and this individual is going to live with that mistake for the rest of one's life. Yes, you cannot say that it is going to be compatible sometime in the future when you know it will not.

Note

1 ABO compatibility is the measure used for ensuring blood donors and recipients are compatible based on antibodies to red blood cell proteins.

11 Science and Technology Amendment Act

While doing my research with the WHO Immunology Research and Training Centre in the late 1970s, I realized we needed a research centre here in Kenya. Fortunately, I had two other supporters, yes, who are now faculty members. We wrote a proposal to the faculty of medicine. So the proposal went to the faculty of medicine for review and then they said there are some fellows here who want to start a research wing of the medical school. My senior colleagues were dismissive, and said, "Wow, this little boy he wants to do this?" And some of the other fellows said, "But why when I have my research in my office?" And another one said, "I also have my laboratory in the office so we don't need this."

We faced stiff resistance and so the faculty of medicine denied it. When it was rebuffed we were feeling gloomy but then I thought to myself and I said, "Now, what are we going to do?" The only thing we are going to do is to ensure that the fire should not die. You see I could not give up. The need to create a research wing of the medical school has failed but in the process I was given a small space, actually it was a sub-department, not a full department. It was a section of the Department of Pathology. It was 40 metres by 60 metres. They said to me, if you want to do any laboratory research, this is where you have to do it. That is what my senior colleagues were telling me.

So what happened, you see, is that I told two of my colleagues, Professor Kihumbu Thairu and Professor Mutuma Mugambi, who were very supportive of me in the faculty of medicine, that we should not lose hope. Because they had bought my idea of creating a research wing in the medical school, yet it had failed. Then all over sudden I remembered that two years previously during my absence from the country a bill had been passed which implemented a law that promoted science and technology in this country. I immediately went to look for that bill because it was very difficult to get some of those official government documents. So I went immediately to the Government Printer to look for a copy. I paid for the copy to be made. You see most of such bills and government matters were published in the Kenya Gazette, or at least most of the official government announcements were published there. They publish all materials related to the implementation of law, formal government appointments, and so on. Even if they are not in the newspapers, you will find they are published in the official gazette. The Government Printer publishes all government documents. So the bill I was looking for had been passed by Parliament, which became CAP 250 of the Laws of Kenya in 1977. It resulted in the creation of the National Council for Science and Technology, or what we call NCST. So I looked at this new act carefully and then I realized that within it, it was possible to amend it to facilitate the creation of a research wing, or even a totally separate research organization within the government.

I talked to my colleagues and suggested that we forget about the medical school as an avenue since they have refused us once, so the only thing that we can do is go in a new direction. I told them that there is this opportunity to create a new organization. We encouraged each other. The three of us then asked ourselves, "How do we do it?" How do we do make changes to the act because the only person who can order such amendments is the Attorney General, which was then Charles Njonjo.[1] Charles Njonjo was a unique fellow. He was behaving like a typical British person, even until today at the age of 97 (born in 1920). He is like that. He has never changed. He never trusts anyone from Kenya and so he had a *mzungu* [/white/] secretary. Yes, he has a unique personality, and he left an indelible mark on the history of Kenya, through the organization of government and also in the passage of certain laws. Yes. We may say he was the real Attorney General. Njonjo. We call him the Prince of Kabeteshire, you see, because he was born in the Kabete area on the outskirts of Nairobi.

And he loves if you call him Sir Charles, yes, he loves it. And he is almost independent politically, which was actually very good for him. Because being a Kikuyu at the time when Kenyatta died, and being the Attorney General, he never listened to what the Kikuyus wanted. Yes. He just followed the law. And he made sure Daniel arap Moi was sworn in as the President of this Republic when Kenyatta died. Yes, although he was sworn in as the acting President because we have an allowance of a 90-day period before the acting President may be officially elected. You see but he made sure Moi took over.

So Thairu, Mugambi and I are discussing how we must amend the Science and Technology Act but how do we reach the Attorney General, a very difficult person? It is impossible even for government ministers to see him. Yes, but then I said, "Now wait a minute! Moi has become the President." I can go to Moi because I had a few friends, relatives who were known to him, and actually we knew each other already. So I decided I must reach the President. You see, at that time I was living along Ngong' Road, yes, along Ngong' Road in a very tiny flat. Yes, which actually was not mine. My sister-in-law had left it for me to stay in for some time. I stayed there for two months. It was actually a bedsit. So I decided to walk to his house to go speak to him about our idea. I walked from my house to his home, it only took me 15 minutes to walk. As I approached, I was found by the *askaris* [/security/]. They said, "Who are you?" And I identified myself. They knew me very briefly since I was not known then like the way I am known today. Then I said, "I want to see the President." They asked, "Why do you want to see the President? Do you have any appointment?" I have no appointment but he is my President. So they talked and then the President said let him come. I walked in. Yes, because he knew of me already when I travelled to the US for my studies.

I had met with him when he was Vice-President because we had visited him in his home as students of the university, because students from the Rift Valley were very few in the university, about 50 students, a small group of Kalenjins studying, and so he invited us to his home. As well, after I was through with Strathmore College I went to teach for a period of time and when I was teaching I wanted him to come and put a laboratory in the school where I was teaching. I wrote to him as the Vice-President and he responded to me. Yes, he said that he was not going to come but he sent the District Commissioner instead. Yes, so you see, I was not a stranger to him. And at one time I had a relative working in his office but I never used that to my advantage much.

So when I went to Moi that one evening and we started getting to know each other again. I started explaining to him what I have been doing, that I had been to these other places for schooling, and so on, because we lost touch in the process even though he knew me earlier on. When I walked into his home he says to me, "So what do we do?" I said,

> There is this thing, Mr President, that you could assist with. You know that we are interested in medical research and we had requested for the faculty of medicine to allow us to create a research unit but the University of Nairobi denied this. Can you please assist us to change a section in the Science and Technology Act to make it possible for medical research to be established in this country?

He said to one of his domestic workers, "Give me the phone, let me call Charles Njonjo." He called him immediately and said to him, "There is this young man called Dr Koech. I know him. This is my young boy. I know him and he is very sharp. So can you please assist him to achieve what he wants?" This is the time I had completed my PhD. So Charles Njonjo said, "Let him come at three o'clock tomorrow." So that is basically what happened.

So I called my two friends and I said, "We have an appointment with Charles Njonjo, we have gotten the opportunity." They said, "What do you mean?" I explained that we had an appointment to see him at three o'clock the following day. So it was now Professor Thairu and Professor Mugambi and then they brought in another person who was dealing with trypanosomiasis, sleeping sickness, called Dr Adrian Njogu. He had run away from Tororo in Uganda to Kenya. He had crossed the border and he didn't have anywhere to stay, you see, to establish his research.

So we went to the Attorney General's office the next day to see Njonjo. We went to the gate of the Attorney General's office and now we are a gang of four. Yes, if you have an appointment with him you must be there and on time because he is very sharp with time. The President had called him and he wants this to be done, period. So we went in. No waiting, we were checked in and taken to his office, I think it was the fourth floor to the Attorney General's chambers. So, reaching there we sat and then he came in and asked, "So who amongst you is Koech?"

"It is me, sir."

"How are you, young man?"

"I am fine, sir."

"And then tell me who these other people are?" I introduced him to the others.

"Sir, this is Professor Kihumbu Thairu. He was formerly the Dean of the Faculty of Medicine at the University of Nairobi."

"And you, he asks?"

"This is Dr Mutuma Mugambi and he is a cardiologist at the Kenyatta National Hospital."

"And you," he points to the last one of us?

"This is Dr Adrian Njogu, sir, who was the Director of East African Trypanosomiasis Research Organization in Tororo, sir. And he has been chased to Kenya following the breakdown of the community."

"Good," he said, "and so what do you want?"

I said to him, "Sir, if you could allow us to explain. We have come here for you to assist us, sir, to amend the Science and Technology Act of 1977 to facilitate the creation of the establishment for medical research because we are interested in promoting research in medicine in this country."

He replied with ease, "Aha? Is that all?"

"Yes, sir."

Then, he called two draftsmen immediately. One was called Arthur Buluma and then another one I can't recall. We also happened to have known each other with these draftsmen at the university because we were students together. Arthur Buluma passed on quite a while ago. So he called them and told them, "Now these doctors here, they want you to amend the Science and Technology Act of 1977 to facilitate the creation of a medical research institute, is it possible?" "Yes, sir," they said. Then one of them said, "Please, excuse me, sir, can we make some further suggestion?" He said, "Can we also use this opportunity in facilitating the creation of other research organizations in this country, sir?" He said, "In which way?"

He explained to him,

> You remember, sir, there was an agriculture and veterinary research unit which was being shared, but we also need an opportunity to create industrial research in this country. This may also be an opportunity to create fisheries in this country, sir.

He was pleased, "Ooh, good, good. That is a very good suggestion, young man." He said to the draftsmen,

> Go and draft this amendment and it should be done as fast as possible! I want it done within two weeks. And remember the organizational structure

> of these research institutions should be such that the chief, the head of that organization, should not be called Director General. There are only few generals in this country. Attorney General, who is me! There is Auditor and Comptroller General who is in charge of auditing our National and Treasury finances, then there are military generals. Those are the only generals I want to see. You get it?

"Yes, sir!" "Anything else?" he asked us. "Nothing, sir. Thank you so much." And we walked out. So when we were out my friends, especially Dr Adrian Njogu, who was the Director General of the East African Research Organization, said now this is good, however good, what are we going to do about the Director General? Because you see we imagined this position to head the medical research unit. Now will the Chief Executive be made Director? I looked at these people and said, "You are all my friends. Are we fools? What is in a name? We wanted some institutions to be created in this country. Now you are fighting over titles. What is in a title? Forget about this nonsense!" And then I looked at my friend and I said, "You are my friend. Actually you are my senior colleague. Whatever you want to be expressed, the fact is you are in charge. You see you are in charge, what is your problem?"

In fact, soon after that the word CEO (chief executive officer) was introduced in this country. So I said to him, "After all, you are an accounting officer. You are the boss whether they call you Chairman, whether they call you General, or Director." What is in a name? Which actually shows the problems we have as institutions where we may be fighting over titles instead of fighting over what we can do? Forget about these titles of yours. You are not here fighting for titles. That one you should go to the political arena and fight for it there. Our roles, my role, here is for us to create institutions to do research in this country, not creating names or titles for ourselves. I am just fighting for the creation of a research institute in this country. So I looked at Njogu and said, "Do you want me to regret why I told you to accompany us?" "No," he said, "let's move forward." Yes, so that is what happened. At times it is unfortunate.

We were working together with the drafters. We were working with the draftsmen to write the bill, especially me, I went there regularly. And, within two weeks, or thereabouts, I can't remember the exact dates, but the draft bill was ready. It was presented in Parliament around late November, actually I think it was in December before the Parliament broke for Christmas recess. It was then tabled and passed by Parliament I think on the 15th of March 1979 and it then became a bill to be presented to the President. It was actually given assent by the President on Wednesday, the 20th of May the same year, 1979. It was the Science and Technology Amendment Act CAP 250 of the Laws of Kenya. So this bill created the National Council for Science and Technology, which facilitated the promotion of science and technology in this country. Yes. It was the Science and Technology Amendment Act, which was actually repealed about two years ago and replaced with the creation of a new bill. In its amended form it led to the creation of research institutes, each with a specific mandate. These included the Kenya Agricultural Research Institute (KARI), Kenya Industrial Research and Development Institute (KIRDI), Kenya Marine and Fisheries Research Institute (KEMFRI), Kenya Trypanosomiasis Research Institute (KEMFRI) and the Kenya Medical Research Institute (KEMRI). The Kenya Forestry Research Institute (KEFRI) was created later through a gazette notice. This act has since been repealed and a new one enacted but it retains the original structure with the focus on the creation of research institutes, with minor amendments. The new act is now called the National Science and Technology and Innovation Act, Number 28 for 2014.

So if there is anything I have done in my career or serious import at that time it was the creation, or facilitation, of these six institutions of research in Kenya. I can credit myself for that and I have no apologies to make and those are my bragging rights. I impressed upon the government for the creation of these research institutions. Although I was going there, I must thank Wanjuki Muchemi and Arthur Buluma, who were in charge of the drafts of the amendments, because I went there thinking only of medical research but by the time I came out, we had included all the other research institutes. There are proper braggers in this case and they are the two draftsmen and then Koech who actually took the proposal to the Attorney General. The Science and Technology Act was amended and it came out as beautiful document which I am so proud to have been involved in creating.

So the Marine Institute did not have much to call an institute. They had some minor facility along the coast, and the industrial research institute did not have much but they were utilizing borrowed facilities. The Kenya Medical Research Institute did not have much in spite of the fact that we were fighting for space and funding. Although we now had an institute, at the end of it we are faced with this reality of not having the facilities to do research in this country. The only facility we had was the Tuberculosis Investigation Centre, which was then a part of the Ministry of Health. The Malaria Unit, which was in Kisumu, was part of the Division of Vector-Borne Diseases of which I happened to have been the boss of at that time.

My attempts to secure an office or laboratory for KEMRI was saved by the fact that I had other positions at the Ministry of Health and at the University of Nairobi. Yes. The first laboratory of KEMRI was actually my own laboratory at the Immunology Department of the University of Nairobi, which had previously been occupied by ILRAD while I was away pursuing graduate studies in the US. So when they vacated the facilities, they left their equipment behind, so we inherited a very beautiful and proper scientific laboratory. Then, number two, is that the field laboratories which the Division of Vector-Borne Diseases had were also converted into field sites for the new Kenya Medical Research Institute in other parts of the country. There was no official administrative headquarters for KEMRI, except the Department of Cardiology where Mutuma Mugambi was the second Director but something happened before then.

Do you know that here in government the fiscal system runs from the 1st of July to the 30th of June. The amendment to the act became law on the 20th of

May and so we had a small window in which to ask for money in order to run the new Kenya Medical Research Institute, just like the other new organizations, especially because we did not have any structure. Nothing, no facilities at all, except these borrowed ones. So what I did was I went to the Government Printer and bought a copy of the Kenya Gazette which contained the new amended law, and then I took that copy of the act to the then Permanent Secretary for the Ministry of Health because, according to the law at that time, all these organizations must be responsible to some parent ministry and we were under the Ministry of Health. I took a copy of the act to the Permanent Secretary for the Ministry of Health, whose title is now Principal Secretary and who is actually the accounting officer in a government ministry. I went to him and I said, "Sir, we would wish that the financial year has not yet come to an end if you could put in some money to help facilitate the Kenya Medical Research Institute." I went with a minor proposal. "If you could put in some money to facilitate even buying basic things to us to start medical research in this country." I told him we needed some funding to support research into tuberculosis, viruses like hepatitis and others. He looked at the act, opened that page, and said, "What do you want? I don't recognize this piece of paper!" And he threw it at me. "If you want money, let that paper give you the money!" In fact it hurt my eye. It actually bled a little bit and became red for some time. Then I walked out. The first Director of the Institute was a person called Dr James Mbogo Gikonyo.[2] He was in the Ministry of Health as one of the Senior Directors in charge of health and some aspects of health services. He had been working in one of the organizations of the East African Medical Research Council and so was identified as a candidate to act as the temporary Director of the new KEMRI. Dr Gikonyo was another interesting person. You could go to him with an idea, and he would give you 1,000 reasons why that idea was not possible to implement, or why it could not happen.

Notes

1 Njonjo joined Jomo Kenyatta's first Cabinet in 1963 as the first African Attorney General, a position he held until 1980.
2 James Mbogo Gikonyo passed 2 February 2010.

12 Daniel arap Moi

I just came from this little village, a boy who had suffered in this world. So that is it, but you see my happiness is that the access I had to President Moi did not interfere with the lives of other people because I never used the relationship for that sort of thing. On the contrary, it assisted this nation. Number one, when I look back at it we built KEMRI, because I had requested President Moi to ask the Japanese for assistance. Then, number two, the research institutes would have been developed but it would not have been as fast during that particular time. We would still be developing research institutes in this country today if it were not for my relationship with Moi, and then, number three is that the development of a structure to regulate university education in this country came not through President Moi, but through the minister at that time. He was willing to listen to me when I explained that it was necessary for us to create a parastatal unit that would regulate university education in this country.

If we allow these private universities to establish themselves without any regulation, our university education system will be of poor quality. So the minister listened and then we primed President Moi so that he could allow the motion to pass through the Cabinet. You see? So President Moi was remotely responsible but mostly he played a role by listening to my recommendations. You see, he could listen to me when I talked with him. When you see him starting to do other things, then you know your time is up. It is time to just wind up your story. Yes, I knew when he was in bad mood. I could monitor it. I could go to him and you see he was talking in Kiswahili. He would say, "People are just coming here to disturb me" and so on. Then I went and said, "Mr President who is this really disturbing you? Let us go out *kumangamanga* [/for a stroll/]. I know where we can go. Let's go *kumangamanga*, let's go and loiter around. Let's get out of this place."

We had to go up to Muranga one afternoon. I said just forget about these things, people coming to disturb you. Let's go. Yes. So you would see him saying, "Let us go" and his officers did not know why he had decided to just leave. Sometimes, he would go to see development projects, some buildings coming up, to see progress in the city, so that is the way you could engage him. Yeah, that is the way one could engage Moi but there are some people who did not understand this. His handlers actually, to some degree, well, they may have not thought about him as a person. They only saw the President as a provider. They are not looking at him as an individual with his own feeling, who needs to relax, and so on. That is why we allowed the court jesters, the fellows who would come and entertain him with rumours. He used to like to be entertained with rumours. "*Mzee*, don't you see it is happening with so and so...." He could laugh and laugh, and laugh and laugh. So when he wanted to be happy, we needed to make him happy. Create funny rumours for him. Yes. Where I could, I tried to make him laugh because people used to go to him always asking for things: "Please assist me to do this .... *Nisaidie hii* ..." [/help me with this/].

But people didn't allow him to be himself. You see, he didn't have any sport to pass time. The only social thing he ever did was to go to church and to go to fundraisers. Even if he goes to fundraisers, there he is expected to cough up some money. Yes. So it happened that he used to have some people who could entertain him until he was going to sleep, because at one point in the 1970s he parted company with his wife. Yes, with Lena, but that is another story. So he was alone from about 1974, the tail-end of his Vice-Presidency, and for his entire 24 years as President. He didn't have a wife, somebody to stay with him. He didn't have a wife who could entertain him or sort out domestic issues for the home.

I felt that many of the people that surrounded him, misused him. They did only for their own benefit. At times they could lie to him and say things like, "I am going to do a fundraising and Mzee we collected a lot of money, yes, thank you ..." but there was not even a single fundraiser! So they made use of him. Yes. Even as we are talking now, he is not like King David where they could look for a woman for him. You remember in the biblical story of King David? They wanted to know whether he was dead, you see, so they looked for a nice young woman to go to entertain him and so the girl came and said the fellow is dead! At this age, of course, his own grandchildren entertain him. Yes. You know when one gets old it can be very lonely, especially a public figure like that. That is why people at times, they want to stay in power until they die because of the fear of being alone. From 1956 or 1955 until the year 2002 he was a leader, a big man, he was the centre of power wherever he went. All those years he has been creating institutions, building Kenya, and all of a sudden you are no longer involved in those things.

I used to have a car, a VW beetle, KJQ 439, so one afternoon I drove to Moi's house. Reaching there the *askari* asked, "Where are you going? Who are you?" I said, "I am Koech." "You want to see the President?" "Yes," I said, "yes, because the President said I can go to his house anytime." But just then as I was talking with the *askari* the President exited the house to go for a walk. So he sees me waiting there and said, "*Daktari*, how are you?"

"I am fine, sir."
"You had come to see me?"
"Yes."
"But I am going for a walk now."

I said, "Okay, I'll come another time."
But then he asked me, "By the way, where do you stay?"
I told him it was near, just up the road.
"Within walking distance?" he asked.
"Yes, sir," was my response.
"Then I am coming to your house for tea."

So I drove slowly, stopping at each bend of the road while he walked with his security detail. He walked to my house for tea. Because he could not get into my car, for it was crowded and tiny, he just walked and then the *askaris* did not even know where we were going. They could see only the President walking, so they followed him. Then reaching the house I told my wife, "Listen, President Moi is coming. He is here." At that time we were staying in an apartment, there were four apartments in the same location, on one acre. Of course, that day we were not expecting President Moi to come to my house. Back then we did not have a modern stove, we were using a *jiko* [/ceramic with charcoal/] to make tea and then we didn't even have any cups to serve the tea in, so I went to my neighbour! I had some cups but not these modern ones, only the ones you see in the villages. They are big mugs, made of iron, painted either green, yellow and so on, but I could not serve tea to the President of the Republic of Kenya in one of those.

My neighbour was a pilot and I knew they had some nice presentable cups, so we went and borrowed his. President Moi was not aware, so we sat down and then we had some tea and my late son, Chang'-Toek, was there then. He went out to the compound, saying, "Moi is in my house!" Of course, because there were no official state vehicles, no one knew he was there. He felt so relaxed with us that he stayed until around 8:30 or 9:00 in the evening. Then the problem was how will the President of the Republic of Kenya get home? He cannot walk along Ngong road and go through all those areas, so my son says to me, "Daddy, you know what, there is a *panya route*" [/short cut/]. These small trails or little openings we call *panya*, which means where the rat runs. These are informal routes, a trail behind the houses. So my son said if we use this route behind the apartments it was much closer. We could come to a field where there are some houses, an estate area, and there are dogs and a hedge that we must duck under. The young boys used to follow this route but I had never used it. So the *askaris* went to examine the route and then said, let us go. But because we have walked to my house during daylight hours, we now did not have any torch (flashlight). So again I went to my neighbour and borrowed a torch. It was quite an adventure! We had to go through just a little opening in the wall, there was a ditch, and then you climb up on the other side, so President Moi had to crawl underneath! The *askaris* said "We will take care of the dogs." I walked back with him on foot until he was home. I said, "Now I have brought you back."

So the following day around 11 in the morning I was at work. President Moi had an assistant who worked in his house and she came directly up to my office and asked, "Where is your house?" So I explained to her but asked why.

President Moi was sending a full sack of *wimbi* [/sorghum/], finger millet food, a full sack of rice, a full sack of this, and a full sack of that. So we had enough food to give to the neighbours. So we were sharing that food with many. We didn't even have anywhere to store those things in that very tiny apartment. Yes. So that's how our relationship was strengthened.

Whatever I could tell him, he could listen. So President Moi kept on coming as a friend to my house. Yes, both in Nairobi and in Kericho. One time he came to my residence in Kericho with eight ministers to have a breakfast in the house. I think he had a meeting in Kericho, and so he said, "We are coming to your house for breakfast." So he arrived with eight ministers and we made them breakfast, and my mother prayed for them. After they just left and said *kwaheri* [/bye/]. You see. Just like that he could come or go.

Yes, and then he started loving me as a person because I never went to him to beg for anything. You see he never gave me a shilling almost in his entire career. He was an extremely generous person, but I wanted to separate my roles: one was friend, and one was professional. I would not go to him to beg for favours or talk ill of any other person in front of him. I would not go to him and ask for land. No, instead, I would go to him and explain the situation and inquire if he could assist. There is a difficulty here please assist, or eventually when I went to do some business I would go to him and say give me this business but do not give it to me for free. You see. I could also return the favour out of the profits I made. So he started having a liking for me because I never went to him asking for two things: I never asked for money. And, number two, I never asked for land or these government properties. Yes. You may see in the corruption reports stories of land misappropriation and so on. My name does not feature anywhere in those reports.

So he knew all along that I would not go to him and ask for favours. I would go to him with a genuine issue and I would visit him at the State House for tea to keep him company, when I have nothing else to do and when he was available. I would see that my family was okay and so I would spend the afternoon with my President. I could go to him but even the gatekeepers knew I was not going to report. They knew exactly who was allowed to see the President and I did not use any of them to make an appointment. I would only tell Moi and I would use a small gate. Yes, and the *askaris* could not deny me. I was never denied access to the State House. I never misused that relationship at all. I was close to Moi and even facilitated the appointment of people in his government. There is one time when he asked me in 1987 to be the Permanent Secretary in the Ministry of Health but I went to him and I told him,

> Mr President, please leave me at KEMRI. I am still young and not yet through with what I am doing. Please leave me out of the public limelight and politics because I know my people. They will come and heap a lot of *fitinas* [/gossip/] about me.

So I never used my relationship with President Moi to manipulate him or to seek favours from him. No. The only favour I received from him was when he appointed me to chair the Commission of Inquiry into the Education System of Kenya. But the beauty is that he was there to listen. We couldn't have created research institutes if it were not for him because he listened to my request to make the amendments to the Science and Technology Act and the request for international funding. KEMRI would not have been developed by JICA (Japanese International Cooperation Agency) if he had not listened to me, we wouldn't have received the money from the Japanese. Yes, he was there to facilitate important developments in Kenya but I did not ask him to enrich myself. I have never asked him to give me any money. No, I have not. And he has not pulled out his pocket to give me money, except one day, when I was going home. I found him at the State House in Nakuru. I stopped there very briefly to greet him and I told him, "Mr President, I am going home." He asked me, "Why don't you wait for lunch?" I said, "You know, if I wait for lunch then what I want to do at home will be delayed for more than two hours and I am strict with my time." So he pulled open his pocket and gave me 1400 KES for lunch. That is the only money he ever gave me. Yes. But he also created opportunities for people to expand. If you approached him without any selfish intentions, he would treat you very well. So that is my relationship with Moi all the way through. Now he has become a little elderly, so we need to give him his freedom to rest.

Moi decided to do away with tribalism. He limited tribal affiliations. He dismantled all tribal affiliations in this country so there was no Kalenjin this or Luo that and so on. There was nothing. President Moi killed it all. There was no

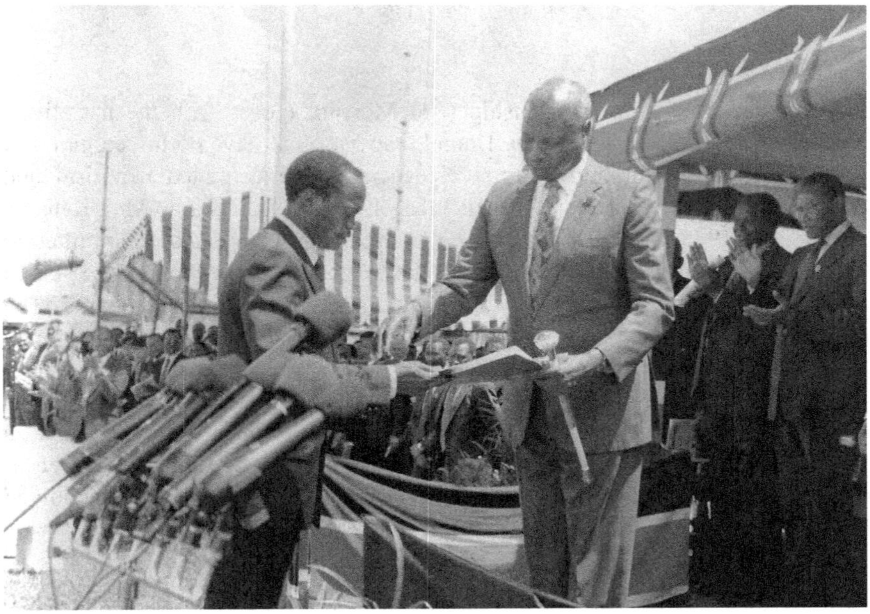

Figure 12.1 Moi and Koech at KEMRI.

vernacular radio or television stations either except on national radio stations where there was time allocation to serve those members of the community who could not understand either Kiswahili or English. He did not want Kenyans to restrict themselves to tribal associations. Yes. He did not favour local tribal associations but when President Kibaki was elected, he allowed it to run their course. President Moi wanted to kill it because at that time the Kalenjin community was one of the minority communities and he decided to strengthen the minority communities, to lift them up, by trying to neutralize tribal affiliations, which I think worked very well. He did this by focusing on education and establishing schools. Everywhere schools, schools. Yes. And that is his legacy – the development of schools in this country. We cannot deny that he did this for our country. You see the education system was very poor in infrastructure. President Moi knew exactly what was happening in this country, what happened in this particular village, for instance. He had an excellent intelligence network. He knew precisely when to strike. Yes.

I have been given three honours or awards (State Investiture) so far from the State. One is the Silver Star of Kenya (SS), awarded in 1984. Another one is the Order of the Grand Warrior (OGW) in 1989 and the other the Moran of the Burning Spear (MBS) in 1998. They were all given in recognition of distinguished service rendered to the nation. So they were given to me but I only went once to the State House to collect them. I was not a fan of being seen with Moi, but I knew we had a genuine friendship. We continued our friendship even though he has left politics because of his age. I go to visit frequently to say hi to him because he acted as my father.

Intermission

Koech's account of his relationship with Moi juxtaposes with the narratives, especially in the West, describing Daniel arap Moi that have portrayed him as a human rights violator and repressive leader, who encouraged nepotism and patronage among his allies and friends.[1] Koech depicts Daniel arap Moi, Kenya's leader from 1978 until 2002, as a man of faith (deeply Christian), committed to educating Kenyans, generous with those he trusted, who was unfairly exploited by those who surrounded him; a lonely man seeking respite and laughter. The stories of Moi walking home late at night along the dirt path, ducking through fences and shrubs, are somewhat endearing. Moi is portrayed as a father figure, treating Koech as a sort of adopted son. Absent from any discussions Koech and I had, even off the record, was mention of the many crimes and egregious acts that Moi and his government have been accused of, though, on more than occasion Koech reported that he had never been publicly accused of being involved in the wrong-doings of Moi.

In an email during the editing phase of this book he clarified:

> Being a friend of Moi doesn't mean I was in the know of everything going on in his presidency. I was not his administrative assistant with government

> secrets. I would therefore not even remotely know of the violence or torture that was going on during Moi's presidency.

Moi authorized detaining citizens without trial (and detained lawyers, oppositional leaders, journalists, activists and academics, among others), he has been accused of rigging the 1992 and 1997 elections, and only allowed multiparty elections after being forced by national demonstrations and international pressure. He banned unions and other organizations under his leadership that supported democracy and human rights, including the Kenya Civil Servants Union and the Universities Academic Union. At one point he closed both Kenyatta and Nairobi universities for a full year. He also further exploited the system of patronage in Kenya whereby he rewarded individuals with leadership roles in Kenya's government, state owned corporations and state institutions (Human Rights Watch 2002). Godwin Murunga (2004), however, points out that Moi did not develop this system of rule (a system of "concentrated power in the presidency"); he perfected that which he had inherited from Kenyatta. These actions were public knowledge during Moi's reign but the financial corruption and violence did not become public knowledge until Moi left the office.

The 2007 WikiLeaks report suggested that Moi, his family (especially sons Gideon and Philip), lawyer and other close associates (like Nicholas Biwott and Joshua Kulei) had laundered and/or hid the equivalent of "billions of US dollars", comparable to Mobutu in then Zaire (see Project KTM by Kroll Associates) through the UK, US, Cayman Islands, Geneva and a range of other nations. The report was damning and reported, for instance, that Philip Moi's wife Rosanna/Zara Moi said he was worth about US$750 million. The family has majority or complete shares in many Kenyan organizations, owns properties around the world and has accounts in many nations known for hiding money.

But the financial corruption and patronage pale in comparison to the reports of torture from the Nyayo House. Moi's 24 years in power became most well known for the violence, detention and torture that occurred in the basement of the Nyayo House from 1982 until the 1990s. A report by Citizens for Justice (2003: X) explains that citizens were:

> blindfolded, driven to the dungeons, thrown into the black or red cells and tortured for days on end. Water would be poured into the cell and cold and then hot dusty air would be pumped alternately into the cells through the ventilation ducts. The victims would be denied food and for days they would be brutally beaten. Others were shot dead as they underwent interrogation. Those who survived this stage ended up in prison or detention after kangaroo trials of sedition or treason. Yet others, after giving names of their friends or relatives, would be allowed to go home.

After the 1 August 1982 attempted *coup d'état,* Moi had political opposition members like Raila Odinga and Otieno Mak'Onyango detained. Naivasha and

Kamiti Maximum Security Prisons were both converted into concentration camps where students, activists, politicians and other "threats" to national security were interrogated and also often tortured.

Note

1 See for example, Human Rights Watch (2002), Hornsby (2012), Murunga (2004), Lynch (2008), Citizens for Justice (2003).

13 National politics

The government at times can be totally ungrateful. Yes. It doesn't matter what you have done. The thing is – it is thankless. I am not even talking about myself. I am talking about others, like the late Professor Joseph Maina Mũngai who helped in the establishment of the Medical School at the University of Nairobi. He was a selfless individual. He even offered to cover my tuition for me so that I could catch up with my colleagues but I said no. It was not his burden but that was the kind of person he was. He eventually became the Vice-Chancellor of the university and later served as the Secretary/Chief Executive of Commission for University Education where I was his Chairman. He established the medical school in 1967. He had to travel across the border to collect cadavers because the use of human cadavers in Kenya had not been allowed at that time. He had to drive using his VW car to collect the cadavers from across the border to bring to the university to teach anatomy! He was professor of anatomy and had completed his PhD in the UK. He passed on a few years ago. Yes. I would have expected the university to honour him too. For instance, they could rename the school the Joseph Mũngai Medical School. The government is such a monster that, immediately once it has made use of you, it dumps you. There are so many individuals that have experienced this here in Kenya. I have asked, please let us honour these individuals, especially people like Mũngai who really worked so hard for our country.

The other one is the late Thomas R. Odhiambo, who was an eminent scientist and entomologist. He was not working for the government but he established ICIPE, the International Centre of Insect Physiology and Ecology. Yes, if you work in Kenya for any amount of time, you will know of him and ICIPE. He passed on in 2003 but people have forgotten about him just like that. There are so many prominent Kenyans who have done a lot of work in this country, yet the government has not even bothered to acknowledge how they have shaped our nation or how we are utilizing their skills, knowledge and legacy. Another person of note is Professor Simeon Ominde. He chaired the first Commission of Inquiry into the Education System of Kenya, which led to the abolition of racial segregation in the schools of Kenya in 1964. This resulted in what we call the Ominde Commission Report, an inquiry into the colonial education system that we inherited from the British.

Under colonialism, you see, there was an English school for the white people, an Asian one for the Asians (Indians), and then one for the black Africans. A totally segregated system. And it was during that period of segregation that I was chased from the Tea Hotel. Strathmore College was the first institution, which opened in 1961, without segregation. When Strathmore opened in 1961, all the schools were segregated. Nairobi School was Prince of Wales for the whites, which used to play rugby with Strathmore. Alliance was only for the African-elite. Africans were also permitted at Mangu and Maseno and probably Shimo La Tewa. Those were for Africans. The Asians attended Allidina Visram in Mombasa and there was another in Nairobi, another one *sijui* [I don't know], I cannot recall the other name. You see? It was a purely segregated system because of the Beecher Report of 1949. My commission on education, the Koech Commission, was the second, although there were committees and reports in between by various individuals. But I really want to urge the government to think twice and to really honour these individuals. They are forgotten the moment they leave or pass.

Outside of my work in medicine and science, I had extra time to play politics. I was basically a political strategist. Even when President Moi appeared to be losing during the multiparty democracy elections, I assisted in changing the tide. Yes, the tide was far too big. And then I told Mr President, "It is time for us to apply the 48 laws of power." Yes. Strike the shepherd, then the sheep will scatter!

Yes. I reflected and thought, okay if there is anything that I can do in order to improve the chances of President Moi retaining his presidency, and the quality of politics in our country, I should. I played the role of an advisor and a strategist. You know the person you see if you watch the television? These are political strategists or political analysts offering commentary and analysis, but if you asked that person if they have ever actually worked for any of the politicians, they would admit no. None of them. I am not a publicity seeker. You may have noticed that. I want to do certain things correctly. I tell the public for those who want to listen. I say this is what has happened.

So during the period, I was through with my active studies outside the country. So I was inside the political system. At that time, we now had a one-party system of government, which was actually a de facto one-party system until 1982. After the attempted coup Kenya became a *de jure* one-party system, dismantled ten years later through international pressure. Section 2A of the Constitution of Kenya was repealed under Moi, which allowed competitive politics or multiparty democracy. Before then, almost everyone was a member of KANU (Kenya African National Union). I think I have a certificate indicating a life membership of KANU somewhere. Yes, that was what we were doing.

But when it came to competitive politics at this time some various strategists came in to assist their own people to venture into national politics. I played a role despite the fact that we were not allowed as public servants to actively participate in party politics, which is why I played a rather silent role. My first participation was during the introduction of multiparty politics between 1990 and

1992. We created a youth movement at that time, we called ourselves the YK' 92 (Youth for KANU 92). You know one of the fellows who was competing for presidency is called Cyrus Jirongo. He was the Chairman. Yes. He was a crowd mover. Our current Deputy President, William Ruto, was one of the active members of the secretariat. So we decided to assist President Moi to win in this new multiparty system, which he encountered for the first time since he took over the presidency. The tide was great and not in his favour, so we designed a strategy to scatter the opposition. Failure to do this, and the tide was going to sweep Moi out of power within five minutes. Yes. So the best strategy was just to create confusion amongst the opposition. So instead of one mass movement running against Moi, we split them into different opposing political groups. We made them disagree and created divisions.[2] In the end, Moi won the election by around 36 per cent. The massive FORD party split its votes, 25 per cent to FORD-Asili, which was led by Kenneth Matiba, and 17 per cent to FORD-Kenya led by Jaramogi Oginga Odinga. The Democratic Party led by Mwai Kibaki garnered 19 per cent but it was not part of the original FORD. There were smaller parties, which garnered less than 1 per cent each. Yes, and you couldn't win the election with less than 25 per cent of the votes cast in at least five of the eight provinces in Kenya.[3] No, to win you needed to get about 25 per cent of the votes in all of those. This was possible for President Moi and it was also possible for those running against him, if they had stayed together, but they found it extremely difficult to garner 25 per cent of the votes cast in five of the provinces. The strategy which we adopted was fairly simple. A youth-like movement was established with a Chairman and the secretariat. The Chairman was reporting to President Moi. I would advise President Moi on several tactics to use. I would go round to meet with the YK' 92 secretariat in private. That is the time I approached President Moi and I told him, "Listen, for this to succeed you must make peace with your opponents."

One of the opposition leaders in 1992 was Jaramogi Oginga Odinga, Raila's father. So Moi said to me, "But how can I go to this fellow who I put under house arrest for several years?" I said it doesn't matter because we are dealing with politics. When we are dealing with politics, those who have been your enemies, you must draw them very close to you. Yes. And the other strong politicians were from the Kikuyu ethnic community. Matiba was a Kikuyu and then Kibaki, who was my Minister for Health, decided to resign from being the minister, creating his own opposition party. So I said the most appropriate person to make peace with in this case is Jaramogi Oginga Odinga. Yes. But Moi asked me, "How can I get him? Will he agree to meet with me? And if he does agree to meet, he is wild, and he is on the opposite side. He will not agree to peace!" Then I said, "Okay, let me have a try." I had a friend who had direct access to Jaramogi, called George Adongo. So I spoke with George and convinced him that Jaramogi and Moi should meet. Adongo agreed and put me in touch with Jaramogi. We told Jaramogi that if you are going to be President, you will need a very strong and friendly opposition leader. President Moi will most likely be the opposition leader in Parliament so the best thing you can do is to meet with him. He agreed, but where? So I arranged for them to meet in my house in Lavington.

I organized the meeting for Moi. I used one of my vehicles, a Peugeot 504, registration number KYP 554, to go to Jaramogi's house, which was very close to Lavington shopping centre; he was living along Mugumo Road, now renamed Margaret Kenyatta Road. I fetched him with my car in the evening, took him to my house, and then I called President Moi to let him know that he (Jaramogi) had come. He asked, "Do you mean it?" I said, "Yes, sir." So within ten minutes, travelling from his house in Kibera, Moi was at my house, meeting with Jaramogi. We made some tea for them and had them meet in one of the living rooms. I provided them with tea and then left, closing the door. The two old men hugged each other for the first time in several years. They were meeting for the first time in a long time, so when they hugged each other, I said to myself that is something. President Moi was the one serving tea to Jaramogi. I stayed outside the room with the security detail. They were together for very close to one hour and, of course, I had talked to President Moi before about precisely what to say to Jaramogi. We had also talked with Jaramogi and so knew precisely what he was going to demand. I encouraged Moi to emphasize their long relationship, that they are brothers. We are contiguous, our boundaries are jelled, we are one people. So I told Moi to appease Jaramogi. Moi said to Jaramogi,

> I know on the basis of your popularity you are likely to win as President. So when you win as the President, I'll be the leader of the minority government in Parliament, so to let's agree that we are going to work together. I am also going to protect you.

Then when they were through, they called for me, "*Daktari!*" [/doctor/].

"Yes, sir?"

So I opened the door and went inside and Moi said, "We have agreed." Then Jaramogi looked at me and said, "Young man…" I said, "Yes sir?" He continued, "I have my son and he is a very stubborn young man. He does not want to listen to me." This is because now Jaramogi and Raila were in the new political outfit that had split from the main FORD party. YK' 92 and other operatives had succeeded in splitting them. Jaramogi said to me, "I want him to see President Moi." I said, "Yes, sir." So I allowed President Moi to leave, and then I took Jaramogi back to his house. The next challenge was to look for Raila and convince him to talk to President Moi because Raila was a difficult person. President Moi had detained him for several years and the pain of being in detention was still in him. And, he is more stubborn than the father. President Moi had put the father under house arrest, then locked the son up because it was believed that he may have participated in the planning for the 1982 attempted coup in Kenya. So Raila had been released but with a lot of fire against the President. So George and I pursued him until he agreed to meet. True to what his father had said, he immediately dismissed our request for him to meet with President Moi. George and I were as persuasive as possible, and then we prayed over it.

Eventually he agreed and so the next meeting was with Raila and President Moi, again at my house. From there, Raila and I, we became friends, so Raila and President Moi, they became friends until they forgot about us. During that particular period when President Moi was campaigning I went to the President and I said to him, "Listen, the best strategy now is that you assist Jaramogi in his campaign against you. He is not as endowed financially as the others from central Kenya. Assist him to campaign against you." Yes. So actually we sponsored Jaramogi, and we sponsored also Raila to some degree, to run against President Moi. YK' 92 succeeded in splitting the opposition into about three or four political outfits.

My rationale was this: the Kikuyus in Central Kenya will definitely not vote for Moi. Kibaki and Matiba were in two different parties. Jaramogi was in a different party. So there were about three or four political outfits that were vying for the presidency. I told President Moi then that these fellows from Central are expensive individuals and they are going to run him dry, and they are not going to give him any votes so treat them as such. They are already splitting their votes. You can manage to retain yourself if you hold on to these other smaller communities all the way from the coast and north Eastern province. I said to him, "You see, what you need to do is to create a fear of a Kikuyu President. Fear amongst them."

So Moi became a very good student of mine, yes, he was of course a smart individual. As an experienced person, he had seen it all and he knew his opponents very well. He had appointed them in his Cabinet and one of them had been his Vice-President. He had other strategic advisors as well, some of them were in his Cabinet. Our role was only to supplement his experience. But he could use some tricks from some of the younger individuals like us. He had, of course, other advisors. I was not the only one. He had other advisors through our youth movement as well. We said to him, "The only thing you need to do is create fear about a Kikuyu presidency, once you have created the fear, people will vote for you." So that fear strategy actually did the trick. But we did not expect one thing – that Kibaki and Matiba had very strong opposing views. Matiba had one party, FORD-Asili, and Kibaki had another party, the Democratic Party, and the two of them both come from central Kenya, and they are Kikuyus, but we knew we had comfortably split them. According to the analysis, each of them would take about 18–20% of the vote, and then Jaramogi who was in FORD-Kenya would also take a proportion of the vote. We had given ourselves, KANU, about 38–40% of the votes, so we had about a ten point advantage.

I told President Moi that he could only finance a few Kikuyu people who were still his friends, knowing that they would not get any votes for him. He had to focus on supporting Jaramogi as the main oppositional candidate. You see, because Luos will vote for him (Jaramogi), no matter what. I told him that among the Luo, in Nyanza, you are going to get no votes at all. He will get a few from the Kisiis, but you will only get 0.9% of the votes from Nyanza. And you could spend a lot of money campaigning but you will never win the Luo vote. We were concerned that because Jaramogi didn't have big financial muscle, he may be inclined to go and join forces with Matiba or Kibaki. If they had all joined forces, Moi would have lost. So Moi actually put a lot of support into Jaramogi's campaign so that he could oppose Moi, and the others. In fact, I said give this to Jaramogi's kitty but let me handle the young MPs [Members of Parliament].

In YK' 92 we used to have the secretariat and then a Chairman who reported to President Moi but they joked and called me the "holy ghost" because I was never seen. I only attended when we were going to see President Moi in his house, but I never attended all those public meetings. I was never there at all. I never appeared, yes. So that is it, eventually, how President Moi came out with over 36 per cent of the votes. As I had predicted, he got less than 1 per cent of the Luo votes. Our trick worked. Yes. So that is it as far as President Moi is concerned.

After Moi I worked for Kibaki. In the 2007 elections is when Mwai Kibaki came in. Yes. So when Kibaki was now trying to fight with Raila is when President Moi told Kibaki,

> If you want to penetrate the Rift Valley, the only person you need to get in touch with is Koech. Yes. He will give you a very nice strategy. He will assist you. And he is capable because at home he is respected. He knows who to approach. He can even reach Ruto himself.

So I went to Kibaki's office because they wanted my assistance. You see, the whole organization was a very mean organization and that is why there were disputed results. He didn't perform as well as the campaign machine of Raila and his team. Yes. It was a poorly managed campaign and Kibaki was not the type of person who could go to the field and then really work. It was a rather poorly organized and a very selfish organization. I went to President Kibaki and told him, "This is not the way to do it." But he did not have too many people, and people were so selfish around him. He could not manage to do anything. And in 2007 Kibaki called me again and I chaired a committee organized to deliver the votes for him from the Rift Valley. This was in September 2007 when I was having my own troubles already at the Kenya Medical Research Institute. If he had managed to listen to what I was telling him, there would not have been post-election violence in 2007. There wouldn't have been. Yes. So it was after that election that we formed a coalition government and then after the coalition government is when Uhuru started fighting with Raila.

As a political strategist I considered how to best organize and how to hit at particular cells in order to gain strategic votes, instead of just going round shouting in the field and having a crowd gather. So Moi knew my ability to do that. Yes. Although it was not known publicly, as a public servant I was the one strategizing for him and on the sidelines telling him don't do this, do this, etcetera. Yes, it was me.

Notes

1 Youth for KANU, or YK' 92 as it is known, included three of Moi's children (Gideon, Jonathan, and June), the now Vice-President William Ruto, and Cyrus Jirongo, among others. Membership was by invitation only. According to Kanyinga and Njoka (2002: 90), "YK' 92 became the main avenue through which the state party disbursed patronage resources to mobilise support for President Moi and KANU in general." For more information on the role of Youth for KANU 92 election and accusations of coercion and bribery see Foeken and Dietz (2000), Kanyinga and Njoka (2002), and Kagwanja (2005). Some suggested that Youth for KANU 92 participated in vote buying and other coercive tactics but its members have denied this and other negative rumours. For more information on Youth for KANU 92, see the film *Sons of Fortune: The story of YK' 92*, available online at www.youtube.com/watch?v=wEYIauUq6tc.

2 The oppositional party members divided into two factions: FORD-Asili under Matiba and Martin Shikuku and FORD-Kenya under Jaramogi Oginga Odinga. And then, Mwai Kibaki left the government and registered the Democratic Party of Kenya.

3 In August 1992 the Constitution of Kenya (Amendment) Bill was passed in Parliament. One of the significant changes made was that it was now compulsory for a winning president to have at least 25% of the votes in at least five of the eight provinces.

14 The Kenya Medical Research Institute

The Kenya Medical Research Institute (KEMRI) developed because my proposal to create a research wing at the University of Nairobi's medical school was rejected, as I have mentioned. Our work on the Science and Technology Amendment Act created KEMRI as an institution but we had no funding and no physical location. We opened its doors officially as KEMRI on Monday, the 5th of November 1979 following the appointment of its Board of Management on 1st November 1979 as published in the *Gazette*. I think that must have been thereabouts on a Thursday because usually *Gazette* notices are published on Thursdays. Then I think KEMRI must have been active immediately. What used to happen was that all government notices used to be published on a Thursday, announcing appointments and so on, and there would also be a radio announcement covering the issues that were announced on that Thursday. For instance, it would indicate the date a bill was effective. But I think the first Chairman and the Board for KEMRI was announced on 1st November.

Fortunately, the first Chairman of our Board was one of the colleagues who had been part of the group that went to ask the Attorney General for the amendment changes on the Science and Technology Act, Professor Kihumbu Thairu. He was our first Chairman of the Board, and Dr James Gikonyo was appointed our first Director. Professor Mutuma Mugambi was appointed to be in charge of the Clinical Research Centre that was being supported by the World Health Organization (WHO). I was appointed as Mugambi's own principal assistant at that particular time. His training was in cardiology, so we did a few studies on cardiovascular diseases because that was his area of research, but I continued laboratory work on parasitology, infectious diseases and pathology. Fortunately, I could utilize other laboratories like those at the Division of Vector-Borne Diseases and of the WHO Immunology Research and Training Centre of the University of Nairobi School of Medicine. We had no physical place yet for KEMRI. You see, there was no department so now we had to look for how to bring in some of the lost departments that were part of the defunct East African Community. The Tuberculosis Investigation Centre joined us with its Director Joseph Aluoch, and then the Virus Research Centre came in with the former head of the unit, a Ugandan called Peter Tukei, and then came the Leprosy centre in Alupe, in Busia County under the leadership of Malachi D. Owili. So we started as a

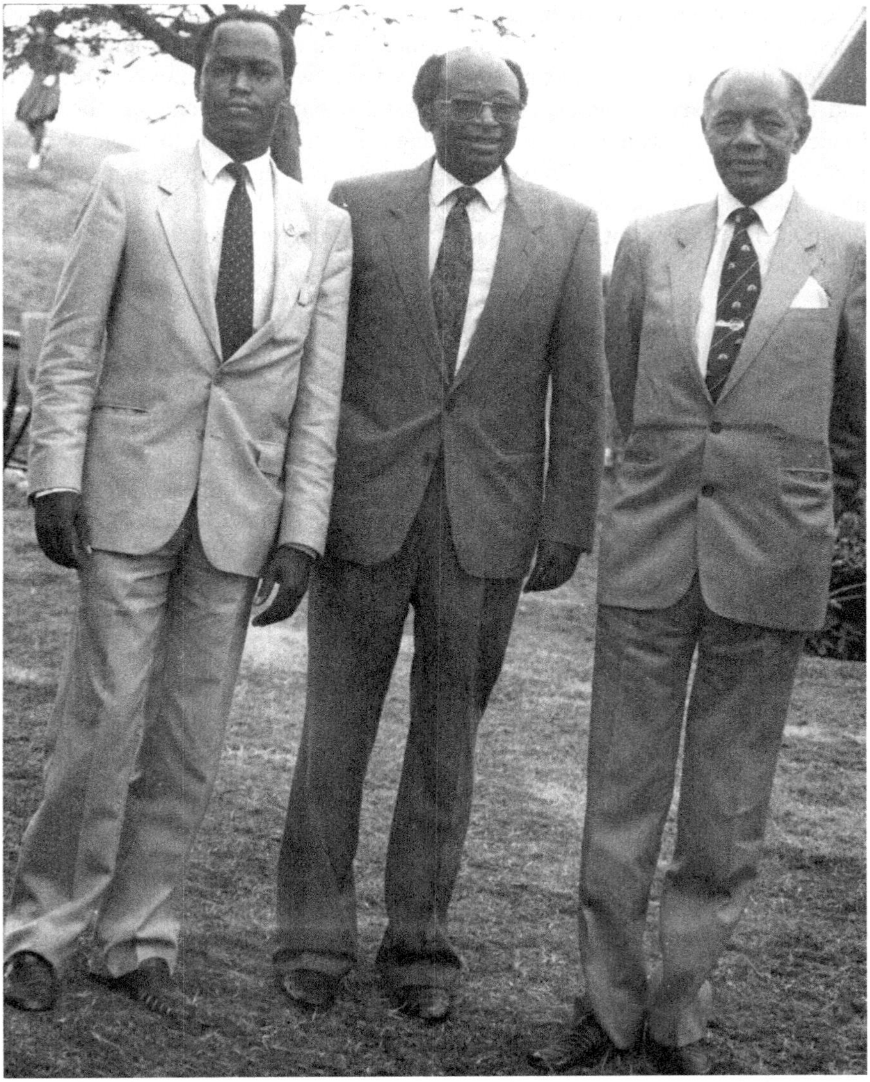

Figure 14.1 Three directors of KEMRI, 1989.

little cluster of people, with little scattered rooms to do some work, and we were still on the payroll of the Ministry of Health, except Mugambi who was on the payroll of the University of Nairobi. We had identified a place where we wanted to establish KEMRI and I had requested the then young President Moi when he was making his first state visit to Japan to consider our request.

I chanced to see Moi during this process. He had travelled for some fund-raising event to Eldoret and then accompanied some of these senior government officials back to Nairobi. I went to the State House and he told me, "Koech, listen, I am making an official trip to Japan." Formally it was his first visit to Japan as the head of state. He asked, "Is there anything that you would wish me to request in your area?" Because he knew I was working in medical research and I was focused on the areas of health and science. I responded, "Sir, *mzee* [/elder/] as you are aware, we are developing medical research in this country so if you can assist us …". Yes. So while people were queuing and begging, saying to him, "Please let me be in your delegation, please let me be this", I was there and the moment his staff saw me they said, "*Daktari* [/doctor/], you are next in line." Because they knew I was going for something very specific, so I told President Moi, "Yes, sir, please what we need in this country is medical research, period."

I noticed that the Japanese had already started funding medical research in Ghana at the Noguchi Memorial Research Institute, which had been founded the year before in 1979. You see, I had visited this Ghanaian institute, established by the Japanese at the University of Accra. I went to see it and then I realized that they were developing research units. It is named after a certain Japanese medical researcher who died I think of yellow fever or something like that, called Noguchi. So it was named after him but it was developed by the Japan International Development Cooperation Agency (JICA). What immediately came into my mind was that President Moi was going to Japan and we also needed to develop medical research in Kenya. So he makes a formal visit to Japan and one of his requests to them is to support the development of medical and scientific research in Kenya. They said yes, and so the moment he returned to Kenya, he called me with the news. There was a lot of paper work to be done but I think by the end of 1979, we were sorted. The next dilemma was where the facilities and office would be located. We didn't have one square inch in the entire republic to put up medical research. So though we had been given an okay to establish KEMRI, there was nowhere to put it.

Most of their aid projects were through JICA. JICA is like CIDA (Canadian International Development Agency), or USAID (United States Agency for International Development), or something like that. But, you see, the Japanese did not give the money directly to KEMRI. For two reasons: one, KEMRI had no infrastructure, not even a bank account to receive money. Nothing. Number two, that is not the way the Japanese operate. The Japanese cost the kind of work they are funding, and then they go and do the job for you. I have known exactly how they work from day one until day X. Yes. They don't give you a cheque or transfer money into your account, which is very good. They will not blame you for the delays. They will not blame you for payment and then poor workmanship. They cost everything out from the beginning and then they tender it out. And, they hire people they know are going to do a good job. They work like this now because they had problems in the past. I asked them internally here and they would not say officially but they have had some bad experience in the Middle East where they gave money and then the people squandered the money for their own enjoyment, or they gave the job to people who made a mess of it. I was not going to embarrass the President.

We didn't have any infrastructure of our own so that is the time now we start lobbying for space and facilities. So fortunately the government brokered with us and gave us the space where KEMRI is standing today. We were allocated that land. It was empty land then, an extension of the Armed Forces Memorial Hospital, which is the neighbour to the institute. The land was lying fallow. People wanted to grab it to put up a housing scheme, or to sell it or something like but we were not interested in that. We were interested in having the land to develop medical research facilities and so they gave us the land. They (JICA) were ready to start building so soon after that they started. Then once they started we wanted to expand from where we had established ourselves. It was empty property, an open space by the road, and then there was an extension of a military hospital, which was close to us, so we thought we wanted to take over that hospital.

So it becomes our clinical research unit of the Institute, then that is the time when the Ministry of Health had asked me to find out whether they could give us some space just off the road here, where they are turning on to the highway along Waiyaki Way. On Waiyaki Way there is the ABC Shopping Centre. Directly opposite it is a plot that was very close to 100 acres, which used to be the orthopaedic and dental units for Kenyatta National Hospital. The new big wing at the Kenyatta National Hospital had just been completed and there was plenty of space so they transferred the orthopaedic and dental units to the main hospital. That is why opposite Waiyaki Way there is an artificial limbs unit because orthopaedics of the Kenyatta National Hospital used to be nearby. So there was plenty of land on Waiyaki Way, so they asked us, it was myself and Professor Mugambi: "If you want to create a medical research institute, why can't we give you that space on the other side?" But then we realized that it was too far. At that time it seemed very far. I wish I knew how Nairobi would grow! We would have gone there directly. It seemed far because we had teaching responsibilities still at the medical school and my colleague had responsibilities in the medical school, and then we were still using some of the facilities in the medical school and so forth. So we said no and instead we took over that small space of 20 acres, where the KEMRI is at the moment, in exchange for 100 acres! Beautiful place. Yes. So because the military had rights to that property, they had to sign it off and with the help of the Department of Defense, I took it upon myself to look for grants to develop the Veterans Administration Hospital along Waiyaki Way so they could release that space for us.

So I was looking for support to develop the hospital, not for KEMRI, but for the military so that they can leave the other place where the Armed Forces Memorial Hospital is located for us. We had exchanged all the papers so the property of Waiyaki Way was now part of the Department of Defense but we had not acquired the other place because they were still occupied there. Shortly after that, together with two military officials, we reached out for assistance from France, from Germany, and then from the UK. The German government said it was willing and we prepared all the papers. The French were a little bit slow. The British was not too willing on the first attempt but the Germans were because they themselves saw the looming danger of an open, all-out war, so they wanted to strengthen some facilities, especially in Africa. Then one morning, and out of the blue, I received a phone call from General Jackson Kimeu Mulinge in the morning saying, “Dr Koech?” He was calling to tell me that the Germans had decided not to sign the aide memoire. Upon his retirement from the military service, General Mulinge joined competitive politics and at one time, he was appointed the Minister for Health under whom I served.

I said, “But why?” I was told, “It is because the Cold War is now warm.” The Germans were no longer interested in investing in military hospitals outside of Germany, especially in Africa, because of an agreement between Margaret Thatcher, Ronald Reagan, and Mikhail Gorbachev. This started a process that soon led to the collapse of the Soviet Union and ended the Cold War. Yes. But we had given the land along Waiyaki Way to the military hospital and so they could not move. It remains there today. So we were restricted in terms of our ability to expand. We could not claim it back because we had already given it. It was part of the military and the military did not know what to do with it until today. It used to be used to train some clerical officers or something like that. There was a time when some space was taken, the military generals started eating some portions, like one acre, who would know. Yes. So that is what happens.

KEMRI was built in two phases. Phase one was the central administration building plus the conference centre, the library and then in the second phase followed by the laboratories. That was the second phase. They came in succession so that you would not be able to know which one came first. But it was actually built in two phases. Yes. And in each phase furnishing followed in quick succession. The moment the construction was completed, you would see the furniture arriving. Then there was a problem initially when we were doing the inspection. I was on the building committee of the institute, which was to set up some small infrastructure, but first we had to give some serious thought about the leadership of the institution because the government felt it necessary to change the directorship of the Institute. Dr James Gikonyo was allowed to continue being the Senior Deputy Director of Medical Services and then a new Director of the Institute had to be appointed. That is what happened now in 1982.

The person who was in charge of clinical research of the institute was then appointed to be the second Director of the Institute, Professor Mutuma Mugambi. He is one of the individuals who accompanied us to the Attorney General. Professor Kihumbu Thairu was already the Chairman of the Institute and so Professor Mutuma Mugambi was the second Director. In fact, today is his birthday but we don’t celebrate some of these things. So Professor Mutuma Mugambi was appointed the new Director of KEMRI. Yes. And then I took over clinical research, and was asked to develop the Clinical Research Centre, which is what is called the founding centre of KEMRI.

We had a small committee, which was made up of some of the founder members of the institute, to oversee what was going on. One of the things that we noticed was that the height of the working benches was lower than what we normally had. In fact, they were about four inches lower so that you were forced to bend over when you were working at a bench. And then we noticed in the bathroom that the toilet seats were also smaller than usual, almost like children's seats. Then we realized that everything was from Japan where they are smaller in stature than many of our tall Kenyan brothers. So the committee requested these be redone. I give credit to the committee for noticing some of the things. We pointed these issues out to the local architects to fix because the Japanese architects had done the drawings for all Japanese funded projects here in Kenya. This is because all projects must pass the authority regulatory mechanisms in Japan before they can start the project here in Kenya. For instance, the KEMRI facilities here in Nairobi have been built to the highest Japanese standards to withstand a major earthquake, I think it must stand up to grade nine on the Richter scale. Yes. Most of their buildings must withstand that.

If you see the way the Japanese Embassy is built here in Nairobi? It is something else but they also need a corresponding local architect to meet our local conditions, so we pointed that out to the architect who actually made those changes. Yes. The Japanese were doing it with precision as far as time was concerned. The infrastructure of the institute, the roads going to the Institute and so on were supposed to be the work of the Kenya government. However, the Kenya government tends to work slow. So the Japanese were concerned that the project was delayed by two weeks so they decided to contribute additional money hopefully to be paid back by the Kenya government when it was available. Yes. So they did that, hoping to finish on time, but in the end they finished the job two weeks ahead of schedule. Yes. I cannot remember the actual period when the construction took place but by 1984 it had been officially completed and then President Moi went there to accept and open the facility.

Yes, Moi officially opened it but we had been using it for more than a year because we were able to move in after phase one was completed. Yes. You see, that is what happened when Mugambi took over as the Director of the Institute, and he was in that post for about six and a half years. Yes, and he did very well. He is the one who actually developed the institute and crafted the critical infrastructure needed for medical research in this country. We were close as friends because, as I mentioned, before I took over to be in charge of the Clinical Research Centre, I was the first designated scientist or lead researcher at the institute. He led the institute competently and extremely well and I am proud of his contribution and we are still good friends. We assisted each other. Yes, he was a dedicated public officer. So during that particular period KEMRI started growing. I was a part of that growth. Although I had a boss, I was the prime force behind it. There are a few things which I wanted him to do but he refused me.

In 1984 I formally moved out of the university laboratory to go and establish my own lab at KEMRI but I continued with my teaching roles within the university. At that time, I also officially vacated my office at the Ministry of Health's Division of Vector-Borne Diseases, which then was still based at Kenyatta National Hospital complex. At KEMRI for the first ten years I would say I was playing the role as scientist. As one of the very few founding scientists of the institute I completely left my role as I said in 1984 at the Division for the Vector-Borne Diseases in the Ministry of Health, where I had been involved in the day-to-day running, to concentrate on KEMRI. I still maintained some of my activities within the Division of Vector-Borne Disease. The next role, which I ceded, was the day-to-day running of the laboratory in the University of Nairobi School of Medicine's Department of Immunology. Yes, although I still retained my laboratory at the medical school even though I was not involved in the day-to-day running of the laboratory. I had also been in charge of the teaching schedules and the timetabling at the University, but I left this also to another person. I vacated those positions somewhere between 1984 and 1985 which is when I said, "Okay, let me now concentrate the rest of my efforts on the establishment and creation of the research institute." Then a number of things happened. One, in which I was directly involved, was the US CDC came to Kenya and their work fell directly under my supervision.

So I stopped being remunerated by the Ministry of Health and then shifted the remuneration to KEMRI because by early 1983 KEMRI had its own individual funding from the Exchequer. I started being on the payroll of the Institute. I transferred my permanent and pensionable terms of the government to the Institute. I was not under contract so I was on permanent and pensionable terms of service with the Institute. In 1989 I was appointed the chief research officer at the institute. As we talk today I have not reached my retirement age. So I am still on those terms in spite of the outstanding legal issues. And then beginning in 1989 I was appointed as Director of the Institute. It was the 13th January 1989. I was appointed as the third Director of the Institute and also Chief Executive Officer. So I had time to do my scientific work but I was also responsible for the administrative work of the Institute. Even though I was both research officer and Director, I was drawing only one salary, which is the salary of the position with the highest remuneration. That should be the Director. I remained in this position and even when I was forced to leave the Institute, the position was occupied only in an acting capacity. The position was finally filled in August 2010, thus ending my position after a record 22 years and making me the longest-serving Chief Executive of a public institution in Kenya's history.

When we finished putting up the structure for KEMRI, despite my own efforts to bring in everything, my own laboratory was not funded by the Japanese. They funded everything else but my laboratory.

Intermission

In October 2009, as KEMRI celebrates its 30-year anniversary, Koech writes a 30-page memoir account called, "I Remember: An eye-witness account of the historical development of the Kenya Medical Research Institute (KEMRI)." As part of that, he has written a detailed timeline of critical events. It is shared here (from Koech 2009: 8–23).

A glance at the past

KEMRI has grown tremendously over the last 19 years from an organization with only a handful of scientists and a few support staff to a world-renowned Institute with activities spread throughout Kenya and with a strong staff base of more than 1,300.

Here are some landmarks in the development of the Institute during the past years.

1979

- In March, the Parliament of the Republic of Kenya passes the Science and Technology (Amendment) Bill of 1979 thereby establishing, among others, the Kenya Medical Research Institute.
- The bill becomes law (Cap. 250 of the Laws of Kenya) on receiving Presidential assent on 23 May. Under the said Act, KEMRI is charged with the responsibility of carrying out health and related sciences research.
- On 14 March, Dr Davy Koech is appointed by the Ministry of Health to assist Prof. Mutuma Mugambi in establishing the Clinical Research Centre, the forerunner to KEMRI.
- The Clinical Research Centre (CRC) is established and becomes the founding centre of KEMRI with Prof. Mutuma Mugambi and Dr Davy Koech as founding scientists. Prof. Mugambi becomes the Director of the Centre.
- Professor Kihumbu Thairu is appointed the Chairman of the first Board of Management. The members of the board appointed at the same time are: Dr Wallace Kahugu, Professor Canute Khamala, Dr David Ombati, Dr Zedekiah Onyango, Professor Ambrose Wasunna, and Mr Eric Kotut.
- Dr James Gikonyo is appointed the first Director of KEMRI.
- On Monday, the 5th of November, KEMRI formally commences its operations.
- The year ends with a total staff of seven plus additional 16 expatriate staff.

1980

- The Kenya Tuberculosis Investigation Centre (KTIC), the Malaria and Other Protozoal Diseases Research Centre (MOPDRC), Virus Research Centre (VRC) and Alupe Leprosy Research Centre (ALRC), all previously under the East African Medical Research Council, are incorporated into KEMRI.
- Dr Joseph Aluoch is appointed to head KTIC, Dr Fabian Kamunvi heads MOPDRC, Dr Peter Tukei heads VRC, and Dr Dundu M. Owili heads ALRC.
- Unsuitable staff members inherited from the defunct East African Community are retrenched. Some have their services terminated while others are taken to the Ministry of Health.

- A memorandum of understanding is signed between the Ministry of Health (on behalf of the CRC representing KEMRI) and the Walter Reed Army Institute of Research (WRAIR) in Washington, DC, thereby facilitating collaborative research between the Institute and WRAIR.
- A similar memorandum is entered between KEMRI and the US Centers for Disease Control (CDC), Atlanta.
- Staff recruitment and training begins.
- In conjunction with the National Council for Science and Technology, the Kenya Trypanosomiasis Research Institute, and the Ministry of Health, KEMRI organizes the first Annual Medical Scientific Conference. These annual conferences have continued to be held uninterrupted ever since.
- The year ends with total staff strength of 30 plus additional 16 expatriate staff members.

1981

- KEMRI Headquarters moves to an office in the former East African Community Regional Headquarters.
- The year ends with total staff strength of 70 plus additional 16 expatriate staff members.

1982

- Professor Mugambi takes over as the second Director of KEMRI replacing Dr Gikonyo, and Dr Koech takes over as the Director of the CRC replacing Prof. Mugambi.
- A conference which outlines KEMRI's research priorities is held in Mombasa. The conference on "Medical Research Priorities" is attended by users of medical research who help formulate research priorities that require urgent attention.
- An agreement between the Kenya Government and the Government of the Netherlands to transfer the Medical Research Centre (MRC), then a department of the Royal Tropical Institute of Amsterdam, to KEMRI is signed. Dr Stephen Kinoti is appointed to head the Centre.
- The year ends with total staff strength of 200 plus additional 17 expatriate staff members.

1983

- KEMRI moves to its first premises, which is a block of pre-fabricated buildings near the National Public Health Laboratories.
- An agreement between the Government of Kenya and Japan for the construction of the KEMRI Headquarters and Central Laboratories Complex is signed. This assistance comes as a result of a request made during a previous visit to Japan by His Excellency President Daniel arap Moi.

- The year ends with total staff strength of 270 plus additional 16 expatriate staff members.

1984

- Mr Dunstan M. Ngumo is appointed Administrative Secretary.
- Phase I of KEMRI Headquarters and Central Laboratories Complex is completed and is occupied.
- Prof. Kihumbu Thairu, the Board Chairman, retires after taking up a post with the Commonwealth Health Secretariat in London.
- Research centres of KEMRI are reorganized. The new centres are:
    - Leprosy and Skin Diseases Research Centre (LSDRC) Busia
    - Biomedical Sciences Research Centre (BSRC)
    - Clinical Research Centre (CRC) (includes the Respiratory Diseases Research Unit, the Reproductive Health Research Unit and the Kilifi Research Unit)
    - Vector Biology and Control Research Centre (VBCRC) Kisumu
    - Virus Research Centre (VRC)
    - Centre for Microbiology Research (CMR)
    - Medical Research Centre (MRC)
    - Traditional Medicines and Drugs Research Centre (TMDRC)
- The Biomedical Sciences Research Centre (BSRC) and the Traditional Medicines and Drugs Research Centre (TMDRC) are established as offshoots of the CRC. Dr Koech moves to head BSRC while Dr Joab Were is appointed to head CRC and Dr Kofi-Tsekpo to head TMDRC.
- The Kenya/Japan Communicable Diseases Project becomes the Centre for Microbiology Research (CMR), a fully fledged KEMRI centre. Dr Peter Waiyaki is appointed to head the centre.
- KTIC becomes the Respiratory Diseases Research Centre (RDRC), MOPDRC becomes Vector Biology and Control Research Centre (VBCRC) and ALRC becomes Alupe Leprosy and Skin Diseases Research Centre (ALSDRC). VRC remains unchanged.
- The year ends with total staff strength of 360 plus additional 18 expatriate staff members.

1985

- Dr Mohamed S. Abdullah is appointed the second Chairman of the Board of Management.
- HLA tissue-typing technology headed by Dr Koech is perfected, opening way to the first living donor-related kidney transplantation in black Africa.
- The Wellcome Trust Research Laboratories start a field research station at Kilifi.

- Phase II of KEMRI Headquarters and Central Laboratories Complex is completed and occupied.
- Construction of Phase I of the Staff Housing Project in KEMRI HQs starts.
- On 23 September, His Excellency President Daniel arap Moi officially opens the KEMRI Headquarters and Central Laboratories Complex built through a grant from the Government of Japan through the Japan International Cooperation Agency (JICA), at a cost of about US$10 million.
- The year ends with total staff strength of 450 plus additional 24 expatriate staff members.

1986

- KEMRI acquires a six-acre plot of land at Kilifi for the development of a research centre along the Coast.
- Construction of Phase II of the Staff Housing Project in the KEMRI HQs starts.
- The renovation of CRC Annex at KNH old block is completed.
- Construction of new premises for the Vector Biology and Control Research Centre starts on a 40-acre plot of land at Kisian near Kisumu. The total cost of the project funded by the government is over KES 35 million.
- Dr M.J. Omwega is appointed to head RDRC following the retirement of Dr Joseph Aluoch from public service.
- The year ends with total staff strength of 700 plus additional 24 expatriate staff members.

1987

- A joint project with KETRI (Kenya Trypanosomiasis Research Institute) commences for the development of staff houses, a nursery school, and other facilities at the Leprosy and Skin Diseases Research Centre, Alupe.
- Phase I of the Vector Biology and Control Research Centre at Kisian, Kisumu is completed and occupied.
- The year ends with total staff strength of 820 plus additional 25 expatriate staff members.

1988

- The Medical Research Centre (MRC), formerly a department of the Royal Tropical Institute of Amsterdam, is fully transferred and integrated into KEMRI.
- Dr Mohamed Abdullah is re-appointed for another term as the Chairman of the Board of Management. Dr David Ombati is also re-appointed as a Board Member for another term while Prof. Haroun Mengech, Prof. Edward Kasili, Dr Joseph Aluoch, Prof. Japheth Kiptoon, and Prof. Walter Gitau are appointed as members of the Board of Management for the first time.

- Phase I of the Staff Housing Project built at a cost of KES 13 million from the Government of Kenya is completed and occupied.
- Phase II of the Staff Housing Project built at a cost of nearly KES 20 million from the Government of Kenya is completed and occupied.
- Dr John Githure is appointed to head VBCRC.
- Prof. Arthur Obel is appointed as Technical Services Coordinator in KEMRI.
- The year ends with total staff strength of 920 plus additional 24 expatriate staff members.

1989

- On 13 January, Dr Davy Koech is appointed the third Director of KEMRI. Dr Koech takes over from Prof. Mutuma Mugambi who retires from Public Service to join a multinational pharmaceutical firm.
- Dr John Githure takes over as head of BSRC to replace Dr Koech while Dr Aggrey Oloo takes over as the head of VBCRC to replace Dr Githure.
- Phase II of Vector Biology and Control Research Centre is completed.
- On the 6th of December, KEMRI celebrates its 10th anniversary.
- The year ends with total staff strength of 1,050 plus additional 25 expatriate staff members.

1990

- On the 5th of June, a drug (Kemron), developed in KEMRI and based on a formulation of low-dose interferon alpha, for oropharyngeal use in the clinical management of HIV infections is registered and launched on the 29th of July.
- The year ends with total staff strength of 1,135 plus additional 25 expatriate staff members.

1991

- Prof. Arthur Obel leaves the service of the Institute to rejoin the University of Nairobi.
- The year ends with total staff strength of 1,200 plus additional 25 expatriate staff members.

1992

- In January, the Malindi Laboratory is completed with the support of JICA and occupied.
- In October, Kilifi staff houses built through funds from the Government of Kenya are opened.
- The year ends with total staff strength of 1,260 plus additional 23 expatriate staff members.

1993

- The year ends with total staff strength of 1,280 plus additional 24 expatriate staff members.

1994

- African Forum for Health Sciences is formed, and KEMRI becomes its first headquarters and Dr Davy Koech is unanimously proclaimed as its first President.
- *African Journal of Health Sciences* is inaugurated. Dr Davy Koech becomes its first Editor-in-Chief.
- In April, the 15th KEMRI/KETRI Annual Scientific Conference converts to African Health Sciences Congress, and constitutes itself as the 15th African Health Sciences Congress.
- The year ends with total staff strength of 1,290 plus additional 25 expatriate staff members.

1995

- In April, the 16th African Health Sciences Congress is held in Nairobi, Kenya.
- The year ends with total staff strength of 1,295 additional 23 expatriate staff members.

1996

- In April, the 17th African Health Sciences Congress is held in Nairobi, Kenya.
- The year ends with total staff strength of 1,300 plus additional 24 expatriate staff members.

1997

- In April, the 18th African Health Sciences Congress is held in Cape Town, South Africa.
- In July, the Director appoints a team of four senior officers (Dr Peter Waiyaki, Dr Mawuli Kofi-Tsekpo, Dr Peter Tukei, and Mr Dunstan Ngumo) to review the current research and related programmes at the Institute with a view to making recommendations on the way the Institute should be structured in order to meet the challenges of the 21st century.
- The report is made available in October whereupon the recommendations are forwarded to the Board of Management for deliberations and further advice and guidance.
- The year ends with total staff strength of 1,300 plus additional 22 expatriate staff members.

1998

- The Board of Management adopts the recommendations of the team, which leads to the renaming of centres for research as well as the appointment of two deputy directors of the Institute and directors of centres.
- On 7 April, the Board of Management made the following major changes at the Institute:

1. Research and Development Department
   Deputy Director: Dr Patrick A. Orege

   Chief Research Officers

   - Dr Peter G. Waiyaki
   - Dr Peter M. Tukei
   - Dr Mawuli W. Kofi-Tsekpo

2. Administration and Finance Department
   Deputy Director: Mr Dunstan M. Ngumo

   Chief Finance Officer

   - Mr Renison K. Kirui

Centres

1 Centre for Biotechnology Research and Development (CBRD)

- Director: Dr Gerald M. Mkoji

2 Centre for Clinical Research (CCR)

- Director: Dr Monique K. Wasunna

3 Centre for Geographic Medicine Research, Coast (CGMRC)

- Director: Dr Norbert M. Peshu

4 Centre for Public Health Research (CPHR)

- Director: Dr David L. Mwaniki

5 Centre for Leprosy and other Skin Diseases Research (CLSDR)

- Director: Dr Nicholas I. Adungo

6 Centre for Microbiology Research (CMR)

- Director: Dr Gabriel G. Mbugua

7 Centre for Respiratory Diseases Research (CRDR)

- Director: Dr Joseph A. Odhiambo

8 Centre for Traditional Medicine and Drug Research (CTMDR)

- Director: Dr Geoffrey M. Rukunga

9 Centre for Vector Biology and Control Research (CVBCR)

- Director: Dr Aggrey J. Oloo

10 Centre for Virus Research (CVR)

- Director: Dr Fred A. Okoth

- In April the 19th African Health Sciences Congress is held in Arusha, Tanzania.
- On 15 May, a contract is executed in Tokyo, Japan by the Director for the establishment of a biosafety laboratory at the level of P3 in KEMRI.
- In October, KEMRI is nominated as one of the three global centres for the strategic control of parasitic diseases in the 21st century, the other two being Noguchi Memorial Institute for Medical Research (NMIMR) in Ghana and Mahidol University in Thailand.
- In November, a new Board of Management of KEMRI is gazetted. Dr Mohamed S. Abdullah is re-appointed as Chairman. Others re-appointed are Dr David G. Ombati, Prof. Onesmo ole MoiYoi, and Prof. Haroun N.K. arap Mengech. New members are Dr Rashid Aman, Prof. Gerishom M. Sande, and Mrs. Monica M. Mutuku.
- The year ends with total staff strength of 1,305 plus additional 20 expatriate staff members.

1999

- In May, Hon. Kipkalya Kones, Minister for Research and Technology inaugurates the new Board of Management.
- In May, the P3 biosafety laboratory is handed over to the Kenya Government by the Government of Japan through H.E. Mr Morihiso Aoki, the Japanese Ambassador to Kenya. Hon. Kipkalya Kones, Minister for Research and Technology, receives the key on behalf of the Government of Kenya.
- In April, the 20th African Health Sciences Congress is held in Accra, Ghana.
- In September, the Government is reorganized and KEMRI is placed under the Ministry of Health.
- The year ends with total staff strength of 1,320 plus additional 23 expatriate staff members.

15 Japan

Japan is relevant here because of their participation in the historical development of the Institute. I have mentioned in the past a discussion about how KEMRI was formally established and the grants that we got which were purely institutional grants and which were generous donations from the people of Japan through JICA. As well, I have mentioned how we developed the program between KEMRI and JICA. In fact, by the time JICA came to Kenya, we had not fully developed infrastructural or human resources and capacity because we didn't have sufficient individuals who were qualified enough to attend to human resource development, the scientific development of the Institute, and the financial management. But with the development of infrastructural facilities that were provided to Kenyans through JICA, we were able to develop those capacities and skills. I want to emphasize today that, despite the fact that they are not featured in most of the places, their contribution to KEMRI is enormous. There is no single donor whose contribution has been as significant as JICA to the development of the Institute, and yet at the same time since the moment they developed it, they never claimed ownership. They would ask permission to use the facilities, even though they provided them.

Yes, their contribution to KEMRI was substantial, despite the fact that it is a small country. Basically, Japan is the size of Kenya's Rift Valley, which is one-third of the size of Kenya. That is Japan for you. And in fact I have a global map where I have inserted these countries together to see exactly how big Africa is compared to Japan. The whole of the US is actually the Saharan desert of Africa so at times we think the US is an enormous country, but it is not. It is just the size of the Sahara. So when you consider this, you see that it is the heart of the people and the willingness to assist that really matters. That tiny country was able now to bring in their infrastructural support to the Institute, to put up actual buildings, and furnish them. Of course, except for my laboratory, which I mentioned was instead funded through a grant from the UK when Margaret Thatcher was in power. So that is it.

I wish to state that during that period they had identified universities for partnership because they had foresight. They wanted to put up infrastructure and let people work and encouraged various individual institutions in Japan to collaborate with the Institute and even extend to collaborate with other institutions in

Kenya depending on the interests of various individuals. There are several universities in every Japanese prefecture. They call it a prefecture, and there are some 47 of them, like our counties in Kenya. So from the Hokkaido Prefecture in the North to the Nagasaki prefecture in the South of Japan, all through there were a few universities which had been identified and whose officers were interested in the area of tropical medicine and tropical diseases. They could come to KEMRI to learn, but they could also bring us new technologies, and then we give them the biological samples. So, yes, the arrangement with Japan was extremely collaborative, despite the fact that they are often shy when you are working with them because of the language barrier. The scientists I have worked with are not extraordinarily talkative and I think that is why they tend to segregate themselves.

I have worked with quite a number of Japanese scientists but I can only mention a few. One of them is Professor Yoshiki Aoki from Nagasaki. We worked together until his retirement. I also visited Nagasaki University when the JICA financial support had ended. JICA gave support for infrastructural and training facilities and then they tapered off their assistance when we were now capable of having direct, or more equal, relationships with the universities in Japan. We were no longer a burden to the Japanese people but we were together working as partners. So we have some degree of partnership with Nagasaki University with folks like Yoshiki Aoki, Shimada, plus a few other colleagues. Within the Tokyo prefecture there were people like Dr Akai. He worked with us for a considerable period of time on parasitic infections. And there was Dr Kawana who was from the Iwate Prefecture; yes, there were several people. Yes.

These are people who have stayed with us for quite a while. When the researchers were departing Kenya, they would introduce somebody else in order to maintain the relationship. I would travel to Japan not for my own training but to go and visit our KEMRI staff that were there for training so that I would be satisfied that our own officers were going to these particular places where facilities were available. Yes, it became a hobby for me to speak Japanese when I went there but otherwise communication was in English. Yes, so there was no problem, although I am usually extremely poor in languages. By the time some of our staff came back to Kenya, especially those who went for actual long-term studies, they could speak Japanese almost fluently. So at the moment we have programs at the Institute that are an offshoot of the relationship between KEMRI and JICA.

There were many Japanese projects here in Kenya that I was responsible for. I was taking my car to the garage the other day and I saw a KEMRI-Nagasaki University program[1] vehicle and I said to myself, it is my signature that brought this vehicle. It was in a garage somewhere close to my neighbourhood. Yes, I am indeed excited about that. In terms of interpersonal relationships, these are people who are down to earth. I think the humiliation they endured from the Second World War is one that changed their character. They colonized part of China, like Professor Shimada, my friend who was working at Nagasaki. His father was a provincial administrator in Shanghai, China during the colonial rule of the Eastern part of China. Imagine that tiny country colonizing the Chinese? Yes. This was before the Second World War. My friend was born in the late 1940s when his father was a colonial administrator in Shanghai. At the end of the Second World War, the bombs of Nagasaki and the last one in Hiroshima, so after that humiliation by the Americans they became very humble. They are humble people; they don't step on anyone's toes.

So in spite of the language barrier we were able to work very well together. They were able to come here and they were speaking better Swahili than us! Because the way you pronounce certain things in Japanese is similar to the way we pronounce it in Kiswahili. And then, they were even having Kenyan names, several of them. You see, like Obama. In fact, it is a small town in Japan. So local African names are similar to some Japanese names but they have different meanings. How it happened we really don't know. It is only when you look at Japanese handwriting does it threaten or worry you. But they have so many different ways of expressing themselves. If they were to write everything in the Roman alphabet, you'd understand very easily.

So I wanted to emphasize their contribution to Kenya and KEMRI because the Japanese are the ones who have provided leadership for the national development of our medical science and research but they also pressured others to do the same. Some of the facilities used by the CDC and Walter Reed were funded and developed by the Japanese people. The Wellcome Trust manged to assist in putting up excellent facilities in Kilifi. They also assisted in the development of our national hospital system. Do you remember the story I told you when I was young, how I broke my leg, how I was hospitalized, and the kind of medical negligence I had to endure? I realized then that we must do something to improve the hospital. This is the hospital at my home in Kericho. JICA offered to fund improvements on the Kericho District Hospital so that it would be a level 5 hospital. So when I was finalizing the negotiation for the support of Kericho District Hospital to a level 5 hospital, there was our Minister for Health, who happened to be a professional colleague and more senior colleague of mine, Professor Sam Ongeri. He is a paediatrician by training and a friend of mine. Professor Sam Ongeri was in government, but before he became a politician, we worked together in the medical school. He was a friend and Moi had assisted him with his political aspirations. So when I was finalizing my request to JICA, he interjected and said, "When you go to discuss Kericho, can you please put in a word also to have a similar facility built in Kisii?" Yes, he wanted me to include Kisii because he comes from Kisii and he wanted his home to also benefit from the assistance from JICA. So I did include Kisii in the discussion as directed but since Kericho was the first in line, the Japanese government said they had already made the commitment to Kericho so it would be a level 5 but they could assist Kisii Hospital in becoming level 4. So everything was finalized.

The Japanese professionals had come to visit Kericho and Kisii and for the purpose of funding requirements and the architectural drawings, and so on but when it came to near the implementation stage, after the Japanese had decided to proceed, there was a change demanded by the Ministry of Health. There had been a political shift during the process whereby the previous minister had moved on to do other things, and so there was a new Permanent Secretary in the Ministry of Health called Hezron Nyangito. So when he saw the paperwork being passed through his office, he said, "No, the level 5 must go to Kisii and the level four to Kericho." So the Japanese consultant said, "We had not planned for that, it is the other way round." The Japanese then called me, telling the Ministry of Health that unless Koech agrees with this, we cannot proceed. This was the beginning of my problems between the Permanent Secretary and myself. I told him that this interference is not the way to do things. I told him you know we have already discussed whatever is going to Kisii goes to Kisii, whatever comes to Kericho goes to Kericho. Yes. After that the Japanese said, "We are sorry but we cannot support this project now." They were threatening to cancel both Kericho and Kisii projects. Then I told the hospital superintendent in Kericho that we had to compromise and that at least this way they would have some improvements, rather than nothing at all. So the Japanese agreed to go ahead as long as I agreed. So I told the hospital superintendent of Kericho to go ahead and agree, and tell the Japanese that I have said it can proceed in this reverse manner. You see. So that is what happened. So I told them it is better to have something rather nothing on the basis of a disagreement about who takes what. That is precisely what happened. Kisii became a level 5 hospital, and Kericho became level 4 until today.

You see the negotiation started thereabout 2004 and it went on for several years negotiating back and forth, back and forth. Yes. You see the Japanese do not rush. They discuss, discuss, discuss, discuss again. Discuss all those things until it becomes a collective agreement. In my experience with them for more than 30 years, it was not routine that they would make a decision on the first meeting. No, because there is a lot of consultation. Even in the writing of our agreements, even changing one comma, they must consult about such a change to the document. Eventually they agreed to the changes requested.

With their financial assistance, we also ended up improving what is called our level 3 biosafety unit at the Institute. Yes, we have a P3 facility for handling viruses because it was needed when HIV/AIDS became a problem in East Africa. HIV was barely known at that particular time, anywhere globally. It was not known as a global disease. No, it was not known at all then. So we kept on improving the facilities so our scientists could focus on HIV. Some of our researchers went for training on such viruses to Japan. The Japanese were with the Institute all the way through. They are the ones who provided the training to most of the officers at the Institute. But that era of Japanese development at KEMRI ended a couple of years ago. But we are still partners with Japan. Yes. I went to Japan several times. It became my second home.

Note

1 Nagasaki University Kenya Research Station NUITM-KEMRI Project has three sites in Kenya: Mbita, Nairobi, and Kwale. See their site for more information: www.tm.nagasaki-u.ac.jp/nairobi/en/

16 Division of Vector-Borne Diseases

I became the Head of the Division of Vector-Borne Diseases (DVBD) in the Ministry of Health in this country in 1980 for about five years. Yes, I was in charge. Because the Institute was growing I was able to develop some additional learning facilities and local laboratory facilities through the Division of Vector-Borne Diseases. Yes, I established laboratories throughout the country. If you go to Kwale, we had a lab there. If you want to go to Busia, there was a laboratory. If you want to go to Turkana, even there we had a laboratory. Wherever you went, we had developed a laboratory. My work at the DVBD further assisted the development of both the Walter Reed Project and the CDC because they both too used the facilities of the Division of Vector-Borne Diseases in Kisumu. That site was the first field laboratory for the US Centers for Disease Control.

Within the Ministry of Health there are the national public health laboratories for diagnostic services in Kenya. All the laboratories in the hospitals were being run by the national public health laboratory services in the Republic of Kenya. Yes. The public health aspect of disease falls within the control of the Division of Vector-Borne Diseases. Yes, so the control of infections such as malaria, leishmaniasis, trypanosomiasis, schistosomiasis, filariasis, you see even river blindness, onchocerciasis, all of those "iasis" fall under the management of the Division of Vector-Borne Diseases. So long as it is transmitted by a vector, whether it is an insect, or a worm like in schistosomiasis, any sort of vector, then it is a vector-borne disease. Yes. These vector-borne diseases were managed by an arm of the government, which used to fall under the main umbrella of national public health laboratory services. It is a public health-related issue but it was removed later on because it required its own specialized facilities. So in all Kenyan hospitals there used to be a laboratory for the monitoring and control of vector-borne diseases. Then there is also a public health laboratory where blood samples, urine samples, stool samples, etcetera, are examined. Those fall under the national public health laboratory system.

Now this unit of the Ministry of Health had a lot of financial support because people used to do a lot of research on these vector-borne diseases. Those external institutions include the London School of Hygiene and Tropical Medicine, the Liverpool School of Tropical Medicine, and the Dutch laboratories. You may have heard of Danish Bilharziasis Laboratory? That was our Danish research partner. And also the Royal Tropical. So these partners all came to Kenya and created a laboratory system that is the Division of Vector-Borne Diseases, a part of the Ministry of Health. So in every Kenyan hospital there is a laboratory where they deal with the control of vector-borne diseases.

It is separate from the Kenya Medical Research Institute. It has existed here since the 1940s, and it was established immediately after the Second World War. Yes, and so I was in charge of DBVD. I was the Director for five years, just as I was establishing KEMRI. So when we had started with KEMRI, it did not have its own laboratories and so we utilized the DBVD laboratories for KEMRI lab activities. So at one time I was in charge of both KEMRI and the Division of Vector-Borne Diseases. I know DBVD inside and out because I built or rehabilitated 45 laboratories across the country between 1974, with a short break in 1975 and 1976 when I was away in the US, and then when I returned I continued putting up the laboratories in the Republic of Kenya within a span of a couple of years. Yes.

I told you that whatever responsibility I am given by whomever, I do it to the best of my ability and that is precisely what I did with the DVBD labs. Yes. We established these labs from Mandera all the way up to Vanga and across up to Sio Port, and further north through Kacheliba, up to Lodwar. From Lodwar up to Marsabit, and everywhere in between. So in every county headquarters we built a laboratory for the surveillance and diagnosis of vector-borne diseases. And these laboratories, I hope, are functional till today. We monitored the outbreaks of disease throughout the country.

I know all of them till today. There is nothing I cannot recall. I know all of them, you see right from Mandera to Wajir, Garisa, Tana River, Mombasa, from Mombasa to Kwale, the border point between Kenya and Tanzania. Yes, and then across to Machakos, Kitui and that is where I did most of my work, in Kitui. Yes, and I went to Embu. You see Embu, Nyeri, Isiolo. Then if you go further north there is Maralal. From Maralal you cross over to Lodwar and then come to Kapenguria. From Kapenguria, you just turn up to Kacheliba, which is close to the border between Kenya and Uganda in West Pokot. You see, and then you come to Kitale. From Kitale you go to Bungoma. Bungoma to Busia. From Busia you go to Sio Port, and then from there you go to Siaya. From Siaya now you come back this way to Kisumu, and then Homa Bay. You see, and then Kisii, straight to Transmara, to Kilgoris. From Kilgoris you go to Narok. Narok to Kajiado. Yes. We set up the labs to consist of basic laboratories, basic equipment for parasitic diseases identification.

So we established these disease control laboratories in all of those places, which became handy when KEMRI was established and we did not have the infrastructure for labs yet. That is part of my legacy of work in Kenya before I joined KEMRI. It was and continues to be under the management of the DVBD. Then I was doubling at the two places, working for both the DVBD and KEMRI, at the same time. In fact, I was in charge of DVBD and I was in charge of the clinical research centre of KEMRI, and I was teaching at the University of Nairobi School of Medicine, in the Department of Immunology in the medical school at the same time. Yes.

Yes, we had to ensure all those laboratories had all the necessary laboratory equipment like microscopes. Yes. So those are some of the things that we did to ensure that every laboratory was very well equipped. Even in Kisumu, which is where we did the first malaria culture in this country. Yes and it was in a laboratory which we created in a room using polythene papers to create a clean space. We were wondering why it was that a certain percentage of people who were exposed to the malaria parasite, even living with the malaria parasite, never get malaria. We realized it was a result of protein A and we all did this work in Kisumu with Harrison Spencer from the CDC in 1980s and Nguyen Fuk, a scholar from the US and Taiwan.

One of the advantages of setting up these labs across the country is that we have been able to graduate now more than 40 PhD and 50 master's students studying vector-borne and communicable diseases and related disciplines, and graduating from both local and overseas universities.

17 The Wellcome Trust

The history of the Wellcome Trust in Kenya is as old as the history of independent Kenya itself because its presence in Kenya was established in 1964 within a year of Kenya's independence. And within ten years of its presence, I became the first Kenyan professional to be employed by the Wellcome Trust Research Laboratories in 1974 here in Kenya. I received my first pay cheque from them. It was a monthly salary of 2,232 KES. I remember then they were writing out the numbers – two thousand, two hundred and thirty-two. There was no automation of cheques. You only rip and write on top of it. They had a clumsy lady administrator who was also white and she wrote the cheques out by hand. Yes. And out of that we created a relationship between KEMRI and the Wellcome Trust following the establishment of KEMRI.

Eventually we found them some space in Kilifi, on the coast, and they put up a wonderful facility. Yes, it is a first-class facility. When it was time for the Wellcome Trust to put up facilities, I actually negotiated with the authorities in the UK. I understood them quite well having been the first Kenyan professional to be employed by the Wellcome Trust.

Then I also opened up ways for Kenyan colleagues to get employed within the Wellcome Trust and I am happy that there are several of them now. Yes. They were doing a lot of work on malaria especially along the coastal line and they wanted some place to put up a facility. At that time we had just acquired a ten-acre property, I think it was ten acres, just adjoining the Kilifi County Hospital. We didn't want to go to Mombasa because they didn't have any land and our philosophy at that time was that since we have these people who are coming to work with us, who are putting up facilities, we should share our land and existing facilities, so that is what happened. And they have put up a wonderful facility. I am happy about what they have done there and I believe they are happy there.

Yes. It is very nice facility. They had a very nice laboratory scientific officer, Bret Lowe, who was there. Yes. He left Kenya to do some activities elsewhere very briefly but later returned to the country. He actually contributed immensely to the design, he assisted the consulting team and the civil engineers and architects in the design and planning of the laboratory. I think this input from a scientist is one of the reasons it is such an excellent lab space. It is a large facility.

Yes. It cost very close to a billion Kenyan shillings to build. I am sure it has increased in value since.

But they also contributed to the Kilifi County Hospital. They moved out of Nairobi because they had been using a very small facility there. Just hardly two acres. It is their property. It is still there. I think they own it. It is their property but it is on government land so they don't have a title for it. Yes. It was sandwiched between a KEMRI facility and the national public health laboratory. Which is an extension of either the national laboratory services or the Ministry of Health, which KEMRI has now acquired. It is close to our Centre for Respiratory Diseases Research, which is also another good facility. It is where we had the baboons and where we were doing the research on schistosomiasis to begin with. That is where I did my schistosomiasis work, which led to my first scientific publication in 1976.

As the Wellcome Trust improved and grew we realized that they would need a new space. Kevin Marsh started working in Kenya in, or around, the 1980s just as I was about to take over as the Institute CEO. He's been here for a long time. It was during the same period and he was a very nice and resourceful friend to me. We worked together on the improvement of the Wellcome Trust, in spite of the individual failures we have heard about recently.[1] But we should look at the positive side of their work here. And if it were not because of people like Kevin Marsh, we would not have such a facility on the coast even to criticize. So back then Kevin and I sat down, and I said to Kevin, "What do we do? The Wellcome Trust is growing." We decided to search for a grant. So we looked at various sources and one of the principal contributors was the Wellcome Trust itself. That is why we called it the KEMRI Wellcome Trust Research Programme. The Wellcome Trust is the major contributor to the establishment of that station. It is the Wellcome Trust Laboratories

It is a private foundation in the UK. It is one of the wealthiest actually in the world. Yes. Because at times we can talk about the Gates Foundation being the largest and most important but the Wellcome Trust is a much older institution. I think it was established in 1936 when Sir Henry Wellcome died. Yes, he worked in pharmaceuticals and left a will for the trust to be established. You see I am used to seeing all these foundations working in Africa. When we have some relationship with them I want to know the history. Anyway, so the Trust has grown substantially into a rather large institution, but without any single person or funder saying this is my foundation. It has taken its own course. It has got its own life. Yes. I told the Wellcome Trust Research Laboratories' Country Director, I said, "Listen, what we need to do is a show. We need to create a show since we are one of the oldest private research units in Kenya." I said, "Why can't we go ahead and do something?" Then we two said to ourselves there is this one-acre back in Nairobi. And then, because the USCDC was focusing its research out towards western Kenya, I suggested the coast where malaria was endemic and there were many public health issues needing to be resolved. Yes. And then it happened that the coast was the place where we had acquired some acreage; I think five or ten acres, something like that. I said, "Why can't we go there?" Yes. So that is the time Kevin and his colleague Bill Watkins actually went to the coast to decide. We negotiated for a very generous grant from the Wellcome Trust and some of the other collaborating institutions in the UK. These are large universities, including both Cambridge and Oxford, and some of the staff members who were with the Wellcome Trust who were actually employees of those institutions but seconded to work with the Wellcome Trust Programme. They also partner with Liverpool and London. The Wellcome Trust still have some offices in Nairobi but the Nairobi offices functions are more like a liaison office.

KEMRI got the land for the Kilifi site from the Government of Kenya. It was a direct allocation by the government but, of course, we paid some money for it to be our own. The allocation of the property started in the mid-1980s so that by the time I took over as the Institute Director there was a question about how to best make use of the facilities that KEMRI had acquired earlier on. That is when I sat down with Kevin Marsh in the late 1980s. We needed to find funding for the construction. Most of these things, they don't take just a single day. It might go for one year or two years, even longer. So in the course of time we identified some architects to come in, and then officers to work with the architects to establish what we need as scientists. Sometime in the 1990s is when we actually started. And then at the beginning of 2000, that is when it was up and running.

Yes, during this particular time we were utilizing facilities at Kilifi County Hospital. We were in there for a couple of years before the new building construction was completed. Yes. So we had our facilities within the hospital itself. So we were working with the hospital and the medical personnel of the Institute were also doubling up as doctors and technicians for the hospital. So were worked very well together. The working relationship between KEMRI and the Kilifi County Hospital was wonderful and continues to be even today.

Then we decided that we wanted Kilifi County Hospital to be a model hospital, which was administratively and clinically efficient. For two reasons: one, we were physically close. We were contiguous. Our property was contiguous with that of the hospital so we just walked across the yard. Two, when we had developed this particular property we decided to surrender most of what we had within the hospital to the hospital itself, but the relationship continued. We were able to map practically every home within that neighbourhood of Kilifi. Yes. So when that person goes to the hospital you know precisely which home that person comes from. Then we created a system whereby we had plotted every home and then because fieldwork was required for the malaria and related research, and some of the other public health issues, we were able to also put that on the map. Yes, everything became digitized so that you would not even go with a piece of paper. It was all within a computerized database, much like the DSS in western Kenya.

So we linked up the hospital and our laboratories, as well as the laboratory in the hospitals and pharmacy. So as a result of that we were able to know a patient's history. The person would come into the hospital and they would be asked, "Have you been in the hospital before? What is your name? Which home do you come from?" With the new system, the staff member would simply search the database and find their number. "You are number so and so." Yes, then we have an ID for that individual and it is linked up with their medical history and other histories of the family members. So the doctors know that the last time they visited the hospital, they had been complaining of malaria. What is the problem today? Mosquitoes bit me. I hurt my leg, or whatever the issue is. We store it in our databank. If they are being sent for an X-ray, laboratory test, it is all recorded in the database. Yes. So it became the first paperless hospital in the country.

It is a fantastic system. So the community themselves, they appreciate what we do and then the hospital itself also appreciates what we do. And at that time some county hospitals had only two or three doctors serving their entire communities but here it was a hospital of 16 doctors. Yes, about 16 doctors because KEMRI contributed to the hospital. All the KEMRI doctors and personnel were also licensed to work in the Kilifi Hospital. Our laboratory scientists were also working in the laboratories and so on. So we never distinguished between the hospital staff and KEMRI staff. We were all working collaboratively, and it is through this that people were able to seek further training and education. They also gained exposure and met trainees from UK institutions and other places. Yes. And it has improved since then. We worked extremely well together. And like other collaborative arrangements with KEMRI the funding of the Wellcome Trust is arranged as such that it goes through the Institute, especially the funding for core staff because all appointments at KWTRP are done by the office of the Director of the Institute. Yes, by KEMRI. Yes.

And so we adopted that administrative arrangement for all collaborating institutions to avoid terms of references for conditions of service being different or lopsided vis-à-vis various collaborating institutions. This was because I recognized early on that some people will say they prefer to be attached to particular programs because maybe they pay more or maybe they pay you extra if you come to work over the weekend, or something like that. I put a stop to that by making all KEMRI appointments uniform, regardless of which site or collaborator you were working with. No, you just work for KEMRI, regardless of whether it is the Wellcome Trust or CDC or the US Army.[2] They are all the same and it worked very well. We were able to get staff stability. The lowest paid officers at that time were those employed by the Exchequer, which is the government, or the National Treasury, but there too we were able to secure funding from other organizations as a grant. Yes.

The Wellcome Trust is a private organization. It is not a state organization or something like the CDC or Walter Reed. It is a private organization. That is why we have we had a lot of flexibility in putting up some buildings with less bureaucracy, because it was a private trust. It has nothing to do with the UK government, although there is a lot of government interest in the private trust. The British High Commission in Nairobi is interested to know what is going on within the Wellcome Trust but that is it.

Notes

1 For more information on these issues, see Elliott 2017.

2 The KEMRI Wellcome Trust Research Program was involved in an important legal case in Kenya when six KEMRI scientists sued KEMRI, the Attorney General and the Ministry of Public Health in 2010 for human rights violations and inequitable labour practices. The courts found in their favour but KEMRI appealed the decision. The case remains stalled in the Kenyan courts.

18 The Walter Reed Project/ US Army Research Unit

The Walter Reed Project joined KEMRI as a result of their research and studies in veterinary medicine, because they had been working in Kenya since 1969. So by the time we brought them in under the umbrella of KEMRI, they had already been working in Kenya for many years and had settled in. I moved them from the veterinary laboratories to KEMRI/DVBD. Yes, they have been here since 1969 doing medical research on trypanosomiasis, which is sleeping sickness, in our veterinary laboratories, or the "vet labs", which is what we call them. This fell under the Ministry of Agriculture, Livestock and Fisheries since sleeping sickness, or Nagana, was common in African cattle. But trypanosomiasis was also spilling over into human health because we have human sleeping sickness as well. We gave an excuse in around 1980 that, since trypanosomiasis and leishmaniasis are caused by flagellates, these are little parasites that are free flowing in blood, the army research unit could be in the DVBD. Yes. Their vectors are tsetse flies and their control is under the mandate of the Division of Vector-Borne Diseases. They are endemic in the Lambwe Valley of Homa Bay County. While I was Director of the Division of Vector-Borne Diseases, I worked to eradicate it so there were very few cases when I was in charge of that in this republic. There were only 13 cases in one year.

So I talked with the researchers at the Walter Reed Project and discussed the many advantages of being associated with KEMRI and the Division of Vector-Borne Diseases. I suggested they could justify a need for more funding and they could justify expansion of their research site and team if they moved into human diseases. There were a few more members at the Walter Reed back then than there were at the DVBD. When it comes to doing certain things, and being military-based, it certainly quickens things up. So we were able to move them to KEMRI and they have grown substantially since then. They agreed to work with both trypanosomiasis and leishmaniasis and they have expanded their involvement to cover malaria and HIV/AIDS. Then I gave them facilities. Initially they were based at the Division of Vector-Borne Diseases where they put up some facilities in Nairobi which when they moved out they surrendered them for the use of DVBD. You see my idea here is that when foreign institutions build facilities, when they leave, the buildings are now Kenyan facilities – this is how we have built such amazing infrastructure for medicine and science in this country.

So then they moved to the KEMRI headquarters here in Nairobi and started building. About this time their American colleagues at the CDC were setting up facilities in Kisian and Kisumu. I asked them, "Don't you see what your friend (CDC) is doing in western Kenya? Let's do something similar." That is when they agreed to help build the Children's Hospital in Kisumu, the one located by the provincial hospital (Jaramogi Oginga Teaching and Referral Hospital).

An interesting thing about the army is that the Walter Reed people were really less fussy about security. I could see a difference during site visitations and inspections. They are more relaxed than the CDC folks. The Walter Reed had also gone through its own team of leaders, just as many as there were at the CDC. At the time I left the position of CEO at KEMRI, the Director of WRP in Kenya was Sam Martin, a native of Cameroon, but now an American national. Sam Martin was a lovely guy but, you see, lovely in the sense that he was not born in the US. He went to the US from Cameroon so he became an American citizen. He did a lot of work here in Kenya, yes, a lot of work. So together we established the Kisumu Children's Hospital, whereby I told Sam Martin, "Listen, how are you going to be remembered?" That is when we decided to build the Children's Hospital in Kisumu. If I remember correctly, it was opened by Kenya's Minister for Health, and commissioned by the then Senator Barack Obama in 2006 when he came to Kenya.

It is located at the far end of Jaramogi Oginga Odinga Teaching and Referral Hospital, what we have called Russia because the initial construction was funded by the former USSR. So when you go to the Russia Hospital, you will find the Walter Reed Project just adjacent to it in Kisumu. So we hived off that space and temporarily called it a KEMRI facility, although the grounds belong to the Ministry of Health. We don't have a title of our own for that property at present. It is an extension of the Provincial Hospital, of Russia. Yes. So in that case we are just strengthening the existing facilities because we do not own them. But the fact remains that it is one: KEMRI and the hospital. They are together a public institution and it is on public land. We wanted to build a public facility for the Kisumu residents. Who knows at some point if those facilities will merge formally? The thing is, the hospital is a public facility and we wanted to improve them. Yes. This Walter Reed Project may not stay forever but the building will remain.

We had a joint venture. We also had to ask the Rotary Club of North Florida to donate money for the facilities. And then we furnished the hospital and then we had very nice work being conducted there. Then, I said "Now, you are my friend and I have some extra space in Kericho so can we set up a facility there as well?" Yes, the largest Walter Reed facility outside of Nairobi is in Kericho. Yes. I will be remembered by my people for my work in KEMRI for this facility in Kericho, because as you know that is my home. I went to the hospital and I negotiated with the hospital to give us some space for the KEMRI-Walter Reed Project. We had new construction there and they helped to improve the existing hospital facilities. But the interest and work in Kericho came directly from the US Army. We had the Deputy Surgeon General of the US Military to open the facility here. And that is why it has done so well. These are top class facilities.

They also have a site at Kombewa, which is in Kisumu County. Kombewa was created as a field laboratory, a small field laboratory. And then we named it the Bruce Weldie/Ishmael Muriithi Laboratory or medical centre because these two were the first to initiate the WRP work in Kenya. Bruce was one of the first technicians to come work there and then he passed on from a heart attack a while back. And Ishmael Murithi was the Director of Veterinary services at that time who helped negotiate and set up the Walter Reed Project in Kenya in 1969.

19 The US Embassy and the CDC

The CDC (US Centers for Disease Control and Prevention) was originally operating using the facilities of the Division of Vector-Borne Diseases of the Ministry of Health when they first came to work in Kenya. That was 1980 when KEMRI was just beginning. And so the CDC fell under my direction within KEMRI and the DVBD, because as you will recall, I was the Director of the DVBD. In part this was because I had the facilities they required since they were doing laboratory and field-based studies then, focusing mainly on malaria studies. Yes, you will see it on record, so I laid the ground rules right from the beginning with CDC. Harrison Spencer was the very first officer and I liked working with him. He passed on recently under unfortunate circumstances.

At the time of his death, he was the head of the American Association of Schools of Public Health, I think, some public health school in the US. He was a great friend of mine, so he and I laid the ground rules for the collaboration with the CDC and KEMRI. As part of the planning to establish the CDC in Kenya, I travelled to Atlanta to meet with the senior CDC officials where we mapped out some working arrangement. I said, "This is how we are going to do it, what we are going to do," and we charted out an expansion plan. CDC was looking for expansion space. They wanted their presence to be felt outside the US. They had been in some countries in South East Asia, and I think they had been working a bit in South America, or something like that, but they had not set their foot in Africa yet so Kenya was the start for them. The name, KEMRI, was still unknown then but for some reason they were willing to work with me. Yes. So we created an expansion plan for CDC to work in Kenya.

So once CDC established itself here, I said to them, "Since 1980, you have been here. I have housed you all along and I have accommodated you. I have given you some political coverage. What are you doing in return? Let's expand these facilities?" So initially when I suggested this, they said they could not manage it. You see they had told me it would be impossible for them to build infrastructure in this country at that time but I said there is always a way of doing it. You see because they are not permitted to fund the construction of infrastructure like buildings or buying land or space to put up facilities. Yes. So I said to them,

> Give me an opportunity to find some physical space or land for you so that you can then run your programs. These are programs they are not infrastructural facilities for CDC. But you know at the end of the day it is ours.

So I considered where should we place the CDC? There was a space here in Nairobi, so we start off from Kisumu. May I tell you among all the CDC people I have worked with, the only person who did some work for the benefit of the CDC and for the benefit of Kenya is Kevin De Cock. Because without him the facilities in Kisumu would not have been put up. Without him the CDC office in Nairobi would not have been put up. Without him the rehabilitation of the old facilities belonging to KEMRI Kisumu would not have been put up. Do you know what I did? I told them that these draft plans for the new facilities are beautiful. These are plans on paper and it will be beautiful when you create these facilities. But then you look at the existing facilities at KEMRI and you could see KEMRI with a roof like this that is getting old. And theirs is very nicely done with tiles and so on. So I said first and foremost you must contribute to improving our existing infrastructure at KEMRI. Then they put up their structure. Kevin and I agreed. We used to agree on most issues because he counted himself as another Kenyan. You see, his wife is Kenyan; his children were Kenyan and everyone else in the family. And he has been here for a long time now so he is one of us. But I knew Kevin before CDC came to KEMRI. We were teaching together at the medical school. He was in the Department of Public Health when I was in the Department of Immunology, directly above each other, so we knew each other when we were teaching at the University of Nairobi. And then he went off the radar and I never saw him again until he was now returning to be the Country Director of CDC in Kenya. We had lost contact you see. I also knew Sopiato, his wife, because we are all in the same profession of medicine and research.

So at the end of the negotiations we allocated them some space outside of Kisumu town, what is known as Kisian, and we were able to improve our facilities at KEMRI. You see we did this by referring to it as "enhancement and improvement". CDC is permitted to contribute to the enhancement of facilities. We were able to complete research enhancement for two KEMRI facilities. However, we were being questioned by the audit unit of the US government as to why we had we spent 11 million dollars to do this and they queried why we were building big structures. CDC told me to provide answers. They improved the facilities that the Kenyan government had previously built by spending more than two million dollars. Yes, two million dollars just to redo the roofing for the laboratories and rehabilitation unit. We could not have the CDC structure looking very fine and then a run-down KEMRI building next to it, so when you go there now they look the same. You see these structures in Kisian look the same. Yes. So I was happy and the next bit that we did was we improved all the facilities in Nairobi.

Yes we did the same thing with the Walter Reed Project. They enhanced our existing facilities. However, there was a time when we needed to recognize their work here in Kenya, especially after the US Embassy bomb blast of 1998 in Nairobi. You see, the first CDC vehicle was mangled into a wreck and it was thrown 1 km away from the blast site. It had just been parked near the US Embassy and one of our officers was badly injured. She went for physiotherapy and was relocated to the US. So after that is when it became apparent that there was need for the Americans in Kenya to be more closely monitored through the US Embassy and it was during that period of change that their security was increased. That is the time when the national Government of the US became more involved in the everyday workings of the CDC, especially during the expansion period. So it was actually my office that was constantly requesting to increase their personnel. They became part and parcel of the US Embassy.

Because they wanted some level of security and so on, they decided to work under the US Embassy in Kenya. This is so they would be given US Embassy status. That is also part of the things that restricted their growth. Everything had to be approved by the US Embassy. Even some minor change like increasing from two to three staff members had to be approved by the US Embassy. Even their vehicles changed their registration number at that time. They became part of the US Embassy. You may see their vehicles having the 29CD. The red license plates? 29CD are the plates designated to the American Embassy in Kenya. They felt this was good for their security and recognition, but it was also bad in the sense that it restricted their growth and movement. Because whenever there was a need, I had to make the request. For instance, I requested that we increase the staff from two to five because they were extremely few until I took over as the Director for the Institute. Then the CDC blossomed. It was a different relationship than that we had with Walter Reed, who I told you already had been in Kenya since 1969 doing trypanosomiasis research, which is sleeping sickness, in veterinary laboratories.

Even most of the monies that the CDC was receiving was through the US Embassy. Although some of the funding that we received was being passed through the US Embassy, they declined to accept some of the monies because it was going to stretch their budget allocation so they said give KEMRI their own allocation. They said, "We are not going to hold this money as part of our money. We receive it and hand it over to you." This played out very well.

I also played a political role negotiating between our government and the Embassy when Moi could not talk with Hempstone. Smith Hempstone was originally a newsman, yes, but he became the US Ambassador to Kenya from 1989 until 1993.[1] These were critical years for Moi and his relationship with the US because of the national protests for multiparty politics. So I asked myself, how can I make these two individuals like each other? There used to be some money for KEMRI. It was sent first to the US Embassy here in Nairobi, then it was sent with a messenger to my office, and then we would take it to the bank and we received this almost on a monthly basis for our operational costs. Then I thought to myself that Moi's government had been denied foreign aid from the US and other countries and that was extremely hurtful to President Moi so receiving even minimal funding, like a couple hundreds of thousands of dollars, was big news. So I created a plan whereby I called Hempstone and I went to see Moi. I said,

> Mr President, sir, you know these Americans are not really bad. In fact they have decided to give KEMRI some money. They have decided to give me about 30 million shillings or so and they are going to give me that every month for a full year.

He asked me, "Is what you are saying true?" I said, "Yes, sir. It is true."

So then I called Hempstone and I told him, instead of sending this money with a messenger, just come with it. And then I planned to call the press. You see little things can create a very big impact. I decided rather than having the money sent by a messenger and being taken to an accountant, let the ambassador come to KEMRI and I called the press. He arrived, the press was there, I shook hands with Hempstone and then I made it a big story for the news. I thanked the US government for assisting KEMRI, for giving us a lot of money, and so on. So after that the relationship between Hempstone and Moi improved. By the time Hempstone left his post, and Aurelia Brazael, an American lady, took over from him, I had actually negotiated a very big breakthrough in terms of Kenya – US relations.

During the period of Aurelia Brazael, I am sorry to digress into politics, but during this era the World Bank Vice-President for Africa had a critical message for Kenya. The Kenya government was not in their good books. Our Minister for Finance was Professor George Saitoti, who was my neighbour just here in Lavington. Just at the road where we met, if you crossed to the other side of the road, yes, he had two plots. He was the Minister for Finance and also had been a long-standing Vice-President in Kenya. He later passed on in a helicopter crash.

Then we were really hurting in terms of the foreign exchange rate and our balance of trade was very bad. You see the US foreign aid to Kenya had been withheld for a number of years because of human rights violations and other accusations levied at Moi. I used my contacts and our relationships within the White House. I also made friends with Brazael.[2] There were operatives within the World Bank and the IMF offices in Kenya who had a personal dislike for President Moi's administration because of their familiarity with the local vocal opposition groups. I had also established some good relationships with officials at the Japanese Embassy in Nairobi. At around the same time, the Japanese ambassador to Kenya was a lady by the name of Sato Ginko. Then I realized in my mind that an opportunity had presented itself. Instead of registering myself as a public lobbyist in my country, like General Flynn who was a lobbyist for the Turkish government or something, I said this is my country and I will approach the US and the Japanese embassies. I am not in a position to disclose the details of the discussions I had with the two embassies as this was privileged and would be unprofessional to disclose. But basically after meetings that I had arranged at my home in Kericho, both the Bretton Woods Institutions and the Japanese government released some substantial aid to Kenya within a span of a few days.

I never tried to approach these embassies without the express authority of President Moi. I called President Moi. I said, "Mr President, sir, please allow me to penetrate into this issue and explore if I can make it work. If it doesn't work, there is nothing you will have lost." "Granted," he said. This was a Thursday. I called Mr Moi around 2 a.m. in the morning, saying, "Mr President, it has happened. It has happened. Keep quiet." And then it was reported in the Sunday papers that Kenya had received some aid. The US government had decided now to give 85 million dollars to Kenya, and the Japanese gave 75 million dollars. Yes, it was public knowledge, nothing was hidden; but of course there are many things that I cannot disclose.

Notes

1 See his biographical account in *Rogue Ambassador: An African Memoir* (Hempstone 1997).

2 Aurelia Brazael was the US Ambassador to Kenya under President Bill Clinton, from 9 August 1993 until 11 September 1996.

20 The Kemron trial

Now we are going to the Kemron story. Although it sounds like a very long story, actually it's a very, very brief story. It is a long story only because of the players involved but they were not part of the scientific project. The story of Kemron is both long and short, it depends on the route we are going to follow. Let us go the long route, which I believe most people would wish to hear.

Yes, yes. So, it so happens that from the beginning matters of science and matters of inventions were really restricted to individuals and institutions outside of Africa. If you hear anything that is coming out of Africa it is usually something negative. I've always wanted to put a stop to that nonsense simply because the persons who talk like this have no idea about Africa. They have no idea about the facilities in Africa. They have no idea about the players in Africa. And it is only a very illiterate mind who would say that a person like me, who has studied in some of the best institutions in this world, can say that just because I come from Africa, just because I did some of the work in Africa, using African populations, using African institutions, that nothing good in science is going to come out of it. I want to prove everyone wrong.

Whatever I'm doing at the moment and in the future is basically to do my own thing. I don't want anyone from outside to teach me how I need to do my science because I've trained enough. And some of the people who are talking about this sort of thing, I beat them in class when I was in their own home institutions. I outperformed them in postgraduate studies. I am proud to be doing what I'm doing and I'm proud to be utilizing the facilities that we have built here in Kenya.

I have done what I would consider as the best any scientist can do anywhere in the world. The story of Kemron dates back to the 1980s when we were working on various modulations in the fight against viral diseases. At the time when this all started we were not bothered about interferons for the treatment of HIV/AIDS, no, we were not bothered about that. We were mainly concerned about exploring how we could utilize some of the known interferons for the management of various clinical conditions as we see it in this part of the world. Since my research background is in the areas of immunology, pharmacology and some areas of pathology, I thought it extremely important to look at various formulations that we use in the treatment of infections. I asked myself some questions based on my observations of local practices: "Why do we do that?" Although you were not born in a rural setting, in my case I was surrounded by quite a number of livestock. We have cattle, we have goats, we have sheep, and so on, but what intrigued me was actually the goats because I have not seen goats being taken to a vet hospital. I have not seen a vet coming to my home to treat a sick goat. We have only seen vets coming to treat cows or pets. So I asked, why not goats?

Yes, even though in my scientific work I have never used the word "why" (even if you look through all my scientific publications, there is not a single time that I have asked "why"), usually it is a qualifying "how come?" So those are some of the things I've asked myself. How come the goats look very healthy? It's because the goats are let loose to go into the bushes and eat leaves and so on. Although at times when we slaughter a goat you might find some intestinal worms present, but seriously there is generally little. So these questions have intrigued me. I concluded that most likely these goats have a way of generating some of the preventative products which nature has instilled in them. We know from history that some of the leaves that the goats consume are the same ones that people have traditionally used as a natural source of medication or treatment. Then I also realized that there is nothing that a goat can take and swallow immediately. It chews slowly which means that there must be something along the oropharyngeal areas of the goats that enables them to absorb some of the medicinal values in the kind of leaves that they are using as a source of food which also work as a form of prevention from infections.

Then I went back to say if that is the case then we must consider the form of drug administration in our treatment of infections. I know from my studies in pharmacology that if you administer the drugs directly into the veins, you use a larger amount of the drug because it can easily be denatured by various enzymes which are flowing in the blood. If you administer the product intramuscularly, you use a smaller amount because it allows the drug to penetrate through the muscles and slowly into the blood stream and so on. If you use the product orally the same process occurs but you must protect that particular product from being digested by the stomach and the intestinal enzymes and the very harsh environment within the gut. So one has to protect the drug. You may see that some medications are covered and protected basically because that method allows the product to go through the stomach and into the intestines where it is absorbed. The intestinal enzymes and the acidity within the stomach is so harsh that nothing can pass through without being denatured by the hostile environment so the outer cover of the capsules, which is coated, protects it so that it can wade through the hostile environment of the stomach before is absorbed in the intestines. So that's basically the nature of it.

So still thinking about the goats, I asked myself, "Is there any other route of administration?" Then I was reminded of the treatment of angina, which is the pain in the chest, because of poor blood circulation within the heart, and so on. There is a product that you give an individual only by mouth that is sublingual. It is placed under the tongue and absorbed quickly. Within minutes the pain in the chest is gone! What does this mean? It means that it is being absorbed within the oral cavity and then the signals are sent with a resultant effect almost instantly. So I realized we have ignored that particular route in terms of drug administration. Then I realized that in the treatment of some of the heavy viral infections, even in hepatitis, that we use some forms of what we call biological response modifiers or cytokines in large quantities. For instance, you would see this in the treatment of hepatitis where you use a heavy dose of the interferon alpha, because there are different types of interferon. You have to use some 18,000 units by venous injection of the product. Then I thought to myself, the body itself produces small quantities of the same product and this small quantity of the same product gives you the desired effect. How then can we replace that effect? We are not going to directly administer it through the blood stream. So it is on that basis that I was trying to find out how best to administer interferon in the treatment of viral infections, all kinds of viral infections.

Though we were aware of HIV, it was not a serious threat at that time. It was gaining some level of endemicity then but it was very new. That was the period of education, trying to explain to people what HIV was and how it was being transmitted and so on. The way it was being depicted was a little scary, however it was not yet a major problem. Even in this country it had not been declared as a disaster at that time, that came much later. I think it was about 1992 or 1993 when it reached the point when we realized we had a medical emergency in this country.

So in the course of this research on drug administration and viral infections, I had a friend who was involved in culturing cells for the production of interferons in large quantities and I also met a friend of a colleague who was staying in Kenya. This was Joe Cummins of Amarillo Cell Culture of Texas. So we got in touch with him and it turned out he was working in association with another group from Japan, Hayashibara Biochemical Laboratories, who were working on the production of interferons as part of a basic research program but not for any particular disease. Yes. So we wondered, "Why can't we try interferons for use in human diseases?" So there were a lot of visitations and consultations back and forth between the Japanese, Joe Cummins and ourselves.

You see, these other partners were experimenting with the use of interferons in feline leukaemia and even in HIV patients. Then they recognized that this product had the effect of increasing weight. As you know, weight loss is one of the clinical manifestations of HIV/AIDS so this was something we were seeing here in Nairobi at that time. Whether this weight loss is due to emaciation of the muscle and cells, or is it due to loss of appetite, or is it due to something else that we did not know, because that was the early onset of HIV, we knew very little of the disease. So we thought even if interferon doesn't do anything else, it is going to cause patients to increase weight. And so we had to do what is called an anecdotal study. So I thought we should try this with humans, not only animals.

I was already working with the Japanese in Kenya through JICA but that research was not in conflict with what we were planning to do with interferons. The Japanese were largely involved in parasitology and some aspects of virology, but even when we first started the work in virology, they were not involved in HIV. They were involved in hepatitis. So I did not foresee a problem in terms of the possibility of overlap or duplication of research work between what I had planned here in Kenya and what the Japanese were doing. That was in 1989.

The discussions among us went on very rapidly. Then I said okay, because interferon is a natural product it cannot be patented or protected. Because interferons occur naturally in the body, like a protein, you cannot patent it. A patent can only apply to something you have designed, or in our case, its production or form of administration. So the patent of interferon for its production in the laboratory setting lay with Hayashibara since they were producing the product I was going to use. But the use of it could not be protected or patented under law. You cannot use interferons at say 18,000 units and protect it because it has been used for several years. But its use in small quantities sublingually is what we were protecting and for a specific use. This was clearly indicated in the patent that we acquired for it. We were not interested in the protection of its production; we were interested in the use of it.

So we decided to try various quantities in a clinical trial, a clinically approved trial whereby our trial protocol was approved by the required authorities. In such a case, the trial required both scientific approval and then ethical approval. So we had our own institutional review committees then, both at the Institute and within the Ministry of Health. In this case we were using both because we were going outside of the Institute to solicit for participants to enter into the clinical trial. So we did like any other clinical trial study and we went through all the processes and procedures.

Yes. So when we found out that this product was likely to be useful to individuals, and with less side effects, we tried to explain this and to justify its use for treating HIV which is why the Ministry of Health got involved. The Director of Medical Services in the Republic of Kenya, which is equivalent to the Surgeon General in the US, received a request from KEMRI to conduct a trial using small doses in the treatment of HIV. We reported on the observations that Amarillo Cell Culture had made regarding its effectiveness in treating animal viral infections. We asked, why couldn't we join forces to explore how we can advance this technology in humans? So it was actually the first time it was ever been tried in humans on a larger scale at that low dose. Yes. So we had to use different doses to figure out what would be the best. And then the method of application was oropharyngeal. Some people want to use it sublingually, but actually it's not technically speaking sublingual, it is an oropharyngeal drug. Sublingual is under the tongue, but here that is not the only place that the product signals are contained. It is the entire wall of oropharyngeal cavity.

When we started, the product was originally in liquid form but we realized that the stability and storage of liquid is not good and the administration may not be welcoming. In the end we went with a powder formula. We tried with the powder in little sachets. It was working fine but the administration and the use of it was a little cumbersome, and then the measurability of what you use because the powder you open will have to be poured away, or it pours out, and so on. So it was very difficult. Yes, so we tried various forms until eventually we said let's try the tablet. So what are we going to suspend it in? And how can we keep it stable? Because this product was going to be prepared in tablet form, there is some level of pressure and heat during that production that may change the drug. So there was a time then when I travelled to Japan, and we tried to discuss with the technical people there how we could prepare it.

Then we considered powder form. Well, it could be stable in the powder form but how were we going to suspend it? So we did the suspension in some kind of sugar, which is an inert sugar that could be used even by diabetics. So we couldn't use glucose to suspend it because it's not very good for diabetics. We had to use maltose to suspend it in, it's a type of sugar but tolerable. So we eventually landed there. After various different forms and formulations. When we first suspended it in the powder form, we realized it is very difficult to administer because it could pour when you are tearing the package open. Then we went onto the tablet. The problem with the tablet initially was how are we going to suspend it and then tableting became an issue of concern because of the generation of heat during the preparation of the tablet. How are we going to create a tablet that can dissolve under the mouth? You see? Yes, because we had to administer it without any use of water. Because it denatures pretty fast when it is exposed to water, pretty fast means minutes, probably within ten minutes or so. It is gone and yet you have not exposed it to the site where it can be absorbed or trigger signals. Yes. So we tried various types of tableting and decided we are not going to coat it because, if you coat it that means you have to swallow it. A coated material will not dissolve in the mouth. So we needed something that dissolves rapidly. If it's coated it has to be a very thin film that immediately dissolves in the mouth, using only saliva to dissolve the tablet.

Yes. So we played around with various methods and you know time was of the essence. We had to do this work rapidly, as fast as possible, so eventually we settled on one particular tableting procedure. We tested it even in our own mouths. By the time you explain it to the patient, you must know what you are doing, yes, you must know. You must have tried it, the stability of it, and how rapidly it is going to dissolve in the mouth. So we did that until we settled on a particular formulation and tablet using different concentrations, or different doses. They were not too many. We had eventually settled on two doses and a placebo, two different doses or levels of interferon, but the same product otherwise. Yes. That's how it was. We differentiated the doses with the foil, which was used to wrap it. White, yellow, and green.

So that's what we did. And then eventually we wrote the final protocol for both the scientific and ethical approval. Which was eventually approved and that's the time we began the study at KEMRI. When you are trying to get the patients there must be inclusion and exclusion criteria in the protocol to determine exactly what sorts of patients are needed. At that time there were serious concerns regarding confidentiality because of stigma around HIV. So you could not just simply call a patient and tell them that they come on this date. So we knew exactly the kind of people who would go to the clinic and then they could now come to us. You see at the Institute do you know we have observation wards? Yes, at KEMRI we have wards. We have a clinic and beds.

But one of the exclusion criteria for our trial was that these people did not have full-blown HIV/AIDS. Yes, as defined by CD4 and clinical observations. So there was a battery of inclusion and exclusion criteria that had to be met for the trial. We had the first patients selected and as is usually done, we randomly selected them to the various treatment regimes and various arms of the study.

Then we were following these patients over time, checking various end points every so often as defined by the scientific protocol: CD4's, viral loads, weight, and we had to monitor liver function and a range of other biochemistry observations. So things like that because we had to be sure about what we were doing. So after a period of three months, we examined the results, considered the patients – how they were responding – and then decided we would continue if there was a positive trend. And we continued following them monthly. And the study went on very beautifully, there was no hitch, there was no problem and then we broke the code at the end of the defined study. At that time we recognized that individuals who were in the treatment regime for both doses of interferon had little change. But clearly there were some changes in the other doses as compared to the placebo arm. They were doing far worse. The interferon arms were maintaining good health. So then we settled on the lower dose for the purposes of the bigger study. Yes. Now why we did this is because the production of interferon is not cheap. Number two is that there was no point giving a heavy dose, if the smaller dose is still capable of producing the same desired effects. Yes. So as you can see in the patent application and protection, it gives you all the various doses and the dose that we settled on and what we used. I think the dose was something like 10 or 15 milligrams per kilogram. But we use 70 kilograms as a standard weight so that we can use either 150 or 200 international units. Yes, it was 150 and 200 international units. I think we settled it down to 100 international units because interferons are tiny, you see. So what other people had been using was 18,000 international units but we only used 100 international units. Which is a very, very big difference. Then we started communicating our data at the scientific meetings, after the small trial, which was in February 1990. The first data were eventually published in the journal *Molecular Biotherapy*.[1]

12 December 2017 Koech adds:

The WHO-sponsored study of Kemron in some research centres in Africa, according to inside information, was poorly instructed. The investigators were reportedly advising the study subjects to take the medication with plenty of water. The product definitely denatured soon after taking it as it was supposed to work within the oropharyngeal cavity. This study was designed to fail *ab initio*. Our observations were frustrated at every step. Nowhere in our scientific communication, reports, speeches or oral communication did we ever make

4 DAILY NATION, SATURDAY, JULY 28, 1990

NATIONAL NEWS

Where to find Kemron

By CHARLES KIMATHI

The Minister for Health, Mr Mwai Kibaki, said Kemron would be available only in Government provincial hospitals and designated private hospitals.

Addressing guests during the launching of the anti-Aids drug, Mr Kibaki said the Ministry would advertise the hospitals where Kemron would be available.

He appealed to Kenyans to report to the police anyone selling it.

"We will not have Kemron sold across the counter, so if any enterprising Kenyans pretend to be selling it, report them to the police," he said.

The Minister urged the public to help by not yielding to the temptation of buying fake Kemron drugs from such unscrupulous people.

It's a moment of joy, says Kibaki

Mr Kibaki, who invited President Moi to address the gathering, said Kenyans had every reason to be proud and joyful for having produced Kemron.

He thanked President Moi for providing an enabling environment, of peace and stability, "where people could work, think genuine and positive thoughts, and address themselves to the problems afflicting humanity".

Mr Kibaki paid tribute to the President for mobilising Kenyans, through Harambees, to provide financial resources for scientific research, and for his keen interest in the activities of the youth.

He said the medical profession in the country was not bothered by the doubts and scepticism expressed in parts of the world over Kemron.

"If one patient is cured of all the symptoms of Aids, that is all we need, nothing else", he said, adding that there were, in fact, 1,300 patients who had been successfully treated.

The Minister for Research Science and Technology, Mr George Muhoho, said Kemron was developed when the Government was directing tremendous emphasis on science and technology.

He said the development of the drug was proof that Kenyan scientists had the capacity to create innovations of great scientific impact.

Mr Muhoho said he expected, before long, to invite the President to launch other innovations and discoveries by Kenyan scientists.

The Minister said it was a source of great pride and joy that Kemron was a product of President Moi's foresight and vision in promoting science and technology in the country.

He said the discovery of Kemron, and other such landmarks, could not have been achieved without peace and stability, which Kenya enjoyed under the leadership of President Moi.

"Such a conducive atmosphere enables our scientists to exploit their talents to the full," he said.

Mr Muhoho presented packed samples of Kemron to the President, who handed them over to Mr Kibaki.

Kemri's chairman, Dr Mohammed Abdalla, decribed the launching of Kemron as "a happy day for mankind", and hinted that there may be "a few more surprises in the pipeline" from Kemri.

He thanked President Moi and the Government for providing an enabling and conducive environment for Kenyan scientists.

Also present were the Vice-President and Minister for Finance, Professor George Saitoti, the Director of Medical Services, Professor Joseph Oliech, the African Regional Director of the World Health Organisation (WHO), Dr Lobe Monekosso, Cabinet Ministers, Assistant Ministers, MPs, diplomats and wananchi.

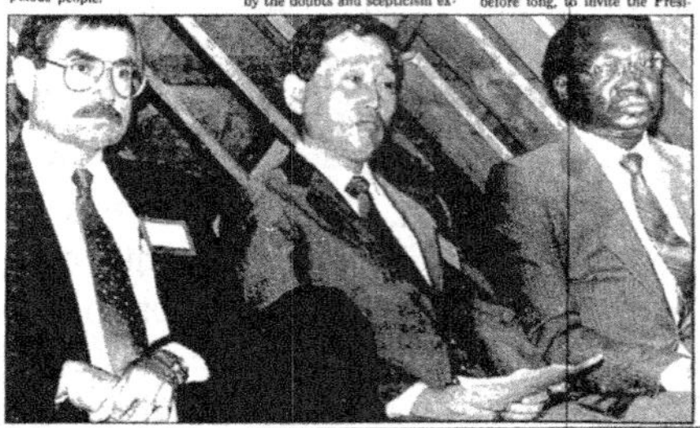

Professor Arthur O. Obel of the Kenya Medical Research Institute (Kemri) (right) with Dr Joseph Cummins of the Amarillo Cell Culture Company of the United States of America (left), and Mr Katsuaki Hayashibara of Hayashibara Biochemical Laboratories, Japan, during yesterday's launching ceremony of the Kenyan developed anti-Aids drug Kemron by President Moi. (Picture by YAHYA MOHAMED)

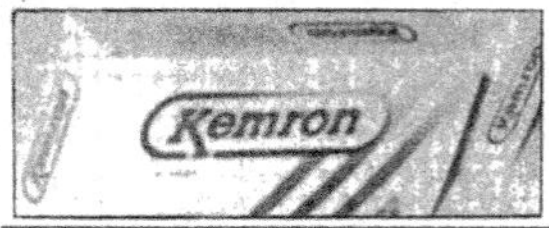

Ayah praises WHO

The Minister for Foreign Affairs and International Co-operation, Mr Wilson Ndolo Ayah, met yesterday with the World Health Organisation (WHO) regional director for Africa, Dr G. L. Monekosso and WHO representative in Kenya Dr Marcella Davis.

Dr Monekosso is in Nairobi to attend the launching of Kemron by President Moi. The WHO regional director said Kemron would be a heritage, not only to Africa, but to all mankind.

He said a new WHO representative would arrive soon to take over from Dr Davis who is due to retire. He praised Kenya for being ahead in WHO activities in many ways.

The Minister thanked WHO for taking Kenyan scientists seriously (KNA)

Anti-Aids drug will cost Sh74 per tablet

By OTULA OWUOR

Kemron, the anti-AIDS drug, will cost Sh74 per tablet and patients may have to take the drug for six months resulting in a total cost of Sh13,320. The price is the cheapest for any Aids drug in the world.

The Director of Medical Services, Professor Joseph Oliech, made the revelation yesterday during a special interview with the local Press.

"Although we have fixed the price of the drug, Kenyans must know that it will only be found in officially recommended health institutions, including all provincial hospitals except Garissa where Aids cases seem lowest," Prof Oliech said.

Experts, including Dr Davy Koech, the principal investigator of the drug, and Prof Arthur Obel, co-investigator, will train health officials from Nairobi, Mombasa and Kisumu on the application of the drug which must be properly taken to have effect.

Yesterday, top health officials from the Preferential Trade Area (PTA) countries and other parts of the world were asking to place large orders of Kemron. But Prof Oliech said: "We are not taking orders today and I request health officials from other countries to formally get in touch with the Ministry in two weeks."

Meanwhile, the Senate of the US state of Texas yesterday congratulated President Moi and the people of Kenya on the launching of Kemron.

A letter from the Senate, signed by the Governor of Texas, Mr William P. Clements, Jr., said in part: "I am pleased to have the opportunity to congratulate you... and to inform you that the flag being flown over the State Capital in Austin, Texas, on July 27, 1990, is being flown in honour of this occasion".

Koech: It's an historic occasion

By OTULA OWUOR

The launching of Kemron is not only a unique and unprecedented achievement in science and technology, but also an historic occasion for those engaged in the global fight against AIDS, Dr Davy Koech said yesterday.

Dr Koech, the principal investigator in the Kemron research and the Director of the Kenya Medical Research Institute, was speaking during the official launching of the drug by President Moi at Kenyatta International Conference Centre.

"Today is a day that offers a ray of hope for the victims of Aids which is the most worrying disease at present," Dr Koech told his audience.

Also present was Dr Lobe Monekosso, the World Health Organisation Director in the African region who helped conduct research on Kemron in other African countries.

He said history showed that major scientific discoveries were initially treated with scepticism, but that those involved in Kemron research, including Professor Arthur Obel who is one of the two co-investigators on Kemron, were not distracted from their quiet scientific work to establish various dimensions of the drug.

There was applause when he said that Kenya's flag was yesterday hoisted in the State of Texas in the United States and Dr Joseph Cummins, the other co-investigator of Kemron who hails from Texas, had brought regards from the Texas Governor.

Dr Cummins is the head of the Amarillo Cell Culture Company which has collaborated with Kemri in certain aspects of the research.

The Kemri Director, who was accompanied by the chairman, Dr Mohammed Abdalla, received further applause when he said that during a recent international health conference held in Montreal, Canada, Kenya was chosen to host the next "International Congress on Infectious Diseases".

Dr Koech said scientists required peace and stability plus moral and material support to enable them make breakthroughs like Kemron.

NATION INFORMATION SERVICE

Lecture: "A People To People Experience; Black Music And The Historical Perspective" a musical dramatic presentation by Anne Hunt Smith at the Paa Ya Paa Arts Centre tomorrow from 3-5pm.

Theatre: Hot Wax Players show, *The Madness of Love* at the Kenya National Theatre from July 23 to July 27 at 7 pm weekdays and 3 pm and 7 pm weekends.

Meeting: Tena Savings and Credit Co-operative Society holds annual general meeting at Khalsa Primary School, Race Course Road at 9 am; The Kenya Commercial Bank hold extra-ordinary meeting at the Kenyatta International Conference Centre at 10 am; Kiambu women hold a meeting at Madaraka Garden, Kiambu at 10 am; The Kenya Women's Finance Trust holds its annual general meeting at YMCA near Minet "Kawangware Hall at 9:30 am.

Exhibition: Poster series entitled "Small Business in America" and "Risk Takers in the Free Enterprise syatem" at the American Centre daily up to end of July.

Works by Frederick Mbugua, Simon Mungai and Stephen Njenga at the Kenya National Museum, Gallery of Contemporary East African Art. 10 am until the first week of August.

PHARMACIES

Kenmart Drug House: New Ngummo Shopping Centre, next to Kenyatta Market. Closes at 10 pm.

Buru Buru Shopping Centre:
Tropical Chemists: Wab Hotel Complex 10 am to 5.30 pm.

Eastleigh:
Ngenda Chemist: Near Sun City Cinema. 9 am to 8 pm.

City Centre:
Avenue Pharmacy: Sundays 9 am to 2.30pm.
City Chemists: 10 am to 1 pm. Holidays 10 am to 4 pm.
Maendeleo Pharmacy: Maendeleo House. 10 am to 6 pm.
Medilife Pharmaceuticals: Utalii House. 9 am to 8 pm.
Olago Pharmacy: Church House, Moi Avenue. 10 am to 2 pm.
Pharmadex: Rahimtulla Trust Towers, Moi Avenue 9 am to 4 pm.
Prestige Pharmacy: Postbank House, Market Street. 8.30 am to 5 pm.
Rawan Chemists: Finance House, Loita Street. 9.30 am to 1 pm.
Rhino Pharmaceuticals: Cotts House, City Hall Way. 8.30 am to 10 pm.
Sega Chemists: Koinange Lane, Shopping Centre, Murang'a Road, 9.30 to 2 pm

Madaraka:
Geotrix Pharmaceuticals: 10 am to 6 pm.
Trichem: Valley Arcade Shopping Centre, Gitanga 9 am to 12.30 pm

Hurlingham:
Yaya Chemists: Yaya Centre. 10 am to 2 pm.

Westlands:
Woodvale Chemists: Pamstech House, Woodvale Grove, 9 am to 3 pm.

Dagoretti Corner:
Kendrug Chemists: Karandini Road. 8 am to 8 pm.

Kikuyu Town:
Africana Chemists: Kikuyu Guest House, next to The Kenya Commercial Bank. 8 am to 8 pm.

Muthaiga Shopping Centre:
Muthaiga Pharmacy: Off Limuru Road. 10 am to 12 noon.

Pangani:
Baraka Chemist: New Pangani Shopping Centre, Murang'a road. Sunday 9.30 am to 2 pm, and 6 pm to 9 pm.
Liberty Pharmacy: Saturday 8 am to 8 pm Sunday 9 am to 6 pm.

Ngara:
Shriji Chemist: Ngara Rd. 10 am to 2 pm, 4 pm to 8 pm.
Madivet Chemists: Ngara Road. 10 am to 4 pm.

Ongata Rongai Town:
Rongai Chemists: 8 am to 8.30 pm.
Magadi Road Chemist: 9 am to 4 pm.

South B Shopping Centre:
Brima Pharmacy: New Plainsview Shopping Centre, Plainsview Road, Shop No. 5. 9.30 pm to 6.30 pm.
Guardian Chemists- South B; Muchumbi Road, Vumira House, Monday to Saturday 8 am to 8.30 pm, Sundays and Public Holidays 9 am to 6 pm.
South B Chemists: Week days 10 am to 12.45 pm. Saturday 10 am to 8 pm. Sunday 10 am to 4 pm.

South 'C' Shopping Centre:
Jamaly Pharmaceuticals Ltd. Sundays 9 am to 6 pm.

Nairobi West:
Jambo Medical Stores, Birongo Square. Sun 11 am to 6 pm.
Benuna Chemists: Mugoya shopping centre, 8.30 am to 9 pm.

Kiambu Township:
Einray Ltd: Kahawa House (opposite Barclays Bank). Monday to Friday, 9 am to 6 pm. Saturday 9 am to 4 pm. Sunday and Public Holidays 9 am to 1 pm.
Vam Pharmacy: Monday to Friday, 8 am to 7 pm.

Saturdays, 8 am to 4 pm. Sundays and Public Holidays, 9 am to 1 pm.

Thika:
Chania Chemists: 8.30 am to 5 pm.
Leo Pharma Ltd: Highridge Shopping Centre, Parklands.
Orchid Pharmacy: Pop-in Centre. Sunday 10 am to 1 pm.

Karatina: Waihenya Chemists. Sunday 10 am to 6 pm.

Kitale:
Cherengani Chemists, Mugua Itari Lodge, Raia Road (Laini Moja), 7.30 am to 9.00 pm.

Ngong Township:
Ngong Hills Medical Stores: Maasai Springs Building. 8 am to 7.30 pm.

Kisumu:
Sifa Chemists Ltd: 8 am to 8.30 pm daily including Sundays.

Kapenguria
Kapepharm Pharmacy: 8 am – 8.30 pm daily

Visiting hours in Nairobi hospitals:
Kenyatta National Hospital: Afternoon 1 pm to 2 pm. Evening 4.30 pm to 5.30 pm.
Nairobi Hospital: Morning 11 am to 12.30 pm. Evening 3.30 pm to 8 pm.
M.P. Shah Hospital: Morning 11 am to 12 noon. Evening 4 pm to 7.30 pm. Maternity 11 am to 12 noon. Husbands 7.30 pm to 8.30 pm and 4 pm to 5.30 pm.
Aga Khan Hospital: Morning 11 am to 1 pm. Evening 4.30 pm to 8.30 pm. Maternity Morning: 11 a.m to 1 pm. Evening 4.30 pm to 8.30 pm. Husbands from morning to 9 pm.
Mater Misericordiae Hospital: Morning: 11 am to 12 noon. Evening: 4.30 pm to 6 pm. Sunday: Morning 10.30 am to 12 noon. Evening 4 pm to 6 pm. Maternity: Morning 11 am to 12 noon. Evening 4 pm to 5 pm.
Guru Nanak Hospital: Morning: 11 am to 12.30 pm. Evening 4 pm to 6 pm.

Mombasa Hospitals:
Coast General Hospital: 12.30 pm to 1 pm.
Aga Khan: Morning 11 am to 12 noon. Evening 4 pm to 5.30 pm.
Pandya Hospital: Morning 11 am to 12 noon. Evening 4 pm to 6 pm.
Mombasa Hospital: Morning 11 a.m. to 12 noon. Evening 4.30 p.m. to 5.30 p.m.

Kisumu: The Aga Khan Hospital Monday to Friday – 11 am to noon, 4.30 to 6 pm, 7.30 to 8.30 pm. Weekenda and public holidays – 10.30 am to 12.30 pm, 4.30 to 6 pm, 7.30 to 8.30 pm.

Shipping: Acceptance period for nominated export cargo at Kilindini Harbour.

Bangla Robi	6/7 –	28/7
Abyot	13/7 –	31/7
J. Amaranto	12/7 –	28/7
CMB Plantin	13/7 –	31/7
Walter Ulbricht	17/7 –	30/7
Ocean Comp	17/7 –	30/7
Gracia Delmar	18/7 –	29/7
Pioneer Wave	19/7 –	30/7
Heroj Paic	20/7 –	6/8
Sandras S.	20/7 –	7/8
Shaula S.	20/7 –	8/8
CMB Merzaria	23/7 –	3/8
CMB Marque	24/7 –	7/8
C/O Liverpool	23/7 –	2/8
N. Linge	23/7 –	31/7
Kota Timur	9/7 –	30/7
Giovanna	26/7 –	7/8
Oyster Bay	17/7 –	31/7
Nacopolo	27/7 –	4/8

Figure 20.1 "Where to find Kemron," Daily Nation, 28 July 1990.

reference to the term or claim "cure". This was the creation of public media and we were criticized for that. I was particularly saddened when a noble study ended up being vilified for no reason of our own. Some media personalities brought politics and business interests into the arena. This was not our intention at all. The reports to the effect that there was some fraud was highly irresponsible and ill-intentioned.

Intermission

In Nairobi, Koech was introduced to Joseph Cummins in 1989, the Texan who had been doing experimental research in the United States on the use of oral interferon. In 1978 Cummins completed a PhD in microbiology at the University of Missouri on a project that explored the use of oral interferon in the treatment of viral respiratory tract diseases in cattle (Cummins and Georgiades 1993). He had experimented in treating his mother-in-law's malignant melanoma with interferon and then treating HIV, somewhat unknowingly, with interferon when a colleague with HIV, Buddy Brandt, asked him in 1986 how he might treat a "big dog with a tumor".[2] Brandt, in fact, had HIV, and made the decision to self-experiment and treat his HIV with pet interferon alpha as he was experiencing increased weight loss and decreasing CD4+ measures (common AIDS markers). In the late 1980s there were few options for the clinical management of HIV and so presumably Brandt was rather desperate to find a treatment. Eventually, Brandt confessed to Cummins that he wasn't treating a dog but himself, and that the treatment resulted in marked clinical improvements: his CD4+ levels improved from 153 to 319, his genital warts regressed, and he gained weight.

As a result, Cummins initiated a double-blinded, placebo-controlled AIDS study at the start of 1989 in collaboration with Texas Tech Health Sciences Center and the local community health department. Although the results were published from this trial, Cummins felt they were not useful given the poor compliance of research subjects in adhering to the drug regimen (see Wright, Hutcheson, and Cummins 1998). Pursuing his research on animal diseases, Cummins travelled to Nairobi in March 1989 where he toured the Kenya Agricultural Research Institute and the Laboratory for Research in Animal Disease. It was during this visit that he was introduced to Koech and shared his story of interferon and Brandt's results. Cummins returned to Kenya in July and shared the data from the clinical trial treating HIV. According to Cummins, he asked Koech to treat HIV-positive patients in Kenya with oral interferon. Koech recalls thinking that it seemed, if nothing else, that interferon was an agent that could deal with wasting syndrome (extreme weight loss) in HIV patients, and so they proceeded with "anecdotal studies".

Given Koech's pre-existing interest in treating viral infections, and an emerging epidemic in East Africa, it seemed a natural scientific question, and this led to a small clinical trial led by Koech and Arthur Obel. Obel, a senior pharmacologist and medical doctor at the University of Nairobi's Department of Clinical Medicine and Therapeutics, was the Chief Research Officer at KEMRI from

1989 until 2004.[3] Like Koech, Obel received training in both Kenya and Western academies (including the University of London, Cambridge University, and Sendai University in Japan). But unlike Koech, Obel somehow escaped the acrimonious accusations that suggested they were corrupt or purposefully deceitful; this is somewhat difficult to explain since Obel went on to claim in 1996 that he had found the cure for HIV with a drug he called "Pearl Omega".

Joe Cummins wrote to me a number of times between 2016 and 2018. He provides additional information on his role in the Kemron controversy in detail and has offered this account (a partial excerpt from a much longer email exchange, dated 14 February 2018):

> Dear Denielle,
>
> In November 1983, Dr. Buddy Brandt, a veterinarian, underwent extensive surgery in Houston with resulting complications requiring multiple blood transfusions. By January 1984, Dr. Brandt developed pneumonia requiring hospitalization. In retrospect, the pneumonia probably was his first Acquired Immunodeficiency Deficiency Syndrome (AIDS)-related illness. Shingles, genital warts, diarrhea, cold sores, mouth ulcers, respiratory infections, and weight loss were chronically experienced by Dr. Brandt. In February, 1986 AIDS-related complex was diagnosed.
>
> In the spring of 1986, Dr. Brandt acquired low-dose oral human interferon (IFN) then approved in Texas as a treatment for dogs with parvovirus and cats with leukemia. Because of Dr. Brandt's success in treating feline leukemia with Pet Interferon Alpha, and because of Buddy's chronic weight loss and depressed CD4+ cell counts (less than 200 cells/cu.mm), Dr. Brandt experimented on himself with oral Pet Interferon Alpha. Four benefits seemed to result: 1) the CD4+ cell count increased from 153 to 319 cells, 2) his genital warts regressed, 3) his appetite improved, and 4) he gained weight. The Pet Interferon Alpha treatment was discussed with his physician who objected to treatment with oral IFN. This physician told Buddy to discontinue oral IFN and take Ribavirin. During 8 months of Ribavirin treatment, Buddy experienced weight loss and inappetence, and his CD4+ cell count decreased.
>
> At the end of January 1987, Dr. Brandt restarted himself on Pet Interferon Alpha oral treatment and claimed he experienced appetite stimulation again; in February 1987, he gained 5 pounds. On February 26, 1987, one month after a previous blood sample, another blood sample was taken and analyzed for CD4+ cell counts; the count was only slightly increased from 189 to 232. From February to April, his CD4+ cell count decreased from 232 to 210, while his CD8+ cell count increased from 549 to 1050. From May to June (after taking bovine IFNα), his CD4+ cell count rose to 520 and his CD8+ cell count increased to 1352. Another blood sample was tested June 29 and confirmed blood cell improvement which seemed to correlate with Dr. Brandt's clinical improvement.

These numerical increases in his blood counts may not have been meaningful; however, Dr. Brandt claimed he felt better than he had in 3 years and attributed his improvement to oral IFN treatment. He was able to continue working full-time, was active in 4-H, and kept a garden. In other words, he was able to maintain the quality of his life for many months, something he was unable to do before. His experience was reported in Lancet, December 26, 1987, p1530-1531. Buddy died when he failed to recover from additional heart surgery.

In October, 1989, ACM (anhydrous crystalline maltose) powder containing IFNα was carried from Japan to Kenya so Dr. Arthur Obel and Dr. Davy Koech could start treating AIDS patients. Dr. Obel reported that the first 6 patients were experiencing nausea.

Because of the nausea, Dr. Obel reduced the treatment to once a day instead of twice a day and reduced the amount of a single dose from "250 IU" to "200 IU". Frankly, it was not known exactly what dose was given because the powdered ACM-IFNα was given in tiny volumes measured by Dr. Koech with the clip off a Bic pen; this amount of powder was then rolled in aluminum foil. Subsequently it was learned that the ACM powder would only keep the IFNα stable if the moisture content stayed below 2%. Exposed to the air, the ACM powder rapidly attracted moisture.

After Dr. Obel reduced the dose in mid-October 1989, he reported remarkable clinical improvement in his patients. Patients with symptoms became asymptomatic and his patients reported improved appetite and increased sexual drive. Even more impressive were the laboratory reports of greatly improved blood counts. The "CD4+ lymphocyte counts," then the most accepted measure of progression of AIDS, were reported to improve from very low counts (<200 CD4+ cells per cu.mm) back to normal (>800 CD4+ cells per cu.mm).

Dr. Koech completed a data set on 42 HIV+ patients (reported in Molecular Biotherapy 2:91-95, 1990). Drs. Koech and Okel, collected such impressive laboratory and clinical data, they had urged him to conduct a blinded, placebo-controlled clinical trial. After all, each patient in his present study knew he or she was receiving IFNα. Perhaps these patients were benefitting from a placebo effect. Dr. Koech agreed that a blinded, placebo-controlled study was needed and Hayashibara Biochemical Labs (HBL) in Okayama, Japan prepared placebo and different doses of HBL IFNα for such a trial. By January 1990, HBL prepared thousands of individually foil-wrapped lozenges containing placebo (white foil), 2 IU per lozenge (blue foil), 20 IU per lozenge (yellow foil) or 200 IU of HBL IFNα per lozenge (green foil), and they were delivered to Kenya. The color-coding was a flaw in the study design. All dose forms should look the same so patients and doctors could be "blinded." Unfortunately, the eventual disposition of these lozenges became a mystery. Some of these placebo and active lozenges became commercially available and were sold in Kenya.

The Kenyan press started carrying bewildering, inaccurate claims attributed by the press to Dr. Koech. KEMRONR was "manufactured in a secret Nairobi laboratory" in one report. In another story, the KEMRONR was "manufactured" and "invented" by Dr. Koech and the country of Kenya was going to benefit from royalties and recognition of this Kenyan invention. Suddenly there was great pride in Kenya that someone in "Black Africa" had developed a "cure" for African AIDS. In the Spring of 1990, stories appeared that KEMRONR was selling for $40 (US) per dose in Africa.

Joe

Notes

1 See Koech and Obel 1990 on the Kemron results.
2 Amarillo Biosciences, "ABI history: History of Oral IFN and AIDS", October 2007, unpublished document.
3 According to news reports, Obel, who at the time was chief scientist for the office of President (under Daniel arap Moi), had suggested that Pearl Omega was the result of research into traditional Luhya herbal medicinal cures. Support among Kenya's senior scientists and political leaders seemed split. Some defended his efforts, others suggested that the drug was simply an ineffective herbal remedy.

21 *Saba Saba* and the Kemron results

In February 1990 we announced the formal results of the Kemron study but there had been rumours to that effect during our tenth-year celebrations for the KEMRI establishment, back in 1989. It was hardly two months before the actual release of scientific data where we mentioned that we had a product with promise. Yes. I have written an article to that effect.

It was during our tenth anniversary celebrations of KEMRI where we were updating the people of Kenya, who mandate us to do scientific research, on our research activities and scientific findings. It was 6 December 1989 when we actually communicated in a formal gathering that we had some products, this is the way we referred to it – "a product" – and we talked about it generally in relation to hepatitis. During that meeting we talked about the KEMRI research in schistosomiasis, we talked about leishmaniasis, we talked about new products in malaria treatment, we talked about so many things. The idea was to talk about the breadth of work we were conducting and to celebrate our achievements. We also announced the work we had done producing the pumps for the control of the transmission of schistosomiasis *haematobium* along the coastal belt of Kenya. In fact we even presented these pumps. We discussed quite a number of our achievements. It was a formal report, a summary of all that we had accomplished in the previous ten years, which we were releasing to the people of Kenya during our celebrations. We barely mentioned Kemron, and we never mentioned it by name. No, we never disclosed what it was. In the report, the discussion of this new product was only half a paragraph.

Even though I only mentioned a product with a code number, that is the interferon trial, in passing, what caught the eye of the press was not what we had done, not all the other details in the six-page report, no just that half a paragraph. You see! So for some very strange reason the following day they forgot all the nice things that we had done and they reported, "KEMRI has got a cure for AIDS!" And we never said we have a cure! What we were reporting on was the *management* of HIV and AIDS. There were so many other products on the market like this; they were not cures, they were just managing the disease. In fact, even the title of the paper is the "management of HIV". I'd not even given it the name Kemron yet. I had not disclosed what it was, just that it worked in the clinical management of HIV. I remember that I presented with my colleagues but I was the lead presenter.

Yes. I've never used the word cure, yes. We never said anything after that. We kept quiet. I told my colleagues that the only thing that we had to do was to keep quiet. We became the centre of attention but we kept quiet: until February 1990 about six or four weeks later, I think six because from there we broke off for Christmas vacation. I wanted us to wait to talk publicly about the results until we could announce them in a more formal scientific forum, during the meeting in February in Nairobi. The Nairobi scientific meeting was a proper scientific conference where scientific information was being communicated. Yes, and it was in that scientific meeting the name "Kemron" was introduced for the first time. There we formally disclosed what we were dealing with. It was in February 1990 at the scientific conference at the Institute headquarters, which was housing the conference.

On that day our presentation was organized with other updates in HIV clinical management globally. As you know at that time there were not too many products on the market. One of the products known then was AZT plus there were a few others. There were very few options for HIV management then, about four or five. This was pre-ART before we had anti-retroviral therapies that worked.

Yes, then a few other products had just been released, which were being manufactured by foreign companies and we gave credit to each one of them in their attempts to clinically manage HIV/AIDS globally. Then we said, "On our part we have also found that low-dose interferon alpha is capable of achieving the same effect with minimum toxicity, and these are the preliminary results." So we gave those results just like all the other people had given their own results. We communicated the information at a scientific conference. It was not in a public rally or something like that which people imply. Once we had announced these results we started the process of trying to make it available to Kenyans living with AIDS.

The first time we actually gave the name Kemron was in February at this African Health Sciences Congress, it was not in a beer party or something like that! It was in a proper scientific conference where several papers were being presented, it was not a single presentation, like a lecture room, no! It was at the African Health Sciences Congress here in Nairobi. During that meeting more than 100 papers were presented.

In view of the need to hasten the provision of and access to the product, we created two separate approaches. One was to grant access to the product as quickly as was possible, then number two was to ensure that we continue with the studies to support our initial operations. So we made all the arrangements, both with Japan and the US, to launch the product later that year, before the end of the first half of 1990. So number one, we focused on the logistics of production, number two, the registration of the product, then distribution. We wanted it to be released first in this country because this was where it was first trialled and registered. So we worked on sorting all of these details. While we were working on it there were also people who were very busy trying to discredit our work.

This did not start immediately, it was not immediately, because people did not know too much about it and they were still trying to find the scientific information behind it and how to access the product and so forth. So there was a lot of drama associated with it coming from the lay press. But we kept our cool and then about March or April we finally managed to have the product registered with the relevant registration authorities. Then, we managed to make arrangements for additional clinical trials; and then last, we had managed to start the necessary preparations for the production of the product. For instance, we had made the design of the label and the packaging, and so on. We had even agreed upon the proceeds of the sales and where they were going. Yes, we agreed upon that and then we had also applied for a patent, I mean protection. This was to be the first patent to be applied for in Kenya.

So we had done everything, a beautiful amount of work. So when it was all systems go, we said when is the best time to do the launch based on the availability of our collaborative institutions, which were Amarillo Cell Culture and Hayashibara. Also, we had to consider the company that was producing and tableting it, and the local company that was doing the distribution. They were receiving the product for the purposes of distribution, which was ITL, Innovative Therapeutics Limited.

So we had done everything in preparation for an official launch. We agreed that we were not going to do any form of distribution before the launch. Yes, at that time KEMRI was under the Ministry of Research, Science, and Technology, not the Ministry of Health as we are today. So we wanted the Ministry of Research, Science, and Technology to allow us to hand over this to the Ministry of Health. We agreed that a senior representative from either ministry should be the guest to launch the drug. Then the only person who was that senior was the Vice-President of the Republic of Kenya, Professor George Saitoti. So we agreed upon that.

He is one of the persons who died in a plane crash, you remember? We said Professor George Saitoti was going to be our guest of honour. We agreed and we even made an application to the secretary of the Vice-President to give us his timetable and we also gave our timetable to allow us to sort possible dates depending on the availability of our Japanese and Americans colleagues. Yes, because this all had to be coordinated. We agreed that the launch would be held in late June but we said it couldn't be early June because I had a meeting out of the country. We agreed on everything, including the venue which would be the Serena Hotel.

Yes, so we all worked towards that date, all aspects of the work: science, logistics, production, transportation of the item, and so on. It so happened that at that particular time in the political history of this country, there were a lot of fights and a clamouring for the opening up of a multiparty political system in this country, which had been abolished by Daniel arap Moi's Parliament following the attempted coup of 1982. There were a lot of demonstrations against the Government of President Moi. People were in the street demonstrating, asking: "Let us express our political wishes through the change of the constitution!"

You see, after the 1982 coup attempt, Moi blocked multiparty democracy and Kenya became a de jure one-party state.

Although in practice, from the collapse of Jaramogi Oginga Odinga's party and then Oginga himself being put in detention by the Jomo Kenyatta administration in 1969, Kenya operated as a *de facto* one-party state. But in 1982–83, Moi outlawed any other party except his, the ruling party. So although it had been basically a one-party state, Moi made it law. You see! So there was a clamour for change of the constitution, clamour for this, clamour for that and so on. There were demonstrations in the city during the first week of June, but I was out of the country at a conference in Montreal. We had our international congress of … I think it was for Protozoology, where I was on its organizing committee.

I was away in Canada and it must have been on 1st June when I was away, I was in Montreal, during the national celebrations, *Madaraka* Day. During *Madaraka* Day in his speech President Moi announced nationally that he would have the honour of launching Kemron later in the year. And so I was informed about this while I was in Canada because I did not know. I became so furious I could not even manage to enjoy my stay in Canada because my program had been distorted. The person who was coming to launch this product as our official guest was the Vice-President, not the President of the Republic of Kenya!

I was annoyed because, number one, it meant that the dates had to be changed for the launch. Then, number two, it was taking on a political angle. I tried to call home but I couldn't get through. Anyway, I got so uncomfortable, I became very unhappy. When I was ready to leave Montreal I could not manage to reach the airport in Canada because the Mohawk Indians had blocked the road because there were some developers who were extending the golf course, on to Mohawk land, and they had blocked the road in demonstrations towards the airport (the Oka Crisis). Actually access to the airport was very restricted and I missed my flight. So I had to reschedule my coming back.

Yes, so that is the time I was actually brokering the transfer of that meeting to Nairobi from Canada. Since I was on the organizing committee, I was pushing for it to be held in Kenya but they were reluctant because they were saying that Kenya was unsafe because of the political demonstrations and so on. But then, I was blocked from going to the airport in Canada, so demonstrations are everywhere! The demonstrations that we had in this country were basically related to multi-partyism. And there in Canada it was an Indigenous community blocking the road because the ancestral land had been taken away by this silly golf club. Yes, I was trying to arrange for the meeting to be held for 1995 in Kenya. So I was trying to impress upon my colleagues who were attending the meeting to vote for Nairobi. Yes, and I succeeded, and I had excellent leadership within the committee. So Nairobi was voted to host the conference in 1995 and then I came back at least with the success of that.

So upon my eventual arrival in Nairobi I went straight to State House and I confronted the President. I said,

> Mr President, with all due fairness whoever asked you to come and officiate in this function was not me, it was not any of my colleagues. Who is it that made you come in when we have made all the other necessary arrangements with Professor Saitoti?

He looked at me and he laughed, and said, "I did!"

But I knew who had convinced him to make this change. It was Hezekiah Oyugi who was a very powerful Permanent Secretary in the Kenyan government in charge of internal security in this country. He could manage to convince President Moi to do certain things. I knew he was the one. Also, I could tell from the way the speech had been drafted. It came from his office, and not from anywhere else. I knew it. Moi eventually disclosed this to me. He said,

> Listen young man! We are living in a political system; we have to use every tool in our hands to show to the rest of the world that despite all these demonstrations in the street, Kenya is still active and doing good business. It is still working as a nation, Kenya is intact, there is no vacuum in the leadership of this country! So we must do the right thing. And also to make sure that whatever we are doing is in the best interest of Kenyans. So you must bear with us.

So President Moi summoned his ministers. George Muhoho (Research, Science, and Technology) and Mwai Kibaki (Health) came and we met at State House. I appealed to the President, and I told him

> You know, Mr President, if you get involved in the launch the attention will be diverted away from the launch of the drug to you and it is going to frustrate our efforts to make these products be seen as they are – properly investigated, therapeutic interventions for the management of HIV/AIDS. But with your direct involvement people are going to misinterpret science to mean politics. So I request that you accept my recommendation that we keep the launch as previously planned and agreed.

So President Moi said: "I have decided that I am going to launch it, is there anything else that you would wish to add on to this? No? So go make arrangements for that day." It ended there!

So to begin with, number one, a new date had to be found, one that was acceptable to both the Japanese and American colleagues. It could not be on the same date that we had previously agreed. Number two, the venue had to change. The President would definitely not go to the Serena Hotel to launch this product. The launch would have to be held somewhere else. Then even the invitations and so on, these things had to change. Because President Moi had said we must honour his decision. If we refused, there wouldn't be any launch! So the task was to make my American and Japanese colleagues find a more accommodating date. Then it was decided it was going to be sometime in July, and the venue was going to be at the Kenyatta International Convention Centre (KICC). And the state took over all the arrangements because it had become a government event. We became secondary, so anyway that is what happened.

On the said date and the venue, the President went to launch the product, 27 July 1990. So the products were launched and we had an open display. We displayed the boxes without the drug because we could not control the access of our product because it is out in the open in this large forum. People would have wanted the drug. Because there were a lot of people clamouring for the drug, we could not have the actual drugs there. You know, KTN was a fresh, private television station in this country and it was the first one in Kenya. That is why it was celebrating 25 years the other day. It was the only private television station in this country, and it was an agent of CNN. So it used to reach a particular time and then the station switched to CNN. So within six hours of our launch, the American news in Washington was already reporting there were empty boxes with no drugs! But of course we would not have real drugs lying around in that venue. So immediately there was a lot of negativity around the launch, and then Kenya's opposition group joined the fray, because they said it was an attempt by President Moi to divert public attention away from politics.

It was a national event with the President, and the leadership of this country was directly involved, all his members of the Cabinet, the permanent secretaries invariably had to be there. It was my day so I can't forget. Also in attendance were a few friends of this country who were in the diplomatic service. And of course our colleagues from this country, and our collaborators from the US, like Joe Cummins, and Japan were there, and recognized. In fact, my daughter Cherop is the one who gave the flowers to welcome the President to the event. There were about 4,000 people in attendance. It filled the plenary hall at the KICC. Yes, it was a lot of people and it was carried live on television. There were lots of local and international journalists. It was very exciting, a lovely day. I think I wore another beige suit. I didn't have my usual dark suit.

Moi in his speech recognized the role of the research in this country. Of course we prepared his basic speech, all the notes and the drafts, and then it was edited and worked on through his office. But essentially he encouraged Kenyans to appreciate the research being conducted. What I wanted to hear from him was a commitment to increase the national of budget for scientific and medical research, but he never mentioned this. From there he started of course talking politics in his speech. But his speech was fairly guarded and very optimistic (see Figure 21.1).

I remember on the 7th of July of that year, there were a lot of demonstrations in town. That is why we call it *Saba Saba*, the seventh of July. *Saba* is seven, so it was seventh day of the seventh month of the year. The launch was hardly three weeks after *Saba Saba* when there was a big demonstration in Nairobi, which eventually led to the change of the constitution to allow multi-partyism in this country. President Moi was being pressured to open up political space in Kenya to allow for multiparty democracy. So with President Moi getting involved in the launch, Kemron was tarnished. Despite my objection to President Moi, he said he was going to launch it. So it took a political angle to the extent that

GABON

Study Shows 1,000 New AIDS Cases Annually

90WE0268B Libreville L'UNION in French
21 May 90 p 3

[Text] The latest survey study done in Libreville and the interior of the country provided an estimate of the number of clinical cases of seropositivity in Gabon. Libreville's study, which involved 386 adults aged 15 to 44 years, showed an HIV-1 seropositivity rate of 2.2 percent, or an increase of 0.4 in 3 years (1.8 percent in February 1986). Since the capital's adult population is estimated at 175,000, there are thus approximately 4,000 seropositives.

In the interior, an average of 0.6 percent of subjects in the adult population, estimated at 500,000, are seropositive, or around 3,000 individuals.

Thus, the incidence in Libreville is 0.13 percent a year. Hypothesizing an identical incidence in the provinces, researchers estimate that the number of new seropositives each year is 250 for Libreville and 650 for the rest of the country. [This makes] a total of 1,000 new seropositives a year: 1990 (8,000); 1991 (9,000); 1992 (10,000); 1993 (11,000); 1994 (12,000); 1995 (13,000).

GHANA

AIDS Cases Rise From 26 to 1,226 in Three Years

AB1608152690 Accra Domestic Service in English
1300 GMT 15 Aug 90

[Excerpt] A National Advisory Council on AIDS was inaugurated in Accra today by the PNDC [Provisional National Defense Council] secretary for health, Nana Ekuaku Sarpong. It seeks to bring new impetus to the program of AIDS control in the country by identifying resources for the prevention and control of AIDS and encouraging research activities relating to AIDS. Nana Yaa Agyeman reports on the inaugural ceremony.

[Begin Agyeman recording] Between 1986 and the end of 1989, reported cases of AIDS have increased from 26 to 1,226. This means that nine out of every 1,000 people in this country have AIDS. In spite of this alarming figure, people appear to be more and more uninterested in the public education campaign against AIDS. That, among other reasons, led to the formation of the National Advisory Council of AIDS representing a broad spectrum of bodies and institutions, both official and unofficial. [passage omitted] [end recording]

KENYA

Kemron Drug Test Results Termed 'Inconclusive'

90WE0255 London AFRICA ANALYSIS in English
8 Jun 90 p 1

[Text] Geneva—The World Health Organisation is preparing a report on the five-nation test of the Kenyan-developed AIDS drugs, kemron (AFRICA ANALYSIS No 93), which President Daniel arap Moi last week announced would be on sale in August. The report, which should be published by next month, covers trials in Nairobi, Abidjan, Brazzaville, Harare and Yaounde—and states that the results were 'inconclusive.'

Although the WHO is maintaining a diplomatic silence over Moi's announcement that kemron is probably the first effective anti-AIDS drug,' officials are known to be furious.

Of particular significance is the fact that scientists in Harare decided on their own initiative to conduct 'double blind' testing, giving one group of patients a harmless placebo and another the recommended dosages of kemron. There was no sign of any dramatic breakthrough.

According to the Kenyan developers of the drug, an interferon which is administered in small doses, there is a 'significant clinical improvement' in most patients after four to six weeks, with signs of a reversal of the disease. The test reports so far submitted—it is understood that Brazzaville has still to report—do not bear out this optimism.

Moi Launches Anti-AIDS Drug

EA2707155090 Nairobi Domestic Service in English
0715 GMT 27 Jul 90

["Live Relay" of speech by President Daniel arap Moi at the Kenyatta International Conference Center in Nairobi]

[Excerpts] Distinguished guests, ladies and gentlemen, as you may recall, during this year's Madaraka Day [1 June], I announced that I would be launching the anti-AIDS drug later in the year. That day has come and it is, therefore, with immense joy that I preside over this auspicious and historic event, in itself a remarkable milestone in the development of science and technology in our land. [passage omitted]

Over the ages, man has, through his unique mental ability and other endowments, realized tremendous achievements for his comfort, welfare, and sustenance of life, but with the advent of the disease AIDS, the clock seems to have been wound backwards, AIDS has struck and assumed epidemic proportions, leaving a trail of death, helplessness, and despair to its victims. It threatens the foundation of human civilization and the existence of mankind, showing how vulnerable man is even with his modern technological advancements.

Figure 21.1 Moi's speech excerpt.

Ladies and gentlemen, AIDS is a very disturbing, bewildering, and devastating disease. One of its most vicious and horrifying aspects is that, by its very nature of transmission, it strikes mainly at those members of the human society who are economically active and useful, thereby unleashing catastrophic consequences in all fronts of human progress. Nasty as it is, the reality must be squarely faced and all possible solutions sought to combat the disease.

It is commendable the way the global community has risen up to this challenge and continues with resolve to search for a cure for the disease. We are happy to be part of the global campaign in the campaign against AIDS.

As soon as the ravages of the disease became known to us, we embarked on a vigorous campaign through public education and information on one front. Clinical surveillance and scientific research on the other to control the spread of the disease. I am gratified that all our efforts in all these fronts have yielded good results.

Today, our national AIDS control program is one of the best programs and a model for many other countries in the world. In the clinical field we continue to monitor closely all those who have tested positive for AIDS as well as to screen all donated blood to ensure that it is free from contamination by the AIDS virus.

On the research front, we are grateful to the Kenya medical Research Institute (Kemri) for its unique contribution in the development of the anti-AIDS drug, now popularly known as Kemron. When the director of Kemri announced in December last year that Kemri with its collaborators, had developed a drug against AIDS, some people could not believe that a country like Kenya with its limited resources, had the human resources and the scientific ability for such a breakthrough. We may not have all the resources at our disposal but we have the courage and determination to direct all our energy and talent to a noble cause that serves to improve human life.

In view of wide and closely monitored clinical trials both in Kenya and in other parts of the world, Kemron has proved to be an effective and safe drug in the treatment and management of AIDS. Used correctly, the drug has minimum side effects of no adverse consequences to human life, and arising from the very encouraging and positive results obtained in the clinical trials, my government has already registered the drug for clinical use.

Ladies and gentlemen, the registration of Kemron for clinical use is a very bold and practical move, Kemron may not be the all out cure for AIDS, but, since it has proved to successfully alleviate the signs and symptoms commonly associated with the disease, we would be doing humanity a disservice if we did not act fast enough and make the drug available for those who need it.

A touch of human compassion should embrace any human mission. We cannot, therefore, afford to wait for an eventual cure or perfection of Kemron when thousands of our fellow men, women, and children are suffering from the disease and when by the grace of god we have a drug that alleviates their suffering and gives them a new lease of life.

As I launch the drug, I would like to express my most profound gratitude and appreciations to Kemri, all the institutions and individual scientists who have participated in the development of Kemron. In particular, I would like to thank the Amarillo Cell Culture Company based in Texas and the Hayashibara Biochemical Laboratories of Japan for their invaluable contribution in the development of the drug. [passage omitted]

You have all done a commendable job, but the struggle is not yet over. And I would like to advise everybody not to get loose simply because Kemron is now available. You must not be complacent, but must continue to fight in the noble task of eradicating this dreaded disease.

Even when the most fulsome cure is found, the saying—prevention is better than cure—will continue to be the surest safeguard against infection. I therefore appeal to all Kenyans that even with Kemron being available, they must not take chances but instead should follow the precautionary guidelines routinely issued by the Ministry of Health in order to protect themselves from this scourge.

NAMIBIA

Nujoma Calls For All To Help Fight AIDS

MB0507090290 Windhoek Domestic Service in Afrikaans 0600 GMT 5 Jul 90

[Text] President Sam Nujoma has called on all institutions, organizations, and especially individuals, to help the Ministry of Health and Social Services in its efforts to prevent the spreading of AIDS.

Speaking at the launch of Namibia's first national AIDS control program last night, Mr. Nujoma said the only weapon against the disease is to inform and educate the public in order to encourage a changed attitude toward intimate relationships, and to bring to their attention that there is no medical cure for AIDS.

The WHO representative in Namibia, Mr. David Tembi, says a worldwide effort similar to the one launched against smallpox in the seventies, is required to combat AIDS, if a human tragedy is to be averted. According to Mr. Tembi, one out of every 50 people in African countries south of the Sahara is already infected with the AIDS virus, while close to 400,000 babies were born with AIDS in Africa during the first half of the current year.

He confirmed that the WHO was giving its full support to Namibia's AIDS control program, and would be contributing financial and technical aid.

Figure 21.1 Continued.

people said it was just a ploy. My own professional colleagues took advantage of that. They belittled Kemron. I remember a friend of mine, he is still a friend of mine today, making an announcement that Kemron was nothing but sugar powder, tableted in Kenya's industrial area. Eventually I looked at him and said, "My friend, what is this you are saying?" I said, "Even you are saying that you do not know the science of it, yet you are an educated physician! You appear

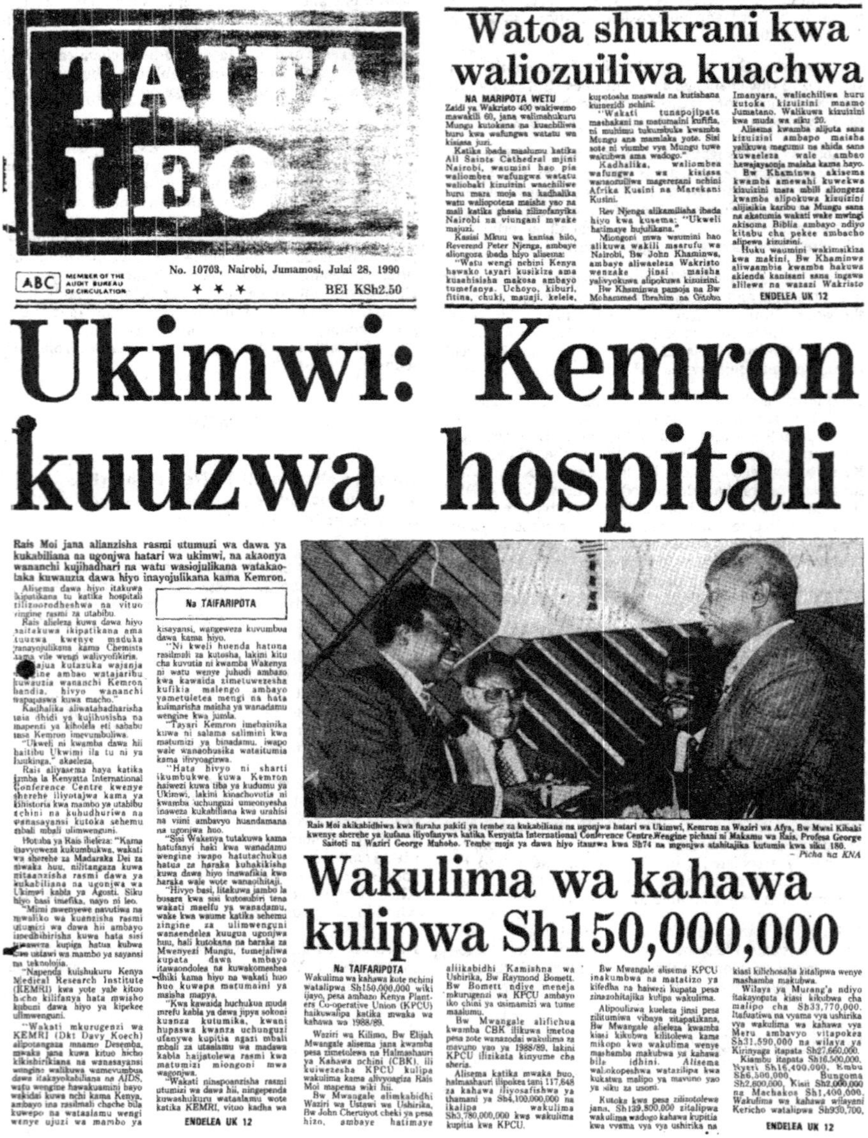

TAIFA LEO

ABC MEMBER OF THE AUDIT BUREAU OF CIRCULATION

No. 10703, Nairobi, Jumamosi, Julai 28, 1990

* * *

BEI KSh2.50

Watoa shukrani kwa waliozuiliwa kuachwa

NA MARIPOTA WETU

Zaidi ya Wakristo 400 wakiwemo mawakili 60, jana walimshukuru Mungu kutokana na kuachiliwa huru kwa wafungwa watatu wa kisiasa juzi.

Katika ibada maalumu katika All Saints Cathedral mjini Nairobi, waumini hao pia waliombea wafungwa watatu waliobaki kizuizini waachiliwe huru mara moja na kadhalika watu waliopoteza maisha yao na mali katika ghasia zilizofanyika Nairobi na viungani mwake majuzi.

Kasisi Mkuu wa kanisa hilo, Reverend Peter Njenga, ambaye aliongoza ibada hiyo alisema:

"Watu wengi nchini Kenya hawako tayari kusikiza ama kusahihisha makosa ambayo tumefanya. Uchoyo, kiburi, fitina, chuki, mauaji, kelele, kupotosha maswala na kutishana kumezidi nchini.

"Wakati tunapojipata mashakani na matumaini kufifia, ni muhimu tukumbuke kwamba Mungu ana mamlaka yote. Sisi sote ni viumbe vya Mungu tuwe wakubwa ama wadogo."

Kadhalika, waliombea wafungwa wa kisiasa wanaozuiliwa magerezani nchini Afrika Kusini na Marekani Kusini.

Rev Njenga alikamilisha ibada hiyo kwa kusema: "Ukweli hatimaye hujulikana."

Miongoni mwa waumini hao alikuwa wakili maarufu wa Nairobi, Bw John Khaminwa, ambaye aliwaeleza Wakristo wenzake jinsi maisha yalivyokuwa alipokuwa kizuizini.

Bw Khaminwa pamoja na Bw Mohammed Ibrahim na Gitobu Imanyara, waliachiliwa huru kutoka kizuizini mnamo Jumatano. Walikuwa kizuizini kwa muda wa siku 20.

Alisema kwamba alijuta sana kizuizini ambapo maisha yalikuwa magumu na shida sana kuwaeleza wale ambao hawajayaonja maisha kama hayo.

Bw Khaminwa akisema kwamba amewahi kuwekwa kizuizini mara mbili aliongeza kwamba alipokuwa kizuizini alijisikia karibu na Mungu sana na akatumia wakati wake mwingi akisoma Biblia ambayo ndiyo kitabu cha pekee ambacho alipewa kizuizini.

Huku waumini wakimsikiza kwa makini, Bw Khaminwa aliwaambia kwamba hakuwa akienda kanisani sana ingawa alilewa na wazazi Wakristo

ENDELEA UK 12

Ukimwi: Kemron kuuzwa hospitali

Rais Moi jana alianzisha rasmi utumuzi wa dawa ya kukabiliana na ugonjwa hatari wa ukimwi, na akaonya wananchi kujihadhari na watu wasiojulikana watakaotaka kuwauzia dawa hiyo inayojulikana kama Kemron.

Na TAIFARIPOTA

Alisema dawa hiyo itakuwa ikipatikana tu katika hospitali zilizoorodheshwa na vituo vingine rasmi za utabibu.

Rais alieleza kuwa dawa hiyo haitakuwa ikipatikana ama kuuzwa kwenye maduka yanayojulikana kama Chemists kama vile wengi walivyofikiria.

"…ajua kutazuka wajanja …ine ambao watajaribu kuwauzia wananchi Kemron handia, hivyo wananchi wapaswa kuwa macho."

Kadhalika aliwatahadharisha raia dhidi ya kujihusisha na mapenzi ya kiholela eti sababu sasa Kemron imevumbuliwa.

"Ukweli ni kwamba dawa hii haitibu Ukwimi ila tu ni ya kuukinga," akaeleza.

Rais aliyasema haya katika jumba la Kenyatta International Conference Centre kwenye sherehe iliyotajwa kama ya kihistoria kwa mambo ya utabibu nchini na kuhudhuriwa na wanasayansi kutoka sehemu mbali mbali ulimwenguni.

Hotuba ya Rais ilieleza: "Kama itavyoweza kukumbukwa, wakati wa sherehe za Madaraka Dei za mwaka huu, nilitangaza kuwa nitaanzisha rasmi dawa ya kukabiliana na ugonjwa wa Ukimwi kabla ya Agosti. Siku hiyo basi imefika, nayo ni leo.

"Mimi mwenyewe navutiwa na mwaliko wa kuanzisha rasmi utumizi wa dawa hii ambayo imedhihirisha kuwa hata sisi tunaweza kupiga hatua kubwa katika ustawi wa mambo ya sayansi na teknolojia.

"Napenda kuishukuru Kenya Medical Research Institute (KEMRI) kwa yote yale kituo hicho kilifanya hata mwisho kubuni dawa hiyo ya kipekee ulimwenguni.

"Wakati mkurugenzi wa KEMRI (Dkt Davy Koech) alipotangaza mnamo Desemba, mwaka jana kuwa kituo hicho kikishirikiana na wanasayansi wengine walikuwa wamevumbua dawa itakayokabiliana na *AIDS*, watu wengine hawakuamini hayo wakidai kuwa nchi kama Kenya, ambayo ina rasilmali chache bila kuwepo na wataalamu wengi wenye ujuzi wa mambo ya kisayansi, wangeweza kuvumbua dawa kama hiyo.

"Ni kweli huenda hatuna rasilmali za kutosha, lakini kitu cha kuvutia ni kwamba Wakenya ni watu wenye juhudi ambazo kwa kawaida zimetuwezesha kufikia malengo ambayo yametuletea mengi na hata kuimarisha maisha ya wanadamu wengine kwa jumla.

"Tayari Kemron imebainika kuwa ni salama salimini kwa matumizi ya binadamu, iwapo wale wanaohusika wataitumia kama ilivyoagizwa.

"Hata hivyo ni sharti ikumbukwe kuwa Kemron haiwezi kuwa tiba ya kudumu ya Ukimwi, lakini kinachovutia ni kwamba uchunguzi umeonyesha inaweza kukabiliana kwa urahisi na viini ambavyo huandamana na ugonjwa huo.

"Sisi Wakenya tutakuwa kama hatufanyi haki kwa wanadamu wengine iwapo hatutachukua hatua za haraka kuhakikisha kuwa dawa hiyo inawafikia kwa haraka wale wote wanaoihitaji.

"Hivyo basi, litakuwa jambo la busara kwa sisi kutosubiri tena wakati maelfu ya wanadamu, wake kwa waume katika sehemu zingine za ulimwenguni wanaendelea kuugua ugonjwa huu, hali kutokana na baraka za Mwenyezi Mungu, tumejaliwa kupata dawa ambayo itawaondolea na kuwakomeshea dhiki kama hiyo na wakati huo huo kuwapa matumaini ya maisha mapya.

"Kwa kawaida huchukua muda mrefu kabla ya dawa jipya sokoni kuanza kutumika, kwani hupaswa kwanza uchunguzi ufanywe kupitia ngazi mbali mbali za utaalamu wa madawa kabla haijatolewa rasmi kwa matumizi miongoni mwa wagonjwa.

"Wakati ninapoanzisha rasmi utumizi wa dawa hii, ningependa kuwashukuru wataalamu wote katika KEMRI, vituo kadha wa

ENDELEA UK 12

Rais Moi akikabidhiwa kwa furaha pakiti ya tembe za kukabiliana na ugonjwa hatari wa Ukimwi, Kemron na Waziri wa Afya, Bw Mwai Kibaki kwenye sherehe ya kufana iliyofanywa katika Kenyatta International Conference Centre.Wengine pichani ni Makamu wa Rais, Profesa George Saitoti na Waziri George Muhoho. Tembe moja ya dawa hiyo itauzwa kwa Sh74 na mgonjwa atahitajika kutumia kwa siku 180. – *Picha na KNA*

Wakulima wa kahawa kulipwa Sh150,000,000

Na TAIFARIPOTA

Wakulima wa kahawa kote nchini watalipwa Sh150,000,000 wiki ijayo, pesa ambazo Kenya Planters Co-operative Union (KPCU) haikuwalipa katika mwaka wa kahawa wa 1988/89.

Waziri wa Kilimo, Bw Elijah Mwangale alisema jana kwamba pesa zimetolewa na Halmashauri ya Kahawa nchini (CBK), ili kuiwezesha KPCU kulipa wakulima kama alivyoagiza Rais Moi mapema wiki hii.

Bw Mwangale alimkabidhi Waziri wa Ustawi wa Ushirika, Bw John Cheruiyot cheki ya pesa hizo, ambaye hatimaye aliikabidhi Kamishna wa Ushirika, Bw Raymond Bomett. Bw Bomett ndiye meneja mkurugenzi wa KPCU ambayo iko chini ya usimamizi wa tume maalumu.

Bw Mwangale alifichua kwamba CBK ilikuwa imetoa pesa zote wanazodai wakulima za mavuno yao ya 1988/89, lakini KPCU ilizikata kinyume cha sheria.

Alisema katika mwaka huo, halmashauri ilipokea tani 117,648 za kahawa iliyosafishwa ya thamani ya Sh4,100,000,000 na ikalipa wakulima Sh3,780,000,000 kwa wakulima kupitia kwa KPCU.

Bw Mwangale alisema KPCU inakumbwa na matatizo ya kifedha na haiwezi kupata pesa zinazohitajika kulipa wakulima.

Alipoulizwa kueleza jinsi pesa zilitumiwa vibaya zitapatikana, Bw Mwangale alieleza kwamba kiasi kikubwa kilitolewa kama mikopo kwa wakulima wenye mashamba makubwa ya kahawa bila idhini. Alisema waliokopeshwa watazilipa kwa kukatwa malipo ya mavuno yao ya siku za usoni.

Kutoka kwa pesa zilizotolewa jana, Sh139,800,000 zitalipwa wakulima wadogo kahawa kupitia kwa vyama vya vya ushirika na kiasi kilichosalia kitalipwa wenye mashamba makubwa.

Wilaya ya Murang'a ndiyo itakayopata kiasi kikubwa cha malipo cha Sh33,770,000. Itafuatiwa na vyama vya ushirika vya wakulima wa kahawa vya Meru ambavyo vitapokea Sh31,590,000 na wilaya ya Kirinyaga itapata Sh27,660,000.

Kiambu itapata Sh16,500,000, Nyeri Sh16,400,000, Embu Sh6,500,000, Bungoma Sh2,600,000, Kisii Sh2,000,000 na Machakos Sh1,400,000. Wakulima wa kahawa wilayani Kericho watalipwa Sh930,700,

ENDELEA UK 12

Figure 21.2 Kemron Kuuzwa Hospitali, 28 July 1990.

more of a sociologist! Why do you, if you do not know anything about it, talk about it?"

You see, other people have reported developing antiviral products in the US, but they have not questioned them, so why when *we* report something do they question us? Does it mean that we are so dumb? We have no science in our heads, we don't know what we were saying, or we don't how we are producing this product? It beats logic! Yes, it beats logic. And especially when some of them who are talking have never gone to school. They may have gone to school but they didn't go to the classroom. Yes so, this is what is very disappointing. Then, second, there was also an attempt within the continent of Africa, my own colleagues who worked to discredit our work.

Intermission

On 13 February 1990, just days before Koech presented the first official results of the Kemron clinical trial in Nairobi, Foreign Minister Robert Ouko, a Luo, was killed in his home outside of Kisumu (about 500 km from the capital, Nairobi).[1] The murderers were not found, and the government responded by stating that Ouko had disappeared, and then they had "found" his body on 16 February. It is unknown what involvement Moi or his government had in the murder but they clearly tried to suppress the facts of the case. Ouko's death rallied opponents across the country, catalysing a year of demonstrations and calls for a return to a multiparty political system.

Before the launch occurred, the pro-democracy demonstrations intensified. Moi had two Kikuyus, Kenneth Matiba and Charles Rubia, arrested on 4 July: both were former Cabinet members who had become key opposition leaders and who, according to rumours, had met with Raila and Oginga Odinga (the Luo opposition leaders). Former Kikuyu ministers increased pressure in the following months and planned a nationwide demonstration against Moi's government for *Saba Saba*, or 7 July, during which protestors demanded the release of Matiba and Rubia. Police attempted to disrupt the demonstrations, which resulted in mass rioting in Nairobi and the surrounding areas, more than 1,000 arrests, and somewhere between 30 and 100 deaths.

I heard many accounts of the KICC launch, described as "surreal" for its grandeur and spectacle, and as "pure theatre" by Western scientists. Moi went all-out. Moi announced at the launch in Nairobi on 27 July 1990 that Kenyan scientists had discovered an "anti-AIDS drug". Moi's speech, like Koech's recounting of Kemron, highlights the geopolitical tensions involved in science by stressing the work of Kenyans and Kenyan science in the "development" of the drug. Moi stated:

> On the research front, we are grateful to the Kenya Medical Research Institute for its unique contribution in the development of the anti-AIDS drug, now popularly known as Kemron. When the Director of KEMRI announced in December last year that KEMRI, with its collaborators, had developed a

> drug against AIDS, some people could not believe that a country like Kenya, with its limited resources, had the human resources and the scientific ability for such a breakthrough. We may not have all the resources at our disposal but we have the courage and determination to direct all our energy and talent to a noble cause that serves to improve human life.
>
> (Foreign Broadcast Information Service 1990)

Moi's speech also framed Kemron as a "national" science project (as does the drug's name, of course). Although Moi didn't call Kemron a "cure", the phrase "anti-AIDS drug" certainly suggested that the drug was curative. As Koech predicted, colleagues used Moi's political interference as an excuse to dismiss the drug as simply a "political ploy", recounting that many Kenyan colleagues and opposition politicians immediately dismissed the claims as an attempt to divert attention from the political unrest.

On 1 April 1992, the National Institute of Allergy and Medicine (NIAID) in the United States published an executive summary that stated there was no evidence to support Koech's claims. NIAID found that although Koech had reported patients being cured of HIV (the disappearance of HIV antibodies, or what had been called "sero-deconversion") in three different reports, their review of evidence from other trials did not support this. The summary stated:

> Unfortunately, subsequent investigations from around the world have not reproduced these striking improvements. In a study involving 108 patients in Cameroon, Congo, Zimbabwe, Kenya and Ivory Coast in which Dr Koech participated, HIV antibodies did not disappear in any patients. In another study conducted in Zimbabwe, with 32 patients enrolled, there was only a non-significant and temporary increase in CD4+ count after four weeks of Kemron
>
> (National Institute of Allergy and Medicine 1992)

Though the World Health Organization (WHO) clinical trial in which Koech participated seemed to have had relatively positive results, it was dismissed based on a problem with clinical trials.

The summary notes that the discrepancy between trial results might have been related to the design of the clinical trial, including differences in dosage, drug formulation, and laboratory testing standards for CD4+ counts. It states:

> Whenever clinical studies are conducted using an open-label design without adequate controls, as in the case of the Koech study, it is difficult to interpret results since a number of factors other than the drug may be responsible for the results observed
>
> (Ibid.)

In the *Journal of the National Medical Association*, a review of three alpha interferon trials suggested that the positive results from the WHO trial were a matter

32 DAILY NATION, FRIDAY, JULY 27, 1990

KEMRON LAUNCHING SUPPLEMENT

US, Japan lend a han

Kemri has collaborated with two other institutions with experience in the field of interferons, in the development of Kemron.

This is in keeping with the universal nature of science.

These are the Amrillo Cell Culture Company in the United States and Hayashibara Biochemical Laboratories of Okayama, Japan.

The Amarillo Cell Culture Company (ACC) was founded about six years ago by Dr Joseph Cummins, a veterinary microbiologist.

ACC's interest lies in the development of oral interferon technology of which its founder Dr Cummins has done some pioneering work.

In this area of oral interferon technology, ACC owns several products related to the use of low dose oral interferon alpha for the treatment of human and animal diseases.

Significant results have been achieved in clinical trials using low dosage oral interferon-alpha therapy in the treatment of cancer and neuromuscular diseases.

Clinical trials have also shown encouraging results with some diseases afflicting dogs, cats, swines, horses and chicken.

The Hayashibara Biochemical Laboratories is a member of the Japanese Hayashibara Group, founded by the Hayashibara family in 1883.

The group is made up of 15 other companies.

Hayashibara Biochemical Laboratories main interest is in biotechnology and has several programmes studying the applications of biological substances in medicine and industry.

An area of special focus has been research into the function of bioactive substances secreted by human cells.

There has also been a drive towards mass production of biological substances, both for commercial and research purchases.

One remarkable result of the company's efforts has been the use of interferon in the development of anti-cancer and antiviral agents.

Dr Yasuichi Nagano, who heads one of the laboratories dealing with interferons at the company, was the first man to record the activity of interferons in 1954.

Mass production of interferons has been achieved using an original innovation which uses a special strain of hamsters.

According to this method, human cells innoculated into hamsters, multiply progressively as the hamsters grow.

This method has been four have an advantage over mass culture methods, i there is a high probability covering other useful bio substances from the in vivo liferated human cells.

About 600 different type human cells are preserved at Fujisaki Cell Centre bank wi the laboratories where resea ers throughout the world have cess to them.

Over 200 institutions wi and outside Japan have recei cells from the centre.

This is in keeping w Hayashibara's idea of establi ing an open research institu

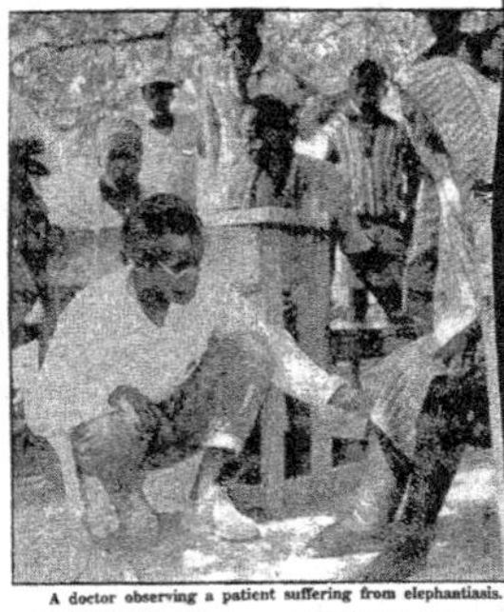

A doctor observing a patient suffering from elephantiasis.

KENYA AGRICULTURAL RESEARCH INSTITUTE (KARI)

The Chairman, Board Members and the entire Staff of
KENYA AGRICULTURAL RESEARCH INSTITUTE
congratulate
H.E. the President
Hon. Daniel T. arap Moi, C.G.H., M.P.,
the entire Government and the
KENYA MEDICAL RESEARCH INSTITUTE
(KEMRI)
on the official launching of the
anti-AIDS drug Kemron.
We take pride in this major medical break-through
in the fight against the dreaded AIDS.

NHIF ***National Hospital Insurance Fund***

Argwing's Kodhek Rd.
Hurlingham
P.O. Box 30443
Nairobi
Tel: 723255

The Directors, Management and
Staff of
NATIONAL HOSPITAL INSURANCE FUND
congratulate
E. the President, Hon. Daniel T. arap Moi, C.G.H., M.P.,
the entire Government and
especially the
KENYA MEDICAL RESEARCH INSTITUTE
on the occasion of the official launching of the
anti-AIDS drug
KEMRON

We mend KEMRI for the researching and development of Kemron
w. s a major contribution to medical research not only in Kenya,
but the entire world.

KNH BETTER HEALTH FOR ALL

KENYATTA NATIONAL HOSPITAL

The Chairman, members of the Board,
Management and Staff of
KENYATTA NATIONAL HOISPITAL
Wish to congratulate
His Exellency the President
Hon. Daniel T. arap Moi, C.G.H., M.P.,
Commander-In-Chief of the Armed Forces,
and
(KEMRI) Kenya Medical Research Institute
on the successful development and the launching of
KEMRON.

Figure 21.3 Kemron Launching Supplement, Daily Nation, 27 July 1990.

of interpretation that had been complicated by the "uncontrolled nature of the trial, the wide range of stages of clinical disease in patients, and the variable use of concomitant therapies, including antibiotics and antifungals" (Jordan 1994). In fact, the WHO results were differently interpreted as inconclusive, positive, and a clear indication of Kemron's ineffectiveness. For instance, an editorial written in the *East African Medical Journal* by then Director of Medical Services Joseph Oliech summarized the conclusions from the WHO report in this way: "The recently concluded WHO Collaborative Study has revealed that there is something immensely valuable in Kemron, irrespective of whatever the entire world thinks" (Oliech 1990).

Note

1 For an excellent account of Robert Ouko's murder and the subsequent failed investigation see Cohen and Odhiambo 2004.

22 Kinshasa and racial politics

Then soon after that the WHO got involved. There was a study that was sponsored by the WHO soon after that to be carried out at a few of the WHO centres in Central and West Africa, and coordinated from the WHO regional office in Brazzaville. HIV/AIDS was more prevalent in areas like the DRC and Congo and so they used some of their collaborating laboratories there. Our role was only to supply the medication. And I remembered when the meeting was being held in Geneva to review the data. One of the investigators in the meeting said, "I went through this, these are my results", and then we asked, "But how did you administer the product?" So he said, "As per protocol", but people in the audience said, "No, he didn't." Then one of the other investigators said, "No, the principle investigator did not advise the patients to allow the product to disintegrate and be absorbed in the mouth." On the contrary, the patients were advised to swallow the product with plenty of water! Because the moment you allow this product to disintegrate in the mouth, you must allow some time for the drug to be absorbed to trigger the signals because we believe then and now that this signalling effect was necessary to effect change. Yes, that is why you require such a little amount of product to create that signal which will then create the subsequent cascade of events, including about 30 different types of events that take place shortly after that.

Yes, so this other investigator, and I don't know who advised him, advised the patients that you must swallow plenty of water with this product. But it was one of the junior officers who was at the meeting who raised his hand and said, "No, that is not what happened. We informed patients that this product must be swallowed, it should not stay in the mouth even for a minute, you swallow it with plenty of water." In such a case, even if you take 100 tablets, it won't do anything. I didn't want to blame anyone but I tend to believe that there was some motive because we had given the protocol to the WHO and they were to go and supervise the investigations in three centres. And they were saying: "We had been advised that this product must be swallowed, it's not crushed in the mouth and you must take plenty of water." Yet the protocol and the administration of the product were so clear – you allow the drug to dissolve in the mouth for a particular period of time and then swallow it using saliva; you can only swallow after about five minutes or something like that. And then you cannot take water

Chinese researchers told to fend for themselves

Beijing. China wants two-thirds of the scientists it now funds to find other sources of support as part of the movement towards a free-enterprise system. But many of the 80,000 researchers at hundreds of government-funded institutes believe that the policy fails to account for the varying appeal to industry of some of their work.

They are concerned that the new policy, if not modified, will mean that researchers in some fields will be forced to abandon their profession. While researchers at the Changchun Institute of Applied Chemistry within the Chinese Academy of Sciences, for example, can be expected to fend for themselves, those at the Geosciences Institute and the Desert Research Institute will have a much harder time of it.

The new philosophy was spelled out in late August by the State Science and Technology Commission. Its goal is to give China a modern research and development network that is well-balanced, efficient and vigorous. Its elements include diversifying talent, stabilizing basic research, increasing the number of high-technology projects, creating high-technology enterprises and preserving existing strengths in basic and applied research.

China's policy-makers believe that new initiatives such as the Climbing programme (see *Nature* **359**, 177; 1992) and the 863 high-technology programme are sufficient to keep China at the forefront of global science. Zhou Guang-Zhao, president of the Chinese Academy of Sciences, is fond of saying that these efforts will allow China "to win gold medals in the world science olympics".

But Zhou's optimism is not shared by most working scientists, who can be overheard at conferences talking about opening restaurants and running shops after state funding is cut off. In an effort to remain viable, the National Geology Library of China has rented out half of its building to a local company, for a fee of 2 million yuan (US$350,000). Unfortunately, the loss of such an important resource can only hurt those left to practise science.

It is not clear whether the new policy is part of a long-term strategy or merely a short-term expedient to withstand the current worldwide recession. Although the government has promised to increase significantly the salaries of those who retain funding, many researchers say that the policy raises questions about the government's commitment to science at any price.

You Qin Li

Japanese increase spending on universities

Tokyo. One per cent of a supplementary budget approved last week by the Japanese cabinet to boost the faltering Japanese economy will be spent on buildings and facilities at government research organizations.

A senior official of Tokyo University, Japan's leading national university, says the supplementary budget is "wonderful news" but that no spending decisions have been made. The universities received a similar windfall in 1987, at the time of the last major supplementary budget, and much of the money was invested in supercomputers and new buildings. The new allocation is for the fiscal year that ends on 31 March 1993.

The biggest beneficiary of science's ¥113 billion (nearly US$1 billion) share of a one-time ¥10,700 billion supplementary budget is the Ministry of Education, Science and Culture, which will get an extra ¥82.5 billion for the national universities, university-related research institutes, private universities, technical colleges and museums. This is separate from ¥20 billion a year for the next five years already set aside in the ministry's budget to rebuild national universities (*Nature* **355**, 99; 1992) with money derived from selling land owned by them.

The Science and Technology Agency (STA) gets an extra ¥17.8 billion, of which ¥5 billion is for buildings and facilities, including ¥1.5 billion for imported scientific equipment. The remaining money will go to several projects, including the world's most powerful synchrotron, Spring-8, being built in Harima science park, installing seismographs 2,000–3,000 metres underground for earthquake prediction, the Japanese contribution to the US space station and STA's marine and radiological research institutes.

The Agency of Industrial Science and Technology, the main research arm of the Ministry of International Trade and Industry, plans to spend its ¥12.7 billion to shorten by one year construction of two institutes in Tsukuba science city that are part of a reorganization of four of the agency's institutes there (*Nature* **351**, 90; 1991). The two institutes — for materials science and life science — had been expected to be completed in fiscal year 1994. Some of the new money will be used for laboratory equipment and cooling systems that do not contain chlorofluorocarbons. **David Swinbanks**

NIH plans trials of controversial AIDS drug

Washington. Bowing to pressure from African-American activist groups, the US National Institutes of Health (NIH) last week agreed to go ahead with government-sponsored clinical trials of oral interferon alpha in AIDS patients.

The government has been accused of ignoring or suppressing evidence that the drug, which goes under the names Kemron, Immunex or Immuviron, is effective in treating AIDS symptoms (see *Nature* **359**, 661; 1992). It has become a cause celèbre for African-American groups, led by the Nation of Islam, after some early uncontrolled clinical trials in Kenya generated reports of dramatic but subsequently unconfirmed results, including serodeconversion.

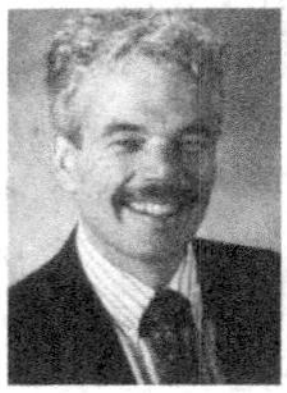

Jack Killen

NIH officials met researchers and African-American doctors who have been working with the drug and announced afterwards that the evidence — both scientific and anecdotal — justified taking interferon alpha to full clinical trial. The next step, according to Jack Killen of the National Institute of Allergy and Infectious Diseases, is a plan to conduct the trials, to be developed in the next few months with help from an advisory panel. Current thinking is for a minimum of three sites at a cost of several million dollars. Barbara Justice and Abdul Alim Muhammad, two doctors affiliated with the Nation of Islam who have been prescribing interferon alpha to their AIDS patients for the last year, are expected to be members of the panel.

Despite NIH's approval, the issue remains controversial. Much of last week's closed meeting, according to participants, was focused not on data but on accusations of "genocide" and racism, some levelled at NIH officials.

NIH based its decision to proceed on data provided by Wilbert Jordon of King-Drew Medical Center in Los Angeles. Jordon reported that, in head-to-head trials of four groups taking AZT, low-dose Kemron, a placebo, or a combination of AZT and Kemron, only the Kemron-only group showed improved CD4 counts after one year. Although the data need further examination, they offer NIH enough evidence to justify taking the next step and relieving, for the moment, the political pressure on the agency. **Christopher Anderson**

Figure 22.1 NIH and Kemron.

by mouth for about 30 minutes. So in our meeting we looked at each other said, "What is going on here?"

We raised that question and then one of the WHO representatives said that is what they were told. By who, we asked? The protocol is there. Maybe there were errors when they translated the English language protocol to French. So, anyway that was one study that we were not responsible for. I felt extremely disappointed about this. It was a WHO officer, and I can't remember the name but I think Jonathan Mann was the programme Director at WHO at that time. He was in charge of the global AIDS program there.

And actually he died on a plane crash, yes, the famous crash of Flight 800, so he was a good friend of mine. But he was not the scientific investigator representing this for the WHO; that was a different person. The administration of the product in any kind of treatment is so critical, more critical than anything else. How do you administer the product? What time do you want to eat? Can you consume food after you take it? Should it be taken with water? These are critical questions in a clinical trial where you are investigating the method of administration. But the WHO did not consider these issues in its follow-up trial.

And then other events took place. Now at home it was almost the same story. So come 1991, 1992 we tried to do the drug distribution as per the guidelines of the Kenyan Ministry of Health and as authorized by our Pharmacy and Poisons Board. Meanwhile, some studies continued but we started being on the defensive because there was one accusation after another. We had battles coming our way, one after the other. They were making derogative remarks, yes, so many derogative remarks. In one particular meeting, outside the country, at the Kinshasa meeting, there was a delegation from the US, I don't know from which department. They asked a few questions as I was doing the presentation and then they tried to make some negative comments and the whole crowd booed them until they had to leave.

Yes, the Americans had to leave the room. Yes, they had no choice … actually it became very chaotic because the rest of the conference participants were listening very keenly, you see. I think I got annoyed at one point during the presentation … yes, I think I said "What are you talking about? I beat you in class!" (Koech laughs). Yes, I mentioned that. I thought no, this is just not right, this is just not right. It's a personal attack on myself, on my person. And then the crowd actually hailed me; yes, they clapped and clapped. And that was the end of the meeting.

My Kenyan colleagues had a change of heart. Some of them had doubted us before, but we had gone there together, and then they had a change of heart. We Africans came out of Kinshasa more united. And then we said, "Now we know what we have been fighting for." It is going to take some time for our work to be recognized, especially if it does not involve the Americans. Yes, you know in global science, you must have some level of affiliation so that you will be recognized. I said, "No, why is this?" And I have decided since that I am not going to include any of those persons in what I'm doing now. They are not going to come in as equals … they will come in as my subordinates for once. Because there is nothing that they can claim to know more about than I do. Let them donate new equipment. Fine, but if it is new equipment, it will take me about three minutes to know how to use it, so they will not be teaching me about the use of that equipment because they are not the ones who did it anyway, they are not the manufacturer, they are not the engineers who developed it, somebody else did.

Then these things continued for some time until one day when there was a problem between Joe Cummins and one of his colleagues. They had some differences. When they had some differences, this other person left the scene. He was not a scientist, I think he was in marketing or something like that. Shortly after 1997, because if you see in the patent protection, it was initially for seven years, and we were now due to renew it, about 1996, 1997. For me, I said I've been fighting over this thing for a long time, the government has not been supporting me, I have used my own personal resources, we have used our own funding, the government never provided us even one cent, and what is this that am fighting for? At that time I had been beaten so hard so that I had no opportunity to even get any reward for investing in it. My main intention was for this product to be available to the patients. So I declined to renew the patent because you must also pay some money and no one assisted me. So I said, just make it open. That is the time that it was being manufactured by another company, under the name of Immunoplex. I said, if there is anyone else who is willing to move on developing it, they can go ahead. So essentially it means that I was not interested in renewing the patent protection. I spent my money even paying for the fees and so on to have this product protected in some of the designated states because when you are protecting it you must list other countries where you also wanted it protected. I said, I said am not going to stand in the way of the progress of this drug.

In May 2003, during the administration of President Kibaki, I was part of the government's delegation to the World Health Assembly in Geneva, led by Charity Ngilu. While there, we were invited for lunch and the Minister for Health, Charity Ngilu, had accepted and told us that there were some people who wanted to share some important medical findings. So we went for lunch at a very nice restaurant in Geneva. We were about seven, nine, maybe ten people. It was the minister and then our Director of Medical Services, then Richard Muga, plus other top officials from the Ministry of Health and myself. Of course, there were also some invited persons from our Embassy in Geneva. So we were together for lunch plus the person who had invited us. After we dined, this person now started addressing the minister, saying, "Madam Minister, we have a product that I want to introduce." This fellow lived in Switzerland. I don't know if it was Geneva or another town but he said, "We have a product and it is very good. It has been registered in 19 African countries for alleviating the symptoms related to HIV and so this is a beautiful product."

So we listened to this presentation and kept quiet and then this fellow produced a booklet that he shared with the minister and the Director of Medical Services. I was seated directly opposite the minister at the far end of the table. I was not close to her. So the minister looked at me and said, "Davy, why are you quiet?" I said, "Please, let me look at that document." So the minister was excited. So she passed over the document to me. I just opened it. So for some minutes I looked at it. I remember I opened to page 101 in the document and then I showed the minister – it read: Koech, Koech, Kemron, Kemron. So after that, the minister said to our host, "Thank you so much. You will hear from us in the next three weeks." Do you know the meeting ended and then from there.... You know this woman can get so hyper. She can get so emotional about certain things. She hits the roof. Something like, "Davy is this Kemron?!" I said, "Yes." So we learned this was a product that had been manufactured and was being distributed by a company in South Africa. She said, "Give me your phone!" You see mobile phones were still not so common at that time. She had just joined the government so she didn't even have a mobile phone with roaming abilities yet. Yes. So she called the State House in Nairobi. She says, "Your Excellency, we have been punishing Koech for nothing and this product, it has been taken over by other people!" So the President asked if we had any course for legal redress. So we went to the Ambassador, Amina Mohammed, who is now our current Cabinet secretary for foreign affairs, and this lady said, "No. No. We cannot allow this thing to go. Let's go take some legal action."

I looked at her and I said,

> Madam *waziri* [minister]. Madam Minister. When the Kenya government decided not to assist me, and made accusations that it was a Moi project even though it had nothing to do with President Moi, when it was due for me to renew the patent I declined because no one would even pay for the patenting fees for protection in various states.

So Ambassador Amina Mohammed asked me, "Is there anything we can do? Are you in a position that we can now return it?" I said, "No, sorry, it is too late. It is going to be active somewhere else. Just let them have it because I tried to talk to you, you did not want to hear. You said it was a ploy." Some of my colleagues were saying it was just chalk powder from the industrial area. I don't want to be associated with that sort of thing. From there Minister Ngilu got annoyed and she kept on talking. We even had a meeting at the Kenya High Commission residence in the evening and she was very focused on this. We had another Kenyan delegation which had gone to Geneva, the ILO, the International Labor Organization, they had their own meeting also in Geneva and even then, she kept on singing and when she says something she wants to sing about it. She is like CNN! They want to repeat the same story, over and over. Yes, but from there we developed a very close relation. This is the same minister who was with me and then she told me that she was being sacked in 2007. And then she was sacked and then I was left with my problems.

The Nation of Islam very strangely came into the picture when there were racial politics associated with it. The Nation of Islam in the US was saying here we have a good product that is coming out of Africa but the Western world is discrediting it because it is from Africa. I never met with the Minister for Health for the Nation of Islam but some young doctor, John, came to meet with me.

LIFESTYLE 6 PEOPLE The Sunday Nation, March 29, 1998

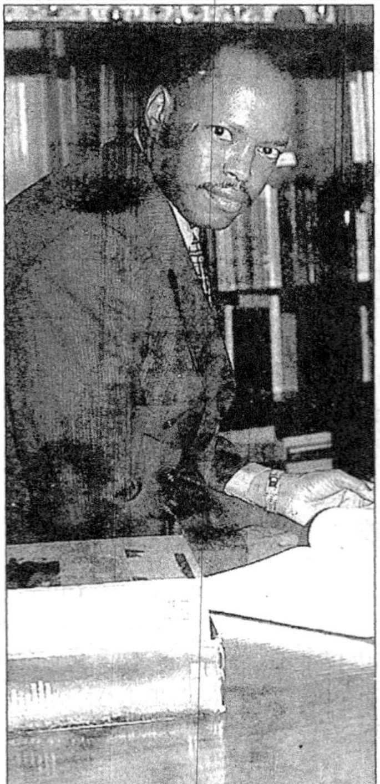

Dr Koech at his Kemri office: "The pessimism and controversy that accompanied the launch of Kemron did not intimidate me. I want my critics to know one day I shall walk up to them and say; I told you!" – *Picture by PETER KARURI.*

Davy Koech: A

By KIPKOECH TANUI

With the ease and precision learned in three decades spent in research laboratories, he squeezed a drop of human blood from a small syringe on to a transparent plastic slide, poured a few drops of staining chemical and studied the cocktail under a powerful electronic microscope.

Dressed in a doctor's coat complete with gloves and a nose cap, Dr Davy Kiprotich Koech — a founder member, chief research officer and director of Kenya Medical Research Institute (KEMRI) — then motions a group of visiting researchers in tropical diseases to move closer and get a view of the virus his prying eye has been able to isolate.

The labs at the headquarters of the state-owned organisation smack of the clinical sterility medical students are taught to uphold in their stations.

Every working day, Dr Koech visits the ultra-modern laboratories of the 19-year-old institution he helped found to further his career as one of Africa's leading researchers.

Born in 1951 and educated at Kericho High School and Strathmore College, Nairobi, Dr Koech's name is today one of the most conspicuous on the lists of Africa's foremost researchers. Apart from publishing 230 peer reviewed scientific papers, he has also spearheaded several breakthroughs in health research.

The Fulbright-Hays scholar and first African scientist at Kemri says he was propelled to this field by a burning desire to get to the bottom of degenerative diseases that depress the body's immune system such as Aids, bilharzia and leishmaniasis (kala-azar).

Dr Koech is a busy man. Apart from his administrative and research work at Kemri, he is the chairman of the Commission for Higher Education and the vice-chairman of Jomo Kenyatta University of Agriculture and Technology's governing council.

"Every year, I sign off at least three or four PhDs and several Masters degrees at University of Nairobi and Kenyatta University's Faculty of Science," he says.

In between the three tasks, he somehow finds time to supervise masters and PhD students at the University of Nairobi's School of Medicine, where he was a student in the early 1970s, and Kenyatta University's Faculty of Science.

A graduate of University of Nairobi and the prestigious Harvard University in the US, Dr Koech is also the editor-in-chief of *African Journal of Medical Sciences* and is the president of the African Forum for Health Sciences. He is also an external examiner at Moi University.

A 1980 recipient of a PhD degree in medical pathology specialising in immunology, Dr Koech holds two Presidential awards and several international honours in medical research.

The man whose name dominated the headlines in 1990 as one of the two pioneers of Kemron, which was then believed to be the world's first Aids cure, says he has perfected the controversial drug and will launch its improved version before the end of the year.

The drug is in use at medical outlets, and remarkable progress has been noted in its role in suppressing the speed with which the killer virus shatters the body's immune system, he says.

In 1985, he pioneered research in perfecting the human leukocyte antigen tissue-typing technique in kidney transplant in Kenya. The technique led to the first living donor-related kidney transplant in the country. Since then, renal transplants are routinely undertaken.

Three years earlier, he had participated in the development of an insulin formulation for use in clinical management of diabetes.

"The pessimism and controversy that accompanied the launch of Kemron did not intimidate me; instead, it gave me courage to do more. I want my critics to know one day I shall walk up to them and say; I told you!".

"The drug (Kemron) is no longer being criticised. It is now being investigated. This is a low-dosed formulation of interferon alpha, it was not new as such. We only pioneered a new dosage and route of administration."

People think Kemri, Kemron and Dr Koech are synonymous. "This is a fallacy; Kemron and Aids form only 10 per cent of our work," he says.

"We must have faith in our own people. We should not be quick to condemn them. Researchers require the goodwill of their peers and the nation to accomplish what they set out to do. We should not treat our researchers as if they are incapable of achieving any-

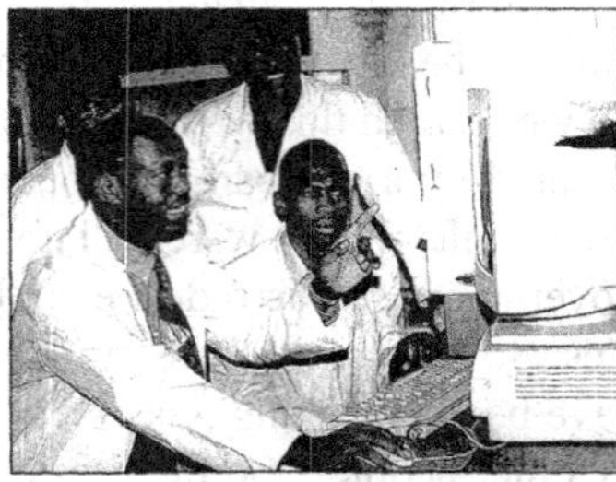

Team worker: Dr Koech with colleagues at the Kemri laboratories.

'If politicians could listen to what we say, the problems facing our countries would be minimised'

What's in a name? For Chinese, everything

Beijing: If your relationship is on the rocks, your career going nowhere and your health in decline, the solution in China is simple: Change your name.

Jin Taochun, 65, takes the idea of transforming bad luck into good through a new name seriously. For the past six years, working out of a tiny office in an old Beijing alleyway, he has been advising clients about the most propitious names for a successful life.

"I came alone last year for the sake of my husband, who despite two operations still had kidney stones," said telecommunications worker Bai Xiunan, 35.

"Jin chose a new name for him which I engraved on a seal. I put it in a pocket of his jacket before his third operation and it was a success," she said with a broad grin.

"It wasn't until afterward that I told him about the seal. He told me he didn't believe in this kind of superstition, but he still carries it around."

Jin says it is not necessary to change one's name on official documents or [illegible] friends, but the mere fact of carry[illegible] new name around engraved on a [illegible]ch or a piece of jewellery can ward off malign influences.

Bai Xiunan was so enthusiastic about the process that she convinced her sister to bring along her six-year-old son, called Yong (brave).

"When was he born, where and at what time?" asks Jin.

"After working out the child's Chinese star sign, as well as his chart based on the ancient Taoist philosophy of yin and yang, Jin calculates the number of strokes the characters OF the boy's name should have.

"He must be called Yufeng, because the words Yu (feather) and Feng (mount) make a good combination," he says.

The consultation lasts no more than five minutes, and the client leaves with her heart filled with hope and her purse lighter by 66 yuan (Sh500).

With 30 to 40 clients a day, six days a week, the business is profitable. But Jin shuns ostentation, and dresses humbly in an old Chairman Mao suit and tennis shoes that have seen better days.

Jin, who claims direct descendance from an 17th-century emperor of the Qing dynasty, does not wish to be seen as a geomancer or a miracle worker.

"My job is half way between science and superstition," he says. "When somebody comes to me with an illness, I scrupulously advise them to also see a doctor."

His grimy office, furnished meagrely with a battered sofa and four wooden benches, welcomes rich and poor alike.

"Many of my clients come to ask advice for the name of a shop or company and some return to say their affairs have prospered," he says. For business clients the price of a consultation goes up to 200 yuan (Sh1,500).

"I also have among my clientele several stars of film, dance and music who want a good artist's name," he adds.

The parents of a boy with heart problems wait patiently for their turn.

"I want my son to have a good first name which will protect him in life," says the boy's father, a teacher.

"I don't see this as superstition. It's above all about giving a moral support, because with couples only allowed to one child, you can't take any chances." – *AFP*

Police trouble for man who castrated himself

A man who apparently castrated himself will be charged with filing a false police report after giving officials three different versions of the event, Bossier City police said.

Ronald Elmore was dropped off at the Bossier Medical Centre emergency room early by an unidentified woman after both his testicles had been cut off, police said.

He first told officers an unknown woman he picked up in a bar castrated him while he was sleeping and he did not realise it until he woke up, police said.

Then he said he and his wife had been taking drugs and when he was unable to perform sexually, he told her to castrate him, which she did, police said. They quoted him as saying they [illegible] put his testicles down a garbage disposal.

The third time Elmore was interviewed, police said, he told them he had castrated himself and put his testicles in a freezer, where police found them.

***

Canada's "Senator Siesta," famous for long bouts of absenteeism in Mexico, has resigned six weeks after he was unceremoniously suspended from the unelected upper house of the Canadian Parliament.

The Senate had stripped Senator Andrew Thompson of his C$64,400 annual salary in February because he had appeared only a handful of times since it began taking attendance in 1990.

But by resigning, Thompson will now be able to collect a C$48,000 annual pension, two years earlier than if he had waited until the mandatory retirement age of 75.

Thompson, 73, had said his chronic absenteeism was due to poor health, though Canadian photographers stalking his residence at La Paz, Mexico, saw a well-tanned man running errands with no apparent difficulty.

Figure 22.2 Davy Koech, The Sunday Nation, 29 March 1998.

He was an MD, PhD and JD. Extremely knowledgeable. He was an extremely smart kid, so he came to meet with me and he was the personal assistant to Louis Farrakhan. Yes, we were together at KEMRI for very close to three weeks. He wrote a story in the Nation of Islam newspaper and then he sent it to me. In fact, I still have a copy. I will go and look for it because you may like it. So that was the period when I had a connection with the Nation of Islam but I never got in touch with them, officially or otherwise. He wanted to know a lot of information about the drug. He was interested in understanding how they could manage to say both that it is a product that they believe in and thus would need to make orders for that product to go to the US.

It didn't surprise me a great deal because I have studied and worked in the US so these issues of race relations were not new to me. Although when I was in the US I never knew that there was the Nation of Islam. I was very busy doing my work so I was not too much involved in American politics and inter-racial politics. Yes. However, it did not surprise me. I said most likely this is an opportunity for them to vent their feelings. I was not too worried because I knew what was going on and because from the beginning AIDS was entangled in these politics of race. They said AIDS was from a particular community, a group of persons, and each time they were talking about it they were shifting their arguments towards persons of colour in the US and globally.

So, as you see, as soon as we produced Kemron it became more of a political story than a scientific story. I look back now and I wonder how I could have handled this differently. But it was difficult to separate politics from science at that time because Kenyan politicians wanted to cash in on a new technology. They wanted to divert the attention from politics of the day and the public demonstrations and so on, and that is why President Moi had to come and launch the product. I had no idea and I told you the story. I had no idea myself that this would happen. They just lie like they did with the Nyayo car. There was a prototype of vehicles that was actually displayed with a very big launch and fan fair and so on: Nyayo 1 and Nyayo 2. Two types of models which Moi also launched.

I was just a simple scientist trying to do my job to the best of my ability. It so happens that somebody was trying to take advantage of my efforts, of our scientific efforts, and so it became a little confused and then from there it took on a life of its own.

Intermission

Following the politicized launch, Koech presented the preliminary clinical trial results at the AIDS in Africa Conference in Kinshasa in October 1990. Although Koech had presented on Kemron in Kenya a few times already, and had published the results, the Kinshasa conference presentation seemed to be the start of the controversy both in Africa and internationally, fed in part by news sources like *Jeune Afrique* which reported, "The greatest controversy at the conference was produced by the 'miracle' drug Kemron developed in Kenya" (Poissonnier 1990).

The Canadian scientist Allan Ronald, now retired, who had been working in Kenya in the 1980s and 1990s and who had attended the conference, recalled that the entire meeting was tense from the moment he and his colleagues stepped off the plane. Kinshasa itself was in a state of transition. It had only been in May of 1990 that President Mobutu had agreed to a multiparty democratic election after widespread opposition in the country. Ronald recalled that there was a concern with security when they arrived at the Kinshasa airport, in part because all the conference participants had been greeted by the local police when they departed the plane and forced to pay US$100 before being allowed to leave. Ronald also recalled that later the police forced conference participants Charlie Gilks and Richard Brindle to give them all their belongings and money. The conference was described as chaotic, and there was a sense of anxiety and tension.

Ronald also recalled that in spite of the concerns about security and political instability in Kinshasa, there was a general "celebratory" sense at the conference. Koech had incredible support. Mark Tyndall, an infectious disease specialist who was part of the Canadian contingent from the University of Manitoba, shared his memories of the moment Koech appeared on stage:

> The African AIDS meeting was held in Kinshasa in the fall of 1990 – I had only arrived in Nairobi in January 1990. There was a pretty big group from Kenya that included a lot of the Kenyan research staff. I hung out mainly with Frank Plummer. There was also this crazy guy from the UK who worked in Uganda – Wilson Carswell. He was a well-known researcher who I met there, and I was sitting with him during the Kemron presentation. The session was chaired by James Curran who was the Director of the HIV/AIDS division at the CDC at the time. PowerPoint was really not around so people used 35 mm slides and most of the presentations were pretty basic. Then Koech comes up on stage with music playing in the background. He was met with a large applause.[1]

Tyndall continued, and reflected critically on Koech's presentation:

> His first slide was Kemron in the same coloring and shape as the ESSO logo. He then presented a series of slides that were said to be a clinical trial. I think that there were about one hundred in the Kemron group and one hundred in the placebo group. Each slide had these columns comparing the two arms of the study. I do remember a slide with all these symptoms listed (cough, diarrhea, headache, fever, etc.) which were all around 100 percent before Kemron and miraculously were all 0 percent following treatment – I think about six weeks of treatment but at the least it was a relatively short course and then it was stopped. There were no effects in the placebo group. It was laughable, but no one was laughing – except Carswell. At the end of the presentation there was a standing ovation for Koech. The first question was by Curran; he said something like, "Well, Dr Koech, if even half of

what you are saying is true you have saved the world from this horrible epidemic." He shouldn't have said that. Immediately there were "boos" from the audience and someone quickly stood up and asked Curran why he didn't think that African scientists could invent such a treatment.

This was a crucial moment in the politicization of Kemron, one that was recounted by other conference participants (including Plummer, Ronald, and Curran) to me. Koech had overwhelming support from a largely African audience and the meeting atmosphere was very congratulatory toward Koech. Some of the conference participants suggested that prior to the conference many Kenyan scientists working in HIV in Nairobi had also voiced scepticism and serious concerns about the clinical trial, but there in Kinshasa the Africans seemed united in their support of Koech. The conference presentation, Ronald recalled, split the audience – Africans against non-Africans – because it was being portrayed as a drug that had been developed by Africans in Africa. Koech explained that earlier tensions in Kenya among African scientists who were suspicious or dismissive of Kemron because of its connection to Moi disappeared in Kinshasa. The conference unified the African scientists politically as they saw themselves marginalized by the international scientific community (even as they worked side-by-side with them in Nairobi).

The Kemron story travelled internationally and, as Dan Royles has explained elsewhere, some African American communities in the United States, including the African American press, took an interest and framed Kemron similarly as an achievement for African science (Royles 2012). An article in the *New York Times* by Bruce Lambert (1990: 42) reported:

> Many of the blacks involved in the debate suggest that white dominated Western news organizations and researchers are playing Kemron [*sic*] down because it poses competition for expensive AIDS medications and because of racially based distrust of African science. "If this had come out of Sweden or somewhere else, it would have been page one everywhere," said Wilbert A. Tatum, the editor in chief of The Amsterdam News. His paper suggested that results had not received a great deal of attention because of a belief that blacks "could not possibly have come up with an effective therapy or cure for AIDS that has eluded white scientists and researchers for the last decade in spite of the billions of dollars poured into research".

A Nation of Islam media source *incorrectly* announced that Koech had met with the Nation of Islam Minister for Health Dr Abdul Alim Muhammad to talk about access to alpha interferon treatment for AIDS (see Muhammad 2002). Muhammad was also the Medical Director of the Abundant Life Clinic in Washington, DC and the national spokesman for Nation of Islam leader Minister Louis Farrakhan. Muhammad was interviewed by the *New Federalist* where he made it clear that he saw the dismissal of Kemron as the result of state interference that continued to deny African Americans treatment.[2] He said,

Dmk

WORLD HEALTH ORGANIZATION ORGANISATION MONDIALE DE LA SANTE

5571095.0302.006

GLOBAL PROGRAMME ON AIDS

WHO sponsored study finds no evidence for KEMRON claims

A WHO sponsored study has concluded that treatment with low dose human interferon alpha (Kemron), does not produce any detectable benefits in symptomatic HIV infection.

The study carried out at the medical school of Makerere University in Kampala, Uganda involved 560 HIV infected people with symptoms of HIV-related disease and CD4 cell counts of less than 300. The patients were divided into two groups of 280. The groups were compatible in age, sex, clinical symptoms, WHO clinical stage of HIV infection, Karnosfsky score, haemoglobin and biochemistry results. One group was given low-dose oral interferon alpha (150 international units per day) while the control group received a placebo. The study lasted 60 weeks.

The researchers found, during and after treatment, that the following parameters were similar in both the treatment and placebo group:

- mortality,
- progression of HIV disease,
- Karnofsky scores (which measure individuals' ability to look after themselves),
- symptom scores,
- body weight and,
- CD4 lymphocyte counts,

None of the patients reverted from being HIV positive to HIV negative.

The study was commissioned by the WHO to follow up on results from a much smaller study three years ago by the Kenyan Medical Research Institute (KEMRI), which suggested that alpha interferon taken orally in very low doses alleviated the symptoms of AIDS.

In the KEMRI study 199 symptomatic and 5 asymptomatic patients were given the drug in wafer form to allow the patient to absorb the drug through the mouth. Treatment was for at least ten weeks. The study did not include a control group.

The KEMRI study reported that within days of taking the oral alpha interferon, AIDS patients' symptoms were reduced; and that within eight to ten weeks, symptoms in all patients were alleviated. The study said eighteen of the patients who had previously tested HIV positive reverted to HIV-seronegativity (tested HIV negative) as a result of the treatment. None of these findings were borne out by the WHO study.

Following the Uganda study, the WHO has concluded that treatment with low dose oral interferon alpha does not benefit HIV infected people. There is no evidence that the drug can eliminate HIV from the body of an infected person.

PRESS CONFERENCE ROOM 6 18³⁰ - 19³⁰

Figure 22.3 NIH plans trials of controversial AIDS Drug, Nature, 5 November 1992.

> In the summer of 1992, when we were able to present our research in the area of alpha interferon to the National Medical Association meeting in San Francisco, and the House of Delegates of the NMA passed a resolution of clinical trials of alpha interferon, we were informed some time later that the National Institutes of Health demanded and got the mailing list of the NMA, and letters were sent to each and every member of the NMA telling them that alpha interferon didn't work and that was not the way to go.[3]

The African American press, African American physicians, and African American patients similarly understood the dismissal of Kemron as a matter of racial politics. The *Capital Spotlight*, published out of Washington, DC, reported: "Black health officials contend that white-dominated news organizations did not publicize the drug because of a racially based distrust of African science."[4] The Nation of Islam, in cooperation with the NMA, demanded that the National Institutes of Health (NIH) seriously consider Kemron and undertake further clinical trials and reviews. They forced the NIH to reconsider its position, and in 1992, the NIH held a meeting agreeing to review the studies on oral interferon alpha.

In 1998, Koech was reported as saying, "The pessimism and controversy that accompanied the launch of Kemron did not intimidate me. I want my critics to know one day I shall walk up to them and say, 'I told you so!'"

Notes

1 Scottish physician portrayed in *The Last King of Scotland* who becomes Idi Aman's doctor.
2 Available online, www.larouchepub.com/eiw/public/1994/eirv21n14-19940401/eirv21n14-19940401_061-dr_abdul_alim_muhammad.pdf
3 NMA was an association of African American doctors.
4 As Karen Booth (2004) notes, even African Americans living in the United States travelled to Kenya for access to the drug for which they paid exorbitant prices.

23 A son's death

So I was there with the Japanese and then one Tuesday evening I received a phone call. This was on 15 January 2002. I received a phone call from my son Kiprop, the second born, and he said, "Daddy, Chang' (Chang'-Toek) has fallen ill. He has been taken to the hospital and he is in the ICU." I said, "What?" And then what immediately rang in my mind, because he was a pilot, I thought he must have crash-landed. He must have had a crash. I asked him, "How did he fall from the plane?" or something like this and my son Kiprop said, "No father." You see, Chang'-Toek and Kiprop were staying together in the US. So I started saying okay which particular hospital has he been taken to? He gave me the contacts and so forth. I just finished talking with the Japanese asking about KEMRI and our work together so in the morning I went to the office. I was not feeling very well. I was feeling very sad but I did the work as usual until evening because I thought he would recover.

Chang' was 26. Yes. I thought to myself, he will be fine. He was in one of the best hospitals in the US. Yes. He was in Fort Lauderdale, Florida. He was a professional pilot and graduate of Embry–Riddle Aeronautical University. So I had meetings the whole day at KEMRI, feeling very bad, yes, feeling very bad. In the evening I rushed back to the house so that I could call the hospital for an update. You see at that time the mobile systems were not efficient. We had not reached the age of mobile phones like today. The mobile system was working but it was not a common affair at that particular time. As I was driving home from the office on the 16th I received a phone call from my house, from my son Yatich. So my son told me, "You know what daddy? I am sorry but the doctors have communicated to us that Chang' is dead." The way the hospital communicated my son's death was so cruel, to say the least, and this was devastating.

What? Just like that. So what I did was I turned the car around. Mama (his wife) was not in the house. She was somewhere in Nairobi and then I called her and I said, "Just come to the house." So she came and then I had to tell her. This saddening aspect is that I tried to call the hospital and when I finally got in touch with the hospital they asked me, "Please let us know where we are going to keep the body." That is the only communication I heard from them! I felt very bad. So I got in touch with my American friend called Stephen Herman. I got in touch with him because he was in Florida. I had been with the boys there and I had

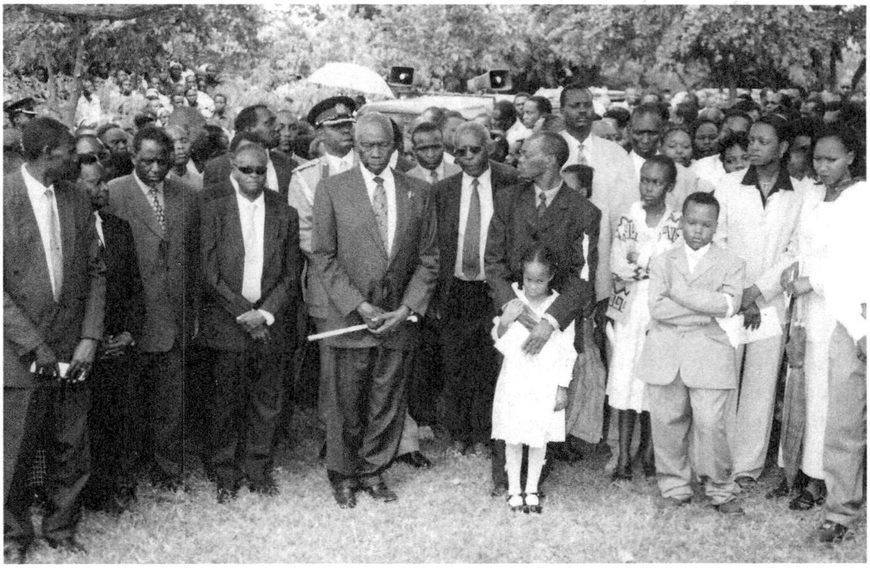

Figure 23.1 Moi and Koech (among others) at the burial of Chang'-Toek, 2002, Nairobi.

taken them to his house so they knew him. I called him and I told him what had happened. He said, "Relax. Leave the rest to me. I can do this and so forth." So I said there is nothing I can do. I could not change anything then and he was there in Florida to assist my son and to process all the necessary papers and that is precisely what he did. Yes.

And I had just been there visiting. You see a couple of months before I was there because I went to visit some institution in Oklahoma and then I went to Texas and stayed in Dallas with some friends of mine. And then I travelled to Fort Lauderdale to visit my sons. You think these things only happen in some movies or something like that. You can't believe that it can happen in real life. I couldn't see it. No, these things you cannot imagine. I am still mourning Chang's death.

24 Collaborative agreements and fiscal irregularities

What happens politically among major powers and the relations between countries affects what goes on in Kenya to some degree. When there was a change in funding in the US, a withdrawal of support, for programs like PEPFAR (President's Emergency Fund for AIDS Relief) and a few other things it affected us. In Kenya, when the US scaled down the activities, it not only affected the CDC but the Walter Reed Project as well. When international bodies change particular policies, it affects us. One clear example, we were not able to put in a military hospital because of the change of politics under Margaret Thatcher and (Ronald) Reagan, as a result of the collapse of the Soviet Union. You see, when it collapsed we lost funding. What was good for the international community was bad for somebody else, us. So what is happening internationally really affects Kenya, including our science and our ability to conduct medical research. Even during the period of structural adjustment programs, which was at the beginning of the 1990s, it affected us because they stopped further employment of staff by various government organizations, including at KEMRI.

Because we were a public institution, we were asked to reduce staff strength by around 10 per cent in response to the International Monetary Fund's (IMF) demands. But I managed to comply without terminating any staff. I made people who were supposed to retire go home. That is how I managed to do it through natural attrition and so we did not lay off any staff members. We were very serious about who to employ and who not to employ and so we didn't have any staff to retrench. Yes. Political happenings and the relationship between nation states also affect us. Like during the early years when there was a really bad relationship between Nairobi and Washington, it affected KEMRI. That was in the early 1990s.

Relations between countries are challenging but it has been my job to negotiate these relations.

You see I am trying to see the full sum of the effects, which *are* positive. I think I have criticized the CDC and I have given them their fair share through all these things when I talk about their lack of coordination, lack of responsibility, or poking their noses into practically everything that goes on, the policy relationships. They will refuse to give us aid money, but then follow up by demanding that we administer their funds, and then tell us we cannot administer it. But you see, they operate within my compounds (KEMRI), so I had to put in some restrictions. The restrictions, which I put in, were strong enough to make sure that everyone was operating in line. Yes, so that no one was having a field day.

But my firm approach with CDC has perhaps caused some of these troubles that I find myself in.

Number one, they (CDC) do not like to be controlled. Number two, when I look at it a little deeper I think it has something to do with misinformation. Everything has to do with misinformation: misinformation, because there was no proper control. The source of the information and the source of the answers were totally different. It was a very simple thing. What happened at that time was extremely simple. We had several accounts at the Institute. We have many accounts and this has been the way since we started doing collaborative research in the 1980s. We have so many collaborators and so we cannot mix your account with the KEMRI general account, and I cannot mix your account with another account. So we end up having different accounts because each agency has different policies for accountability. Yes. As a leader and a head of the Institution, I have a large degree of responsibility. For example, by the time I left KEMRI we had total staff strength of slightly more than 3,000, probably closer to 3,500.

These people are employed from many different sources. The core staff of the Institute are employed through funds from the Exchequer, that means from the National Treasury. So that money comes to KEMRI through the parent ministry. If we are responsible to the Ministry of Health for the purpose of research, that is it. We started from regional development and then we went to the Ministry of Research, Science and Technology, and then we went back to the Ministry of Health, then to science, we went back to this and so on. These shifts back and forth depend on the feelings of the state and the presiding President. When it happens that way the National Treasury brings in our allocation. We use what is called "one-twelfth allocation". This means if the government has approved a certain amount of money for the year, it does not give you the full amount at once. Instead, they pay it out monthly, so that is why we used to call it one-twelfth. KEMRI would receive its allocation on a month-to-month basis in part because of the way the state receives money from taxpayers. The funds for KEMRI and other parastatals come from what is called the consolidated account.

The consolidated account of the government is where the monies from taxation are held. From there it is distributed but people don't pay tax on the same day. They pay taxes and levies as they go along so the National Treasury cannot give you the money for the entire year because of the possibility of misuse. So it leaves you with the basic principle of one-twelfth. The National Treasury prepares the payroll but they don't give you the actual money. They give you what is called "issues". The issue comes from the National Treasury. It comes to the ministry and then the ministry gives it to KEMRI. So the money does not actually leave the Central Bank. All government departments and all government ministries have their accounts with the Central Bank. The only agencies that have their accounts outside of the Central Bank are parastatals like KEMRI. Yes.

Parastatals like KEMRI have different signatories than the ministries. Accounting officers of the Ministries are called Principal Secretaries. The Ministers are not the accounting officers. They are policy makers and they guide policies but of course they can overrule on certain decisions. So by the time we have an issue for a cheque from KEMRI for example, it is probably during the first week of the month. If we were to depend on that to pay salaries we would be paying salaries on the tenth of the month. You get me? But I created a formula that we know how much money we are receiving from the parent ministry, and all the other various grants, and I must pay people on the same day. I must pay them on the same day whether you are receiving the salary from the National Treasury (the Exchequer), or the Wellcome Trust, Walter Reed, or CDC.... They are all paid on the same day. It is usually the last Friday of the month, and your salary must be in your account. Usually we operate on "salary in arrears". That means that you get paid for work done. Staff are not paid in advance of work, which happens in many places, and is like the payment of rent. If you are paying rent, you pay in advance. But we pay salary pay in arrears. So that is the official policy and then I also created a policy of harmonization of pay for all officers of the same grade regardless of where your money comes from. At the end of the day it is my office that issues salaries.

Under my policy of harmonization, if you have the same qualifications and same experience, even if one staff works for, let us say Walter Reed, and another staff member works for the national government, your salaries should be equitable. In order to do this though I had to find some extra money to make sure that people are earning the same pay for having the same qualifications for similar work and experience. People are usually graded which indicates their salary level. If you are on grade five, you will be paid the same as someone on grade five at another agency. But when we started these international collaborations, there were some granting agencies that had different pay scales so during the negotiations of the collaborative agreements, we call it a "Coag", we harmonized pay for equity out of the KEMRI office since it is the office of the CEO that issues letters of appointment. Yes. The allowance must also be the same. Housing allowance too. If there is any difference, because maybe my granting organization pays less for the same grade, I secure what is called "supplementary money" from elsewhere so at the end of the day, your salary is harmonized. That is what harmonization is all about. And rationalization.

You see, we did not want our staff saying, "I want to work for CDC because they have higher salary" and so under the harmonization policy they are paid equally. I wanted this to avoid staff disenchantment. So the government usually used to pay less than the foreign agencies and so to guarantee harmonization, I used funds from the overheads that I am getting from all these other granting institutions. I have some extra money left and I use part of that to harmonize the salaries, for salary supplementation. This was necessary because people used to write requests for transfers, asking to leave KEMRI to work instead for the Walter Reed Project: "Please transfer me." I said we had to solve this nonsense.

Yes. So this is what happened. But it is a very expensive thing. So then I said this is not sustainable. Yes.

We can't do this so I started harmonizing letters of appointment as well so they were all issued by the same office – mine. I discussed this issue with all of the granting agencies. I said all employees must be employed by KEMRI unless this office is not paying them. But otherwise let them be employees of the Institute, with the same letter of appointment, because labour issues, for instance, had to be handled by my office since we are in Kenya even if I never issued letters of appointment for staff working for CDC or Walter Reed, for instance. So I said, no this nonsense must stop. Yes. They are working in my compound and then they were earning different salaries, and then who knows their pay, what day they are being paid, and so on. No, and then these foreign agencies are still using my electricity and water and so on, so we made it a uniform requirement for all our collaborators. All the staff must be paid by one office so I know the conditions of the offers and so that I will be able to take care of the labour disputes. Because it is my office that knows what is allowed and what is not allowed, even when it comes to leave and other conditions of service. So we harmonized that so that at the end of the day it is one letter issued by one office, KEMRI, with conditions, but then at the end of it staff will be attached to specific programs like the CDC KEMRI, Walter Reed Project, UCSF program, or the Wellcome Trust. Yes. I put a stop to the nonsense between programs. It has actually worked very well.

It also worked well for monthly fiscal management. Under this arrangement I could borrow money from the grants account and put it onto the payroll. When the money comes now on about the tenth of the month from the National Treasury, I return the money. I did the same for balancing the research budgets. For instance, if one project is running low on funds, I can cover you until your next instalment is received.

So this is what happened with other activities too. For example, if I am supposed to pay for water and the account for payment of water is not ready, I did not wait for the water to be disconnected because it is going to affect all of us, so I borrow money from this account until the funds are received. Funds do not always come when you expect them, there are delays and so on, so we need back-up plans. This is what happens also in research grants. If you see the research is going on but you have exhausted this account, you have not received the money, then you just scan around and if there is a project that is also going on well with funds, you know you are going to get the money on time and you put that money into this and the program continues. You see? So that is what happens until today. So one day when we were planning a meeting in South Africa with funding from global health but we had some shortfall, I looked at the other grants and there was some money from the Walter Reed Project and we also had some money from the CDC account. I transferred some funds to cover the other that would be replaced once the other funds were received. We do it all the time. Yes. So this one time, CDC was making a lot of noise and they didn't even know what was going on. They didn't realize it was routine reporting, and that we are doing it all the time. You see this is why I say it is about misinformation. Yes.

I don't think Jono[1] knew exactly what he was doing. He was making routine reports to Atlanta and then eventually they said that I had taken money. We had taken it but this is what we were doing daily, and we would do tomorrow. It is the way that information was mishandled and then they said *ati* [/that/] I stole some money but I did not. They checked everywhere but it never went into my account. Eventually the other funding authority gave me the money, and we replaced it in the account as we have always done. I told them that their money was there. It was the most unfortunate event during the particular political climate in the country during that time because even the permanent secretary received that letter from the CDC. Then it was not even from the relevant offices. You see at times they say that it was the US Embassy who was unhappy but CDC was not even concerned. There was somebody who wanted a promotion in Atlanta. Yes. Do you know, there are some people who can be a pain in the arse. I am sorry to say that, but it is true. There was a person from Atlanta who called me about ten times. I told him, give me 30 minutes and then he calls me back after three minutes, as if that 30 minutes is gone. So there was a person who was doing that from Atlanta. I was attending a meeting in London and he was calling me. I said, "I am in London, my brother. Can you please wait until I go to find out whether we have received the money from the other funders?" And we had 22 different grant accounts. Yes, 22!

I had recognized in March of 2007 that it was time for me to vacate my office so that I would be able to groom somebody else to take over the leadership of the Institute. I had decided that it was now time for me to go back to my lab and concentrate on my research because I wasn't going to stay in that office forever. It is a public office and I had served for more than 20 years. I said let me give myself a maximum of two more years serving in this office. The only thing I need to do is to identify someone to replace me. Slowly I'll be able to mentor the individual and introduce them into the position. I called a special Board meeting in March 2007. It was in March, I remember it very well. I told the Board of Management, "Please, I have called you because I want to step down as the CEO of the Institute but not today. I am not resigning but I want to assist the Board to look for a replacement." So the Board Members deliberated on it and then they refused. They said, "No, we don't want you to go." I said,

> If there is nothing I have done all these years, then there is nothing I would do for the remaining years. I have served you long enough. It is time for me to go back to my laboratory to concentrate and to assist it in any other capacity.

Yes. We had the deliberation and then the Board asked, "Do you have anyone in mind?" I said,

> No. It is up to the Board, but I can guide the Board while we are looking for someone. When we have identified somebody else to take over then I will be able to take that person round to meet all the granting agencies so that we have a smooth transition.

At that time we were living largely on grants. About 92 per cent of our recurrent expenditure came from grants and the remaining 8 per cent from the Exchequer; that is from the national government. Because of this heavy reliance on foreign grants and these complex collaborations, it was not possible for the Board to quickly appoint one person today and then tomorrow make an announcement. No. So after the meeting the representative of the Permanent Secretary, as is routinely required, went to the Permanent Secretary and told him, "Listen, Koech is planning to retire from office and the Board has agreed to look for somebody to be trained, to learn the ropes, to walk those very slender ropes over time." Then three days later the Permanent Secretary calls me.

Because that office is the one that, in terms of policy, is responsible for the affairs of the other parastatals within the ministry. Yes. So he calls me, "I hear you want to go? I have somebody in mind." I said, "Oh, who is this person?" I think he said he was a lecturer in one of the universities, then I told him, "Listen now this office is very tricky. Could I see the C.V. of this individual? And then the Board will discuss." This individual must be introduced to so many other people. I told him that my deputy in charge of the scientific development would not qualify because of age. He is older than me. He is in his late sixties. The Permanent Secretary tells me then that the individual that he has in mind has passed retirement age yet he can serve as a CEO. But I explained to him that someone that age will not bring anything new and we need a much younger individual. Yes. He said no. I'll give you the name. I said that is fine. So when I told him that we could not have someone old, he took offence. He thought I would say, "Okay, go ahead and recommend that person to the Board." Because usually the appointment is done by the minister with the recommendation of the Board and the CEO. Yes. So the CEO is not appointed by the Board, neither can that person be sacked by the Board. That started in March and then about June/ July he started picking on me, picking on me, picking on me. And then I grew weary of this, so I went to him and I told him,

> Listen, this office you are holding I was given by President Moi 20 years ago! I would have done it in 1987. This is the year 2007. Exactly 20 years ago! If I were you I would not be handling this office in this way. I have a duty as the CEO. Part of my mandate is to advise you and this is precisely what I am saying.

I told him, "You have been in the service for hardly a few months. So my responsibility is to advise you about what you need to do for KEMRI. I would be failing in my duty if I never advised you." Yes. And he asked me, "You mean you would have held this office?" I said, "Yes!" I declined because it is a more of a political office and I would have been sacked long ago due to possible political interference. I was not ready for it. I was more concerned about developing KEMRI than holding an office such as this.

Yes. I said to him, this is my office and I have plans for my office. I told him that I had several serving officers who would knew the art of walking the ropes at the Institute. They know the intricacies of getting money from various sources, they know how to use the money, and they know the main players, etcetera. So it went on like that and then he received this solitary letter from some officer at CDC in Atlanta. He said, "I hear there is money, which was lost." I said, "There is no money lost, there is no money lost!" He could not understand. "There is money that got lost there and we are going to lose a lot of money from the US government, we are going to blah, blah, blah, blah…" You see? And then he immediately wrote a letter suspending me.

Intermission

Koech's story forces us to consider patterns of accusations, or who is accusing whom of being corrupt. As Jean and John Comaroff (2013) have illustrated, Africa has been constructed as the epitome of corruption, as if the very same practices don't exist in Western nations, or that postcolonial African nations didn't learn and inherit such practices from the colonial actors that governed them. Koech's stories help us understand how state actors navigate the complex state arrangements that encourage corruption among the elite, and how Western states accept, and sometimes encourage or benefit, from such practices and certainly by such accusations. Such stories of corruption levied at African elites are definitely not new (see Smith 2007), but what is interesting are the sources and

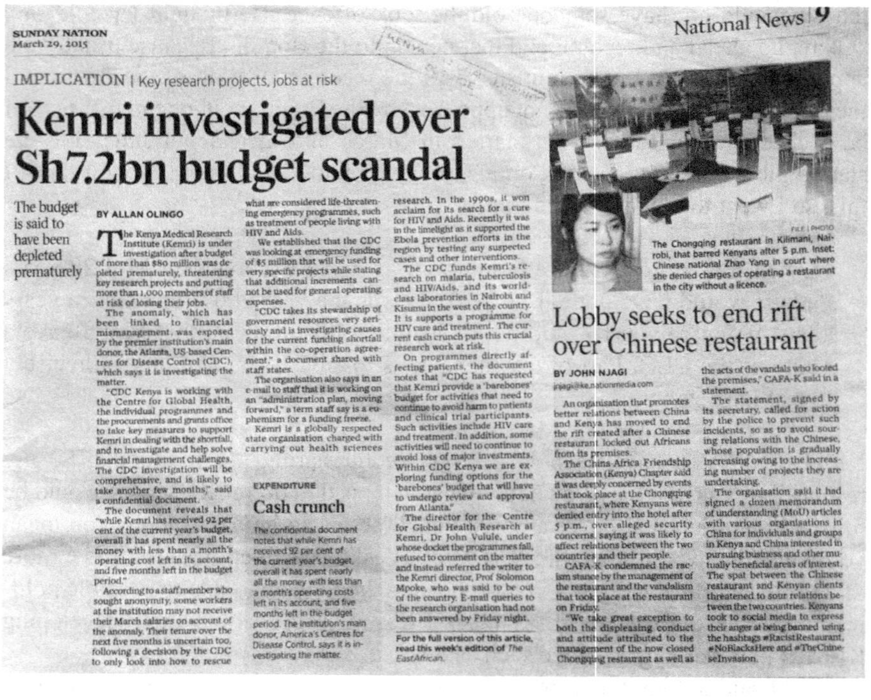

SUNDAY NATION
March 29, 2015

National News | 9

IMPLICATION | Key research projects, jobs at risk

Kemri investigated over Sh7.2bn budget scandal

The budget is said to have been depleted prematurely

BY ALLAN OLINGO

The Kenya Medical Research Institute (Kemri) is under investigation after a budget of more than $80 million was depleted prematurely, threatening key research projects and putting more than 1,000 members of staff at risk of losing their jobs.

The anomaly, which has been linked to financial mismanagement, was exposed by the premier institution's main donor, the Atlanta, US-based Centres for Disease Control (CDC), which says it is investigating the matter.

"CDC Kenya is working with the Centre for Global Health, the individual programmes and the procurements and grants office to take key measures to support Kemri in dealing with the shortfall, and to investigate and help solve financial management challenges. The CDC investigation will be comprehensive, and is likely to take another few months," said a confidential document.

The document reveals that "while Kemri has received 92 per cent of the current year's budget, overall it has spent nearly all the money with less than a month's operating cost left in its account, and five months left in the budget period."

According to a staff member who sought anonymity, some workers at the institution may not receive their March salaries on account of the anomaly. Their tenure over the next five months is uncertain too, following a decision by the CDC to only look into how to rescue what are considered life-threatening emergency programmes, such as treatment of people living with HIV and Aids.

We established that the CDC was looking at emergency funding of $5 million that will be used for very specific projects while stating that additional increments cannot be used for general operating expenses.

"CDC takes its stewardship of government resources very seriously and is investigating causes for the current funding shortfall within the co-operation agreement," a document shared with staff states.

The organisation also says in an e-mail to staff that it is working on an "administration plan, moving forward," a term staff say is a euphemism for a funding freeze.

Kemri is a globally respected state organisation charged with carrying out health sciences research. In the 1990s, it won acclaim for its search for a cure for HIV and Aids. Recently it was in the limelight as it supported the Ebola prevention efforts in the region by testing any suspected cases and other interventions.

The CDC funds Kemri's research on malaria, tuberculosis and HIV/Aids, and its world-class laboratories in Nairobi and Kisumu in the west of the country. It is supports a programme for HIV care and treatment. The current cash crunch puts this crucial research work at risk.

On programmes directly affecting patients, the document notes that "CDC has requested that Kemri provide a 'barebones' budget for activities that need to continue to avoid harm to patients and clinical trial participants. Such activities include HIV care and treatment. In addition, some activities will need to continue to avoid loss of major investments. Within CDC Kenya we are exploring funding options for the 'barebones' budget that will have to undergo review and approval from Atlanta."

The director for the Centre for Global Health Research at Kemri, Dr John Vulule, under whose docket the programmes fall, refused to comment on the matter and instead referred the writer to the Kemri director, Prof Solomon Mpoke, who was said to be out of the country. E-mail queries to the research organisation had not been answered by Friday night.

For the full version of this article, read this week's edition of *The EastAfrican*.

EXPENDITURE

Cash crunch

The confidential document notes that while Kemri has received 92 per cent of the current year's budget, overall it has spent nearly all the money with less than a month's operating costs left in its account, and five months left in the budget period. The institution's main donor, America's Centres for Disease Control, says it is investigating the matter.

FILE | PHOTO

The Chongqing restaurant in Kilimani, Nairobi, that barred Kenyans after 5 p.m. Inset: Chinese national Zhao Yang in court where she denied charges of operating a restaurant in the city without a licence.

Lobby seeks to end rift over Chinese restaurant

BY JOHN NJAGI
jnjagi@ke.nationmedia.com

An organisation that promotes better relations between China and Kenya has moved to end the rift created after a Chinese restaurant locked out Africans from its premises.

The China-Africa Friendship Association (Kenya) Chapter said it was deeply concerned by events that took place at the Chongqing restaurant, where Kenyans were denied entry into the hotel after 5 p.m., over alleged security concerns, saying it was likely to affect relations between the two countries and their people.

CAFA-K condemned the racism stance by the management of the restaurant and the vandalism that took place at the restaurant on Friday.

"We take great exception to both the displeasing conduct and attitude attributed to the management of the now closed Chongqing restaurant as well as the acts of the vandals who looted the premises," CAFA-K said in a statement.

The statement, signed by its secretary, called for action by the police to prevent such incidents, so as to avoid souring relations with the Chinese, whose population is gradually increasing owing to the increasing number of projects they are undertaking.

The organisation said it had signed a dozen memorandum of understanding (MoU) articles with various organisations in China for individuals and groups in Kenya and China interested in pursuing business and other mutually beneficial areas of interest.

The spat between the Chinese restaurant and Kenyan clients threatened to sour relations between the two countries. Kenyans took to social media to express their anger at being banned using the hashtags #RacistRestaurant, #NoBlacksHere and #TheChineseInvasion.

Figure 24.1 KEMRI investigated, Daily Nation, 29 March 2015.

patterns of rumours about corruption in medical science. The allegations against Koech were only the first in a series levied by the Americans against KEMRI senior management. In 2015 the Centers for Disease Control again accused KEMRI officials of stealing money. *The East African* reported (Olingo 2015):

> The Kenya Medical Research Institute (KEMRI) is under investigation after a budget of more than $80 million was depleted prematurely, threatening key research projects and putting more than 1,000 members of staff at risk of losing their jobs. The anomaly, which has been linked to financial mismanagement, was exposed by the premier institution's main donor, the Atlanta, US-based Centres for Disease Control (CDC), which says it is investigating the matter.

This too resulted in a senior official, John Vulule, being forced to step down as Director of the Centre for Global Health Research at KEMRI. The man who took over from Koech as the new Director of KEMRI, Solomon Mpoke, was also sent on compulsory leave in December of 2015 in response to the CDC's charge of "missing funds". An American financial auditor came to Kenya to investigate, and a colleague reported to me that it seemed the funds weren't missing after all. In 2016, Elizabeth Bukusi, then Deputy Director of KEMRI, and her colleagues were also questioned about possible fraudulent practices and a conflict of interest after they started the Research Care and Training Program in Kisumu, a collaborative project with the University of California San Francisco (Psirmoi 2016). Gathii (2009) explains that elite politically connected Kenyans often use the judiciary, through slander suits, to prevent accusations of corruption from the Kenyan state or others. In this way it is also as scholars Ireri (2016) and Gathii (2011) note: the Kenyan state and judicial system are used to both deter and support fraudulent and corrupt practices and other misuses of offices of the state.

Koech's stories demand that we consider why it is that only the CDC continues to report missing funds, not the US Army Research Unit, JICA, the Wellcome Trust, or the other nearly 60 organizations the KEMRI is working with at any one time? His account of the moral ambiguity that pervades global health research and national science asks us to think about how accusations of fraud, corruption, and illegal activities are used against Africans to discredit and challenge their contributions. And how such patterns of accusation create persistent narratives and maintain racist logics. I frequently heard Americans who were conducting clinical trials speak about widespread corruption in procurement in Kenya. It was considered "a necessary evil" of working in East Africa, without acknowledging the same practices occur within European and North American governments. Kenyans too speak frequently in everyday conversations about the problems of corruption, such as police officers pulling cars over simply because they want a bribe.[2] Accusations and charges that focus on Koech as a fraudulent scientist or corrupt state actor diverts our attention away from a complex system involving elite politicians, international actors, and state institutions from Kenya and abroad that permit, encourage, sometimes demand, creative acts in fiscal

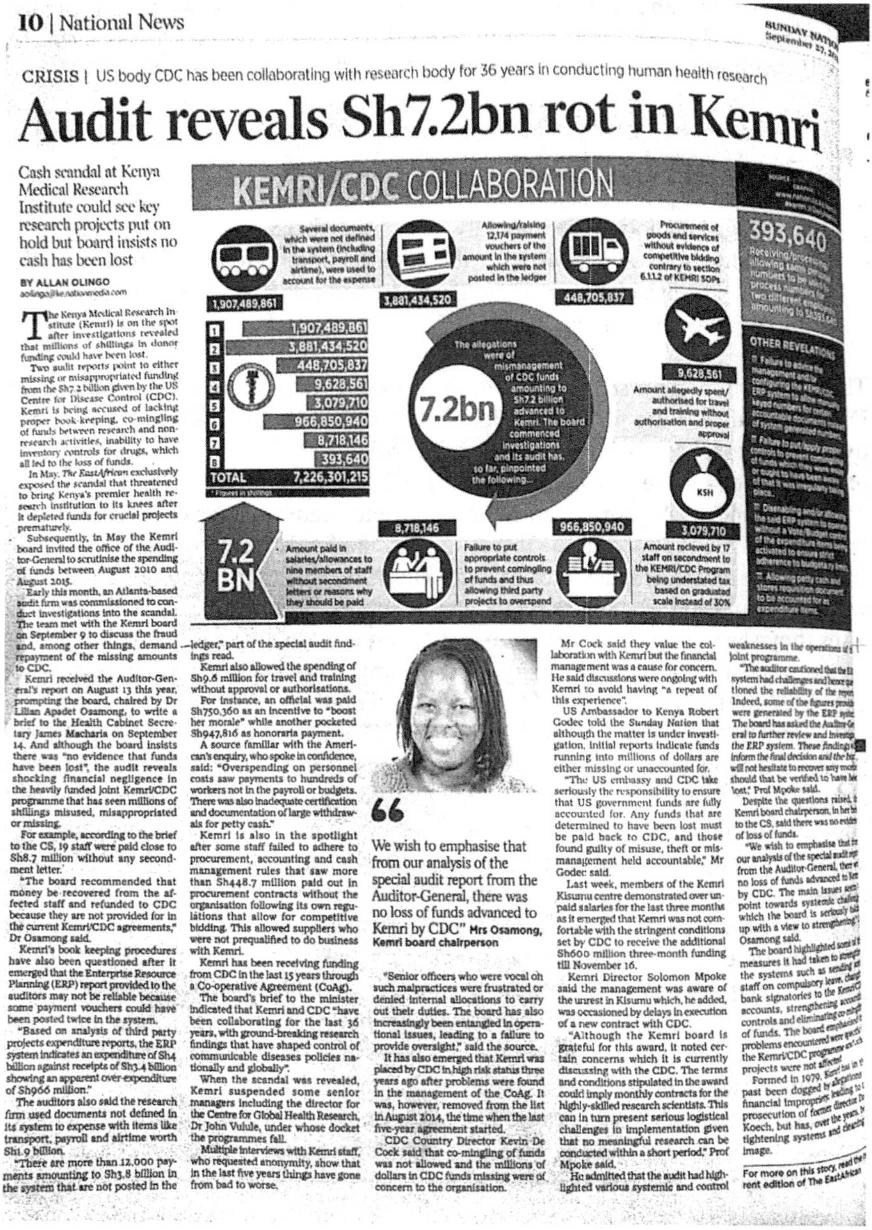

10 | National News

SUNDAY NATION September 27, 20

CRISIS | US body CDC has been collaborating with research body for 36 years in conducting human health research

Audit reveals Sh7.2bn rot in Kemri

Cash scandal at Kenya Medical Research Institute could see key research projects put on hold but board insists no cash has been lost

BY ALLAN OLINGO
aolingo@ke.nationmedia.com

KEMRI/CDC COLLABORATION

1,907,489,861 — Several documents, which were not defined in the system (including transport, payroll and airtime), were used to account for the expense

3,881,434,520 — Allowing/raising 12,174 payment vouchers of the amount in the system which were not posted in the ledger

448,705,837 — Procurement of goods and services without evidence of competitive bidding contrary to section 6.1.1.2 of KEMRI SOPs

9,628,561 — Amount allegedly spent/ authorised for travel and training without authorisation and proper approval

3,079,710 — Amount recieved by 17 staff on secondment to the KEMRI/CDC Program being understated tax based on graduated scale instead of 30%

966,850,940 — Failure to put appropriate controls to prevent comingling of funds and thus allowing third party projects to overspend

8,718,146 — Amount paid in salaries/allowances to nine members of staff without secondment letters or reasons why they should be paid

1	1,907,489,861
2	3,881,434,520
3	448,705,837
4	9,628,561
5	3,079,710
6	966,850,940
7	8,718,146
8	393,640
TOTAL	7,226,301,215

* Figures in shillings

7.2bn — The allegations were of mismanagement of CDC funds amounting to Sh7.2 billion advanced to Kemri. The board commenced investigations and its audit has, so far, pinpointed the following...

7.2 BN

393,640 — Receiving/processing/ allowing same person numbers to be used to process numbers for two different employees amounting to Sh393,640

OTHER REVELATIONS

- Failure to advice the management and/or configuring the KEMRI/CDC ERP system to allow manually keyed numbers for certain accountable documents instead of system generated numbers.
- Failure to put/apply proper controls to prevent comingling of funds which they were aware or ought to have been aware of that it was irregularly taking place.
- Disenabling and/or allowing the said ERP system to operate without a Vote/Budget control of the expenditure items being activated to ensure strict adherence to budgetary limits.
- Allowing petty cash and stores requisition document to be accounted for as expenditure items.

The Kenya Medical Research Institute (Kemri) is on the spot after investigations revealed that millions of shillings in donor funding could have been lost.

Two audit reports point to either missing or misappropriated funding from the Sh7.2 billion given by the US Centre for Disease Control (CDC). Kemri is being accused of lacking proper book-keeping, co-mingling of funds between research and non-research activities, inability to have inventory controls for drugs, which all led to the loss of funds.

In May, *The EastAfrican* exclusively exposed the scandal that threatened to bring Kenya's premier health research institution to its knees after it depleted funds for crucial projects prematurely.

Subsequently, in May the Kemri board invited the office of the Auditor-General to scrutinise the spending of funds between August 2010 and August 2015.

Early this month, an Atlanta-based audit firm was commissioned to conduct investigations into the scandal. The team met with the Kemri board on September 9 to discuss the fraud and, among other things, demand repayment of the missing amounts to CDC.

Kemri received the Auditor-General's report on August 13 this year, prompting the board, chaired by Dr Lilian Apadet Osamong, to write a brief to the Health Cabinet Secretary James Macharia on September 14. And although the board insists there was "no evidence that funds have been lost", the audit reveals shocking financial negligence in the heavily funded joint Kemri/CDC programme that has seen millions of shillings misused, misappropriated or missing.

For example, according to the brief to the CS, 19 staff were paid close to Sh8.7 million without any secondment letter.

"The board recommended that money be recovered from the affected staff and refunded to CDC because they are not provided for in the current Kemri/CDC agreements," Dr Osamong said.

Kemri's book keeping procedures have also been questioned after it emerged that the Enterprise Resource Planning (ERP) report provided to the auditors may not be reliable because some payment vouchers could have been posted twice in the system.

"Based on analysis of third party projects expenditure reports, the ERP system indicates an expenditure of Sh4 billion against receipts of Sh3.4 billion showing an apparent over-expenditure of Sh966 million."

The auditors also said the research firm used documents not defined in its system to expense with items like transport, payroll and airtime worth Sh1.9 billion.

"There are more than 12,000 payments amounting to Sh3.8 billion in the system that are not posted in the ledger," part of the special audit findings read.

Kemri also allowed the spending of Sh9.6 million for travel and training without approval or authorisations.

For instance, an official was paid Sh750,360 as an incentive to "boost her morale" while another pocketed Sh947,816 as honoraria payment.

A source familiar with the American's enquiry, who spoke in confidence, said: "Overspending on personnel costs saw payments to hundreds of workers not in the payroll or budgets. There was also inadequate certification and documentation of large withdrawals for petty cash."

Kemri is also in the spotlight after some staff failed to adhere to procurement, accounting and cash management rules that saw more than Sh448.7 million paid out in procurement contracts without the organisation following its own regulations that allow for competitive bidding. This allowed suppliers who were not prequalified to do business with Kemri.

Kemri has been receiving funding from CDC in the last 15 years through a Co-operative Agreement (CoAg).

The board's brief to the minister indicated that Kemri and CDC "have been collaborating for the last 36 years, with ground-breaking research findings that have shaped control of communicable diseases policies nationally and globally".

When the scandal was revealed, Kemri suspended some senior managers including the director for the Centre for Global Health Research, Dr John Vulule, under whose docket the programmes fall.

Multiple interviews with Kemri staff, who requested anonymity, show that in the last five years things have gone from bad to worse.

> We wish to emphasise that from our analysis of the special audit report from the Auditor-General, there was no loss of funds advanced to Kemri by CDC" **Mrs Osamong, Kemri board chairperson**

"Senior officers who were vocal on such malpractices were frustrated or denied internal allocations to carry out their duties. The board has also increasingly been entangled in operational issues, leading to a failure to provide oversight," said the source.

It has also emerged that Kemri was placed by CDC in high risk status three years ago after problems were found in the management of the CoAg. It was, however, removed from the list in August 2014, the time when the last five-year agreement started.

CDC Country Director Kevin De Cock said that co-mingling of funds was not allowed and the millions of dollars in CDC funds missing were of concern to the organisation.

Mr Cock said they value the collaboration with Kemri but the financial management was a cause for concern. He said discussions were ongoing with Kemri to avoid having "a repeat of this experience".

US Ambassador to Kenya Robert Godec told the *Sunday Nation* that although the matter is under investigation, initial reports indicate funds running into millions of dollars are either missing or unaccounted for.

"The US embassy and CDC take seriously the responsibility to ensure that US government funds are fully accounted for. Any funds that are determined to have been lost must be paid back to CDC, and those found guilty of misuse, theft or mismanagement held accountable," Mr Godec said.

Last week, members of the Kemri Kisumu centre demonstrated over unpaid salaries for the last three months as it emerged that Kemri was not comfortable with the stringent conditions set by CDC to receive the additional Sh600 million three-month funding till November 16.

Kemri Director Solomon Mpoke said the management was aware of the unrest in Kisumu which, he added, was occasioned by delays in execution of a new contract with CDC.

"Although the Kemri board is grateful for this award, it noted certain concerns which it is currently discussing with the CDC. The terms and conditions stipulated in the award could imply monthly contracts for the highly-skilled research scientists. This can in turn present serious logistical challenges in implementation given that no meaningful research can be conducted within a short period," Prof Mpoke said.

He admitted that the audit had highlighted various systemic and control weaknesses in the operations of the joint programme.

"The auditor cautioned that the ERP system had challenges and hence questioned the reliability of the report. Indeed, some of the figures provided were generated by the ERP system. The board has asked the Auditor-General to further review and investigate *the ERP system. These findings will inform the final decision and the board* will not hesitate to recover any money should that be verified to have been lost," Prof Mpoke said.

Despite the questions raised, the Kemri board chairperson, in her brief to the CS, said there was no evidence of loss of funds.

"We wish to emphasise that from our analysis of the special audit report from the Auditor-General, there was no loss of funds advanced to Kemri by CDC. The main issues seem to point towards systemic challenges which the board is seriously taking up with a view to strengthening," Dr Osamong said.

The board highlighted some of the measures it had taken to strengthen the systems such as sending staff on compulsory leave, changing bank signatories to the Kemri/CDC accounts, strengthening accounting controls and eliminating co-mingling of funds. The board emphasised that problems encountered were specific to the Kemri/CDC programme and other projects were not affected.

Formed in 1979, Kemri has in the past been dogged by allegations of financial impropriety, leading to the prosecution of former director Dr Koech, but has, over the years, been tightening systems and cleaning its image.

For more on this story, read the current edition of The EastAfrican

Figure 24.2 Audit reveals rot in KEMRI, The Sunday Nation, 27 September 2015.

management, public procurement, and contract negotiations (Smith 2010). Though the Penal Code and the Anti-Corruption and Economic Crimes Act 2003 criminalize bribery, money laundering, abuse of power, extortion, and conflict of interest, Koech's stories reveal how such shadowy practices are continually negotiated and contested in the global health industry, international politics, and within the national context of Kenyan politics.

Notes

1 Jonathan Mermin, CDC Country Director in Kenya from 2006–2009.
2 Transparency International (2015) reports that 75% of Kenyans believe the police are corrupt.

25 The accusations

I travelled to Kisumu where we were celebrating something with the CDC at the Kisian field station. So we have been doing some very good work with Jonathan Mermin (Jono). Of course, a few things we managed to do right. I travelled to Kisumu to the event with CDC where they gave me a plaque in my honour. It is a souvenir given by the CDC. I have it on my table. Yes. They said, "We are giving this to you because of the services you have given to us for all these years…" And actually it wasn't from the local office here but from Atlanta. But then on the same day I received a letter saying that I needed to report to Nairobi. I thought it was some joke. I called the Permanent Secretary. CDC Kenya was not the one complaining. This guy in Atlanta was writing a routine memo and then somebody used it because … I don't know sometimes you don't know what to believe and what not to believe.… This happened in August 2007.

The day Hezron Nyangito, the Permanent Secretary, wrote the letter suspending me I was very busy in Kisian with the CDC. It does not make the slightest sense because even the money he was talking about, we know that it had been transferred from one account to the other account and the money had been returned. You see? So the money was borrowed, it was used, and then returned when the other funds were received. Yes. And the office knew about it. And all of this was made public. So I went to him and said, "What you are talking about? It is such a small amount! Even today, as we are talking, there have been other borrowings from other accounts. Why restrict yourself to this account? This is not the only account we have!" So he saw actually there was nothing to be lost from the US government. It had nothing to do with the CDC Kenya. It is the way Jono handled the information. And also the way Atlanta was thinking. The supposed missing amount was 18 million KES but we had a budget of ten billion KES. If I were interested in stealing money, I would have swindled more than 18 million, surely.

This is where there has been a problem with the chain of command and information gathering. This is something that I have said right from the beginning. The USCDC was patronizing towards us, not trusting us with accounting. So this is where the problem has been lying. The fact is if you trust me enough to give me that amount of money, why don't you trust me to manage it for you? Then if you are concerned about an account that I am managing for you, you ask

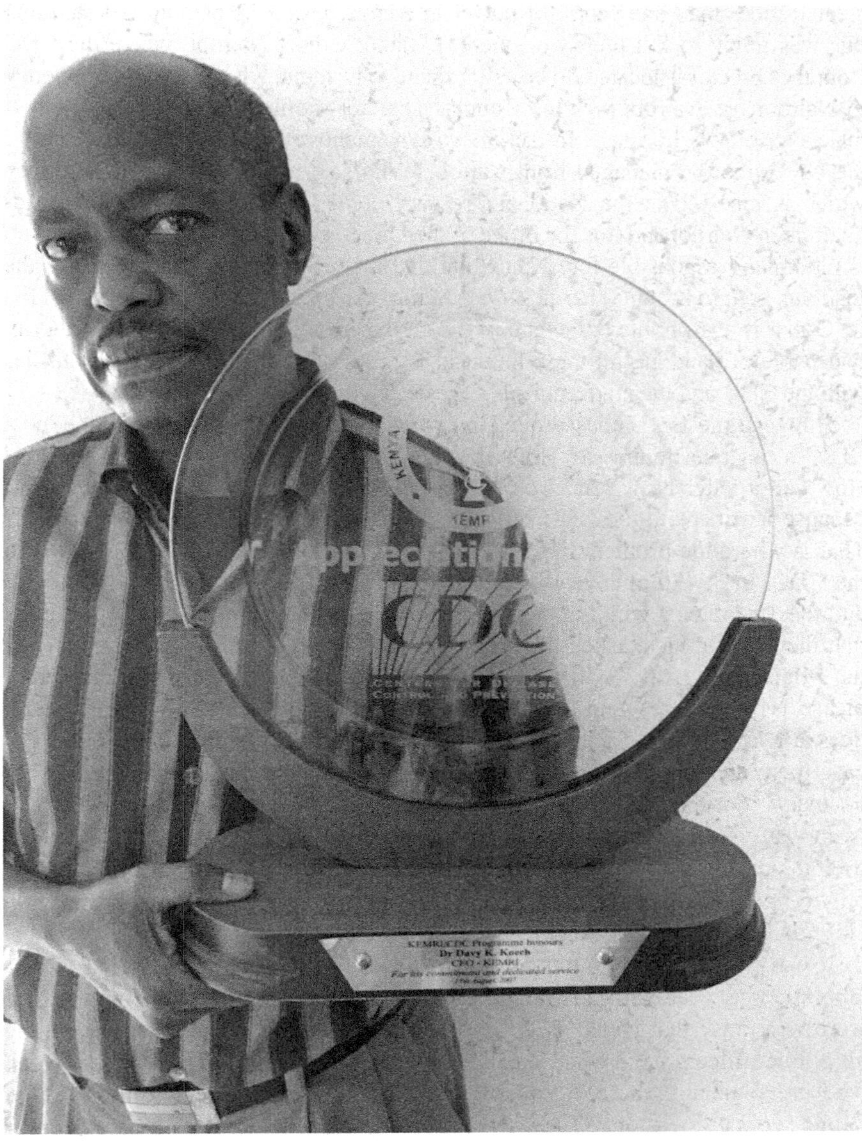

Figure 25.1 Koech in 2017 with the CDC award he was given in 2007.

me about it, you don't go and ask somebody else. And actually there was a point that I was thinking of taking the bank to court for entertaining strangers, that is the CDC. Yes, strangers. I cannot explore or inspect your account because I am not the signatory. I am not authorized. But CDC was doing that on and on and on and on to the point that they had different information.

This was one of the problems, but the other problem was that the CDC had created more than one centre of power in Kenya. From the beginning I said that this was going to kill their work here. I cannot expect Nairobi, where the CDC Country Director is located, to be subordinate to Kisumu. Kisian was giving money to Nairobi but Nairobi was the Country Director's office. It makes no sense. It makes absolutely no sense. In fact, they say somehow the money that comes from the US cannot be managed from Nairobi. Who said it? In fact KEMRI's money which is received at the National Treasury comes direct to the KEMRI headquarters in Nairobi and it is the office of the Director of the Institute, the CEO, who is ultimately responsible for channelling that money to the various centres of the Institute, be it in Kisumu, Busia, Kwale, Kilifi, and so on. Yes. It is the office of the CEO that is answerable at the end of the day. Yes, and then a legitimate authority is capable of handling all these financial issues so that is where the problem lies with the CDC and the management of these supposed missing funds.

How can the US Embassy question what goes on in the CDC when the local CDC is not questioning it? How can they say the US Embassy is doing this? How can a letter be written from Atlanta, Georgia asking me certain questions because I work with the CDC office? Why are all these letters floating around? That is where the problem has been. There is no proper chain of command with the CDC. In my 20 plus years working as the Director of KEMRI, we have not had these problems with our other collaborators. What should have happened is that they should have asked me directly or queried the Ministry of Health. Then the Ministry of Health will come to me and say "We have received this letter, please assist us to respond to it" because they have no way of knowing our practices at KEMRI. Those are the actions of a responsible authority. But now in my case there are too many players. It is just like playing football. If you do not have any coordination it cannot work. Unless there is proper coordination there is no way you are going to get information properly. This is the problem and I tried to correct it. You see it does not make any sense. In fact, 18 million KES is only 50 per cent of the money we are spending *per day* because we spend very close to 30 million KES a day.

It was the month of August in 2007. We were celebrating the period of collaboration between KEMRI and the CDC. I think 25 years or thereabouts and we were very busy that week. The Kenyan government created a system whereby all public officers have what is called a performance contract and so that week we were evaluating the performance contracts among the serving officers in the public service. I was one of the persons who had been appointed by the government under the Office of the President to be involved with, even to chair, some of the committees evaluating public officials of the government, even those outside of KEMRI, so during that period I was extremely busy. KEMRI was also being examined but by somebody else of course so there was no conflict of interest and I had appeared before them to defend the Institute. Yes, it was an extremely busy week.

I think it was Friday, the 15th of August, or thereabouts, maybe a Wednesday, I travelled to Kisumu for a very big celebration that we had organized with the Americans. CDC recognized and acknowledged my work for facilitating their coming to Kenya, maintaining their stay, and making sure that their projects were complete. So on the same day that I received a gift from the CDC for years of service and good work that I performed with them, ironically, I was also accused of stealing money! When I arrived back in Nairobi on Monday I found a letter from the Permanent Secretary of the Ministry of Health telling me that some funds had been misappropriated. They were talking about 18.5 million KES. I was forced to leave the office on the 23rd of August. The letter indicated I must leave the office with immediate effect. Yes. I was being sent home because I have supposedly stolen money from the CDC but they have just given me an award. I could not understand this. Those transactions were open and I told the CDC what had occurred and that the money was coming.

The Permanent Secretary, totally unprocedurally and without reference to any rules, removed me from office. You see, number one, it is the function of the Board of Management who would now see if there was any problem raised by the Permanent Secretary in the Ministry of Health regarding public servants, and especially for CEOs like me, and they would have forwarded the complaint to the Chairman of the Board of Management of the Institute so that they can now examine the issue and do their own investigation if necessary, and conclude whether I was right or wrong. They would then make a recommendation to the Permanent Secretary. In my case, without any reference to those other bodies, the Permanent Secretary sent the letter directly to me and then copied it to the Kenya Anti-Corruption Authority and the Chairman of the Board. Yes. So I just found this letter on the Monday after I had arrived from Kisumu, then it was followed with all kinds of complaints and accusations that I stole some money! Yes.

Yet, they knew from the records that I never stole even a single cent. That is the normal operation in the Institute. I saw in one of the projects that it was going very well and it was recommended to me by my own officers that because this project was going very well and we were going to receive some money in about one or two months, that we could borrow from this other grant because they have sufficient funds which we can utilize. I said go ahead because that is what we do daily and because every month we borrow from external grants to cover the Exchequer funds. The Exchequer funds come from the treasury government funds.

Some 1,000 staff members were on the government payroll and then another 2,000 staff members were being funded by external grants. Now we pay all officers on the same day but the funds are transferred to our accounts on different dates, sometimes months later. Officers will not know who is paying them. So when it is time to do the payroll we prepare all payrolls at the same time. So at the end of the day the officers get their money in their own various bank accounts and it is left to the management, my office, to regularize those payments and that is precisely what we do. When one research account is down, you borrow money from another account so you can continue the research and other services of the Institute. It is done every day then and even now, and I would do the same thing tomorrow. Yes.

It happens then that I made an appointment and I went to see this guy, Hezron Nyangito, who has accused me, and I asked him,

> By the way, what is the problem? This is not theft because it is on record. The trail is there for the money, which you purport is stolen. When you take money, you destroy the records so that you are not monitored! But this is open. You see. Why do you accuse me?

I really do not know why he accused me. I never knew then and I don't know now because I had no opportunity to question this fellow. He was the first complainant in the charge sheet so when the court went to hear the case he was supposed to have been the very first person to come to be grilled in court, but he was not available. He never came to court, and then he died.

That was also the time when the minister became very furious, a lady minister who has just been elected as the Governor of Kitui County, Charity Ngilu. She is a friend and we had a meeting. You will see that on the record is the letter that I wrote to the Attorney General because I don't change my stories. Yes, if you are trying to lie, you tell one story today, then the following day you don't remember what story you told, but my story is there on record and is consistent. So I reported the matter to the Minister for Health and then she called me for a meeting. I received the letter Monday and I booked an appointment with her on a Tuesday. When we met on Tuesday the Minister gave instructions to the Permanent Secretary to withdraw the letter. She gave instructions telling him that this is not the way to handle matters like these. We are dealing with an extremely senior person in the government who has really done a lot of work for this country and beyond. This is not the way to treat him. She was very sympathetic to my case. She gave instructions on the same day and told the Permanent Secretary to withdraw that letter. Yes, because he had copied the letter to different offices. He said, "But I have released the letter!" She said, "Yes, it is the same letter that you wrote! It is you who is still going to write a withdrawal to those letters!" "He said, 'Yes ma'am.' "

So after that meeting, she kept on monitoring the situation. He said, "I have drafted the letter but I am yet to sign." He was delaying. I went to the minister and she told me, "You know what? The President is likely to sack me!" She told me this, "You see what I have in the office?" It was a small box. She said, "This is my only personal item in this office." She was already prepared to be sacked. Because the previous weekend she had gone to attend a rally belonging to the opposition party using a government vehicle with a flag. The elections were in four months so there was a lot of movement of persons in the government. I think the following day she was relieved of her duties as minister and so she vacated the office. She called me and said, "*Daktari* [/doctor/] …" I said, "Yes ma'am?" She continued, "You know you are a fighter and I am now going out to go and fight my own battles. I am leaving you with yours." Yes. That is precisely what happened. I kept monitoring the progress but the Permanent Secretary stood his ground. He said, "No. I am not withdrawing the letter." And so August passed, and then the following month or something like that, and he was transferred from the Ministry of Health to be the Deputy Governor of the Central Bank of Kenya. Then the person who was brought into the Ministry of Health to replace him was actually a fellow from home (a Kalenjin) who could not even touch a fly because of lack of confidence. This was during the Kibaki administration. Yes, and now Moi gets furious, well, he didn't get furious, but he got concerned.

During this time, I was involved in the strategic committee. I was meeting with President Kibaki and it was a campaign period. And may I tell you the situation, being what it is, unless someone has an interest, unless there is something they are going to get out of that particular situation, no one will bother to assist you. You will end up spending a lot of time and resources trying to chase these politicians. Fortunately for me I have seen how they work. I'd seen people lying. I said I don't want to solve it this way. I don't want to because it will mar the truth from politics.

In October I met with President Kibaki in his office. Charity Ngilu had been removed by President Kibaki and he brought in a fellow from home (a Kalenjin), called Paul Sang', whom he told to go and sort out Koech's problem. So when I met with him he said, "I want to go to Kibaki to find out what needs to be done." I thought he must be naive! I told him,

> You have the authority to make decisions. So do not go back yet when you have been given detailed instructions to come and sort out my problem! You have to ask how you are going to sort it out? You know the law is on your side and it is so clear! Section 19, number 1, I think, has given you the power to hire and fire the CEO so make use of it.

I even showed him the act within the constitution. We were not able to agree. I met him just the other day again and we greeted each other. He was there for only two months as the minister.

So this fellow, the Permanent Secretary, was the ruler in chief in the Ministry when Minister Ngilu left the office. He could not listen to anyone. He even called the various granting authorities and told them not to deal with me. Yes. Then they came to report to me that the Permanent Secretary for Health advised that we should not talk to you!

So I left the office. Yes. I had to hand over some of the basic things. And do you know when I was leaving the office I never touched anything because I thought in my mind I would be returning very soon. There was nothing I had done so why should I start migrating from the office? Yes. I left my personal things within the Institute, which I had there for more than 33 years. Yes, the whole office was mine, with many personal documents, photographs and such. I left that day basically with what I could carry. At that time when I was handing over the keys, I thought I was going out for about three weeks. Now it has taken more than ten years. It is coming to the 10th year.[1]

Then it appears as if it was a grand plan to destroy me. Either they wanted to destroy me physically or they wanted someone else to destroy me. Even now I do not know who was after me. You see? Even the complainant in court was not KEMRI. Usually when you are charged, there is that somebody who must make the complaint, but it was not KEMRI. It was an individual, this Permanent Secretary of Health, Hezron Nyangito, as the official complainant in the court case. And then this all stopped me from doing my own research. My research has really suffered over time. There is nothing that I did professionally that warranted asking me to go home, yet I was and still am on permanent and pensionable terms of employment. So whatever they did was wrong, *ab initio* as they say in law. Yes, right from the beginning. Right from the beginning and then they were not after my position because I was requesting to leave anyway. You see? Why punish me for requesting to leave? Is it because I said this is the procedure to follow in looking for a replacement? I have a duty, so it became a purely personal vendetta. From the time I left, there has never been a truly stable leadership at the Institute.

The Permanent Secretary asked for an investigation to be completed within three weeks. This person was also from his community, he was a Kisii. He sent three persons to do the investigations at the Institute. They were from his community and then the person they appointed as the special prosecutor was also from the same community. Are you getting me? So when you consider this, it appeared as if this person wanted to speed up the agenda which I cannot understand because I know that even with that community we have no differences. With them we are very friendly, you see. The Kipsigis and Kisii people, we have no problem. That is why I am saying I never tried at any one period of time to seek a political solution. You see usually I could figure out the truth. And I wanted to separate the truth from politics. Yes. I wanted to know the truth of what was happening and why, not the politics.

Like the way you see it in the local press at the moment. Some people are taken to court the following day they have changed political camps. They say now this government is rotten and so on. How can a minister in the government of Uhuru Kenyatta say now that Uhuru's government is worse than has ever existed? I did not want that because in this country the moment you touch an officer they read mischief, they read it as a political thing. It had nothing to do with the minister, she had not been informed about it. She only heard about it when I reported it to her. The Board was not informed about it. It was only one person involved. It was just one person.

When you look at my letter to the Attorney General you'll be able to see. You will be able to understand that when I left the office I thought I was going for three weeks. I thought that I was leaving the office for three weeks, only it is now ten years. There was a makeshift arrangement for someone to fill in for me, but so, even that they had not thought about carefully. So upon my dismissal we lost about three to five billion KES within one week because of lack of contract agreements and poor management. So it becomes very messy, yes, extremely messy.

The government and its institutions are thankless employers. I see some people who have contributed so much but they are being run down the drain because he or she forgot to put a full stop in a sentence. They ignore everything that the individual has done. Yes. Just because this fellow came late one morning? For example, 18.5 million that I never took? It is what cast me out of the Institute because some fellow accuses me? Come on! Can they really say I have stolen 18 million and yet it is there? You get me? If I were put in that situation again, I would do precisely the same thing again because I did it in the interest of science. Here I have a project and we are ready to get very good results but it is low in budget, yet there is this other money which is in this other project and so I transfer this money as a loan. It is done daily, including in fact as we are talking! How does KEMRI pay their staff when they have not received their salary from the National Treasury? Where? They borrow. Yes. It is a standard practice all over; you borrow from this account so long as you may return the money. You see it is not like I walked around with a gunny bag of money. But some people have been reported with that kind of money at night. Yes, I mean, is 18 million shillings just a few dollars that you just put in your pocket and walk away? Come on.

Note

1 This excerpt is from a 2015 interview. As this goes to press in January 2018, it has been 11 years.

26 Ethics and Anti-Corruption Commission[1]

It is just like you are driving and then you crash in an accident but you have survived, living on life support machines, and you have lost everything in the process. It is as if you are told one day to go home immediately without advance notice by the master whom you have served for decades, but you have not made arrangements. So that is fine for me. For my case, in particular, I can bear that, but for the rest of the family, it was very traumatic. Very traumatic. Yes. You are together but you are doing nothing. You are just looking at each other's faces, sitting in the house. So there had to be some level of adjustment. Even if you try to adjust, what do you do in the process? It is difficult. You adjust. How do you adjust? You are living in a home and the best thing is that I own my home. That is one fortunate thing – that by the time I was relieved of my duties I had no mortgage to pay and I had no rent to pay except the statutory payments. So I landed into a comfort zone. I had my own home and I didn't have any mortgage so the only struggle was the payment of water and electricity, and the general maintenance of the home. I am not getting paid a salary even now.[2]

On the morning of 27 January the EACC officials were knocking my gate. The EACC is the anti-corruption commission. Yes, EACC. We used to call it the Kenya Anti-Corruption Authority. They changed the name now to the Ethics and Anti-Corruption Commission. There is a controversial history to the Ethics and Anti-Corruption Commission. It was formed a while ago as the Anti-Corruption Squad. It has been evolving. You see it was something else when it began and then some people were taken to court when they realized that it was unconstitutional and so it was disbanded during Moi's regime. Yes. Some of these anti-corruption fellows had been hiding taxes and then some people were arrested. They were close to Moi and they made a constitutional reference and then it was realized that the authority was illegal. It was unconstitutional and so it was disbanded. When it was disbanded, the Kenya Anti-Corruption Commission (KACC) came in. Then the courts also disbanded the Kenya Anti-Corruption Authority saying it too was unconstitutional. Even right now Parliament passed a bill trying to sack everyone at EACC, you see. I don't think President Uhuru will assent because they are even trying to sack the CEO of the EACC. The new Director of the EACC is some guy called Waqo. I think he is an investigator. I really do not know. They have been having their own problems. After some time they found out that he was involved in some deal so they tried to remove him as well, so not all of them are clean. The Chairman who was trying to sort the secretariat was bundled out. A new Chairman was brought in early in 2017. So it has been very difficult for them to get the correct person. The corruption commissioners and the secretariat are corrupt.

So they came to my house. I'd just come back that morning from dropping one of my children to school. The moment I dropped into the house, I parked the car and when I was getting out I saw some fellows walking in. I asked the *askari* [/the guard/], "Who are these people?" He said, "I thought you had told them to come." So the *askari* was concerned and they didn't know that he was petrified because they were being accompanied by police officers in uniform with automatic rifles. Two stayed at the gate and two walked in. Yes. I said, "What is going on?" So they showed me a court order for search and seizure. I called my lawyer and said, "Please come, the police are here." The lawyer was a little bit concerned and he didn't take a keen interest, but he came.

So they took my documents, some things. I am an organized person. I am the head of the family. They went to my private office, they went through all the bedrooms, and you see they were looking down the beds to see whether they can find any hidden money. It was a comedy but it really shook the family. It scared the family because some of the family members were still in bed, because they came early in the morning so no one was really awake. Yes, they came early in the morning without notice and they went into the bedrooms. Some people were still asleep and these fellows are looking under the beds, opening the drawers, and so on. So they found my computer on the table, it was in my office, so then I asked them, "There is vital amount of work in this machine. Can I back it up?" But they said no. But my son's "A" Level assignments were on the laptop. They said they would return the computer in two weeks. They said they had gurus and experts who knew what they were doing so I shouldn't worry. But I asked again, "Please allow me to back it up." And they said,

> No, no, you may be deleting information. We are just police officers. We do not know but we have been given some assurance that you are going to have your computer back in two weeks. We have no interest in your machine. Since we found it we are going to take it.

So they took it. After two weeks I asked them for it and explained that my son's homework was on it. Eventually because they would not release it, I told my son, "Listen, the best thing is we do the work again. Let's repeat the assignment because otherwise you will not be able to hand in your work." He said, "Daddy but how?" So he even went into a depression because of this. Imagine the police coming to this kid with automatic AK47 rifles, going through every room? Then they departed the search with nothing but my laptop and some documents.

How could they come to my residence with four fully armed police officers, or detectives, with big boots and intimidate members of my family? Going into every room, even when some of the family members were asleep? Mama had not even taken her shower and was half-naked! Looking in all of the cupboards to see if we have hidden money. If there is cash! Which money? Later, they went into my bank account and all the money I had was 5,000 KES. Yes. Then they checked any account that I was associated with, even private companies and the foundation. They never found any hidden money. They took the cheque books and the counterfoils. And I said what are you looking for? This money that you are describing is money that was probably lost following the collapse of a government investment company that had started ailing before I became Director of the Institute!

I had received a lot of money for a grant, millions of shillings worth of research, sometime in between when I left the institute in 2007 and early in 2009. You see, I continued working on my research. So I was working on this research and they decided to take my computer. It was on the 27th of January 2009. It had important work that I had organized, plus there was a project that I was going to launch on 20th September, the same year 2009, and which had cost more than 800 million KES. I had to start all over again by contacting the funders and redoing some parts of the research.

But on a more personal level the people most affected were members of my family. At that time I had four children studying in the UK and then a number of them studying locally. Yes. In the universities and colleges and high school. Malakween was still young. He didn't know exactly what was going on but he ended up following the case very keenly. I had no resources and I had to make some adjustments. I had nothing to sell because they were holding my properties. If they had given me my properties I would have sold some of them to make sure my children finished school. One of my sons was in the UK doing his master's degree in wireless communication technology, and is currently working with Google. So he had to come home because I could not pay the fees. I was sponsoring him. He came home and then my daughter also came home. Then I had another son at the University of Southampton doing engineering. He was slightly affected and then he went into a temporary depression for some time and we had to manage that. He had to come home. I had my daughter who was in one of the schools. I had others who were finishing their secondary education and trying to find them a university placement. And so it interfered with what they were all doing. Yes, so even the payment of school fees was a problem. In fact, some of them had to be home-schooled. Yes. I could not manage to pay fees for some terms.

So it happened that I became a part-time teacher in mathematics and sciences, even of history and English at home. Even my daughter – her school was just outside the door but she couldn't attend. She had to register to do her "O" Level secondary education privately. Then she went to sit for them and still she passed very well. She was admitted to the university and now she is in her final year. You see my son, Malakween, also had to do partly home-based learning and he did very well. He did very well and it is because I was there with him. I told my children that this is one of the things that you go through in life and you must be prepared. You must be patient in life. You know, I said, there are two alternatives in these situations. Either you lose out in this world or you become strong and wait it out. Yes. I gave them various examples of people who have gone through challenges in life, some of them were politically instigated, some of them were not, and who decided to give up. You may give up at a time just when you are about to make a breakthrough. I told them life is full of challenges. But my son got a job, my other son is doing an apprenticeship in the UK, both my daughters got jobs and so people are moving on.

Two officers were at the gate and two were inside. Even at a murderer's home they don't go in with that much force! They searched everywhere, all my accounts. Nothing at all. Nothing at all. They finally left the house at around three or four o'clock in the afternoon. They were basically here for the whole day searching everywhere. I gave them some tea while they continued to search. Then I realized later on that they had broken the law. It was an illegal search. Then very close to one year after that, I was taken to court.

It was a big embarrassment and it was a lot of stress. Yes, I tell you – a lot of psychological stress. There was a friend of mine who was in charge of one of the institutions who went through the same circumstances as me. His experience was less traumatic but he couldn't stand it. He went into depression and he died one night. So it was very sad. Dr Cyrus Ndiritu who was the CEO of the Kenya Agricultural Research Institute from around 1989 until 2000. He had left the service and then he was going to take up a job in the Netherlands for some international agricultural body; I guess it was INSAR. He had already decided to go. So somebody within the system who didn't want him to go wrote a letter that said he was being investigated for swindling more than two billion KES, which belonged to some organization. They were trumped-up charges and so he ended up not getting the international position in the Netherlands and he remained doing a few things here in Kenya but I think that stress took a big toll on his mental health. One has to make every attempt at all times to be sane. Yes, because you have to as the head of the family. You have a responsibility to the children going to school. They must go to school; you have to pay school fees. You must feed them and you must clothe them. You and they are accustomed to a particular lifestyle. You are accustomed and then it is over all of a sudden. May I tell you that money is the source of all happiness and all evil. When there are no resources, you can't go on leave; you can't get basic things. You see, you find they have disconnected the power because you have not paid the bill. At times the power is disconnected since you have no money so even to charge the phones you must go to a neighbour or you must go to some other place to charge the phone.

They took everything, even what I inherited from my own parents. It couldn't have been acquired through corrupt practices and then they have raided my accounts where there is no money and then they have taken all certificates. We call them "MemoArts" … that means the Memorandum and Articles of Association, the certificates of registration of companies, any company, that was in my custody, whether or not I was associated with. Some of them I was just keeping for my relatives and friends. Yes. So I have had no access to those things until today.

I also realized during this period that some people are very weak and can be manipulated, or manipulative themselves, so that there are even close relatives who say, "Oh yah, we don't want to be associated with him" and so on, so they wanted to distance themselves from me. Then, there are other friends who used to call me, several times in a day, asking "Where are you? Let us meet," and when I left the Institute they disappeared. Yes. They disappeared but you see I'll not forget. Some abandon you. They don't stick with you. When you try to call them, they don't want to take your calls. Either they think that I want to ask them for money or I want to beg for something. They don't want to be seen associating with me. I met somebody recently and he said, "Oh, I have been looking for you all this time." I thought, what is it that you are after? My numbers have not changed; you could have called me. But then there were others who were not even directly associated with me and whenever I would see them, they were lovely and gracious. So I made new friendships. Yes, the initial impact was devastating but as you go along you realize this was not that important. You see, I would have killed myself because of this but here I am, and I want to thank, if not all, some members of the family who have been very supportive.

Then it was not until the 14th of July when I was called to go and finally collect my computer. So I went to pick up my computer and that is when they arrested me. They said, "We are taking you to court." I said, "You want to take me to court? Take me there right now. It is still early, take me. Go and charge me." They said, "No, no, you must sleep in the police station until the following day." I said, "Come on! *Kumbe!* [/alas!/]" And it turned out, while I was waiting inside there, they called both local and international media so when I exited the building I assumed the President was near because it had attracted so much attention!

Intermission

Koech wrote a letter to the Attorney General, documenting his concerns. This is an excerpt from that letter where he offers an explanation to the charges:

Complaint against the Kenya Anti-Corruption Commission ACC22/2009 and ACC1/2010

(Criminal Case Number 22 of 2009): The KEMRI/CDC Account

1. KEMRI has a number of organizations and institutions who support some research and operational activities of various types. These organizations operate independently and have independent accounts which are not subject to the control of KEMRI. Such organizations include but are not limited to Nagasaki University, Institute of Virological Research (IVR), ICAP, DNDi, Case Western/DVBD/KEMRI and African Medical Services Trust (AMSET). These organizations have been supporting research for a number of years and they have independent audit systems. AMSET has been supporting certain research and related activities in KEMRI since 1995. Its bank account only happened to have been maintained in the same bank as the KEMRI/CDC Account, the Standard Chartered Bank of Kenya Ltd.
2. The KEMRI/CDC operational account is maintained at the Kisumu Branch of the Standard Chartered Bank. This account is being serviced on a

reimbursement basis by the Kipande House Branch of KCB where all other accounts of the Institute are held.

3. Operational difficulties were noticed in the handling of activities being supported through the account in Kisumu. It was observed that some of the KEMRI/CDC activities are also in Nairobi and being serviced from the funds from Kisumu. This posed some logistical difficulties since the funds could either be withdrawn from the Kisumu account and the cash physically transported to Nairobi or other more secure mechanisms could be found. Since I had been a signatory to some accounts at the Standard Chartered Bank in Nairobi, it was found prudent to include my signature for the Kisumu account so that an accountant from KEMRI/CDC office (one Leonard) could be sent a cheque with one signature. The accountant could then ask me to accompany him to the bank where I could countersign the cheque before the cash could be released to the accountant. The accountant is not an employee of the Institute, but of CDC; hence he could not act as a signatory to the Kisumu account. This arrangement posed some difficulties because I had to be in Nairobi when the cheque for Nairobi operations was being sent from Kisumu. On occasions, the funds being required in Nairobi, which at times could run to more than KES three (3) million at a time, could not be supported by the balance in the account in Kisumu at the time of drawings. I could then borrow from the African Medical Services Trust (AMSET) account to which I had access in order enable the accountant to collect the cash required for the operations at KEMRI/CDC Nairobi. This was on the understanding that reconciliations of the accounts could be done later.
4. It was during these occasions that some funds were borrowed and in good faith from the KEMRI/CDC Account to AMSET account. As a matter of routine reporting, I informed my CDC colleagues and assured them that reconciliations and reversals could be made as soon as practicable. There was no evidence that the funds were deliberately diverted because if it were, I could not have made the effort myself to report on the same. But before reversals could be done, and for bank purposes, we had to regularize the transfers with the bank as bonafide.
5. The sums transferred were KES 800,000; KES 6,000,000 and KES 12,500,000. Initially, these figures could not be fully supported by documents and were simply treated as accounts receivable in our KEMRI books.
6. It is important to note that CDC does not have direct access to the account details being held at KEMRI. The CDC relies on the information received from the KEMRI authorities, or by their independent auditors. In this particular case, the report was made by me as a matter of course.
7. The funds transferred was spent in supporting the 28th African Health Sciences Congress in Durban, South Africa where more than 100 staff members of KEMRI participated. I am the President of the Congress and of KEMRI houses, the secretariat. We had also supported another meeting on the Forum for African Medical Editors (FAME) of which I am its Secretary. The funds were paid to travel agents, plus cash per diems for congress

participants. The Trust had supported previous congresses before in Egypt, Arusha, Nairobi, Kampala, and Ethiopia.

8. The Principal Funder of AMSET was informed of the borrowings and the Funder started making extra arrangements to remit the funds to cover the debit. The initial KES 800,000 was remitted to the KEMRI/CDC Account while the balance was being awaited. Since I had already left the Institute, the balance of these funds was received in July 2008 through the advocates of AMSET and arrangements for the reversals made for purpose of restoring the KEMRI/CDC Account. However, the completion of reversal was frustrated by the management for lack of cooperation. It formed a wall of inaccessibility even by itself to the extent that it has not been possible to regularize the account, yet the funds have all along been held in the account of AMSET's advocates. AMSET lawyers had been instructed to communicate with the Institute management on how the funds can be remitted to the relevant CDC account held at KEMRI.
9. It is important to note that while the funds to regularize the accounts at the Institute were received from the funders of AMSET in July 2008, the KACC officers, in blatant violation of the law and of my constitutional rights, raided my houses on 27 January 2009 and later my office on 2 February 2009 purportedly executing a warrant of search and seizure granted to them through a Kibera Miscellaneous Application Number 54 of 26 January 2009 and took some vital documents and a lap top containing sensitive scientific data. Six months later, on 14 July 2009, the same KACC officers came to my house and requested me to accompany them to their offices under the pretext of going to hand back my laptop. Shockingly, they arrested me outside their offices and in blatant violation of the law, compromised my line of defence by condemning me before local and international press which they had called for a press briefing, even before being charged in a court of law. I was remanded at the Kilimani Police Station until the following day (15 July 2009) when I was taken to court and charged.
10. AMSET was incorporated as a charitable trust in 1995 and has sponsored a number of successful research projects at KEMRI, the notable ones being:

    a) Approved Research Protocol Number 557: Dose Range Determination of Trioxolane KE091/ATX (Alphamir) for Efficacy, Safety and Tolerance in Individuals with Asymptomatic HIV-1 Infections in Kenya. The Principal Investigator for this study was Dr Juma Rashid.
    b) Approved Research Protocol Number 558: Determination of the Efficacy of Trioxolane (Arthromir) in the Management of Patients with Rheumatoid Arthritis. The Principal Investigator for this study was Dr Monique Wasunna.
    c) Approved Research Protocol Number 559: Laboratory and Clinical Evaluation of Therapeutic Potential of Trioxolane KE091/ATX in the Management of Acute Upper Airway Viral Infections in Kenya. This study was headed by Dr Jeremiah C. Muhwa.

11. Each principal investigator received directly from AMSET an honorarium of KES 100,000 per month during the period of the study. In addition, other investigators got sums ranging from KES 50,000 to KES 20,000 per month depending on the extent of their participation in the study. All the research material was sourced and disbursed by AMSET.
12. Before the clinical trials were undertaken, the background studies on the products had taken more than 14 years under the sponsorship of different donors at a cost of more than KES 150 million over the period. Some of the sponsors were Biochem Solutions, Inc. (USA) and Mirable, Inc. (USA). AMSET came in as a sponsor during the clinical trials stage with the support of both Biochem Solutions, Inc. and Mirable Inc.
13. These studies led to the development of two drugs trade named Alphamir for the treatment of HIV/AIDS and Arthromir for the treatment of Rheumatoid Arthritis. These were subsequently registered as drugs for specified functions by the Ministry of Health's Pharmacy and Poisons Board initially in 2001 and registration renewed in June 2006 under registration numbers 13945 (Arthromir Solution) and 13946 (Alphamir Solution). The application for registration was sponsored by Molecular Technologies Ltd, a company registered by the funders for this purpose. The continued monitoring of the efficacy of these products, as required by the Pharmacy & Poisons Board, has been frustrated by my absence from KEMRI.

(Criminal Case Number 1 of 2010): The KEMRI Retirement Benefits Scheme

1. The reasons behind this case do not address the real issues surrounding the custody and management of the pension contributions by members and the employer. The persons who made the adverse report did not discuss this issue with me, nor with the external auditors of the scheme, nor with the actuarial consultants. Picking records of contributions alone without an audit report does not amount to any meaningful conclusion. I made several attempts (both verbally and in writing) to advise the chairman on this issue, but he ignored my advice.
2. In order to understand the true situation, it may be necessary to briefly summarize the historical aspects of the scheme, from its inception. This summary is not new because records as well as the audit reports of the Controller & Auditor General together with Public Investment Committee (PIC) reports are available and are in the public domain:

1984–1996	Name of Scheme: KEMRI Staff Pension and Life Assurance Scheme. Contributions made to the Kenya National Assurance Company Limited (KNAC) to manage.

1996	KNAC went under receivership with more than KES 150 million (inclusive of interest) belonging to KEMRI staff members. Staff retiring or leaving the service of the Institute for whatever reason had not been paid.
1996	KEMRI engaged the services of an actuarial expert (Actuarial and Benefit Consultants Ltd, headed by a Mr. Leslie Okudo) to determine the true value of KEMRI's investment at the defunct KNAC.
1996	The actuarial consultant advises KEMRI to internally administer its own pay-outs to deserving cases because a new law was underway that would regulate pensions contribution and investments in the country. This law was to eventually usher in the Retirement Benefits Authority (RBA) Act.
1996–2001	KEMRI internally administered its own pension scheme while awaiting the new law to take effect. The administration was restricted to paying out those overdue benefits which would have otherwise been settled by KNAC. Since Exchequer funds could not cover the essential needs of the leavers, it was necessary at that time to secure extra funding from non-exchequer sources in order not to badly inconvenience retirees and other leavers.
2001	KEMRI Board of Management appointed Board of Trustees to develop Trust Deed and Rules for the new KEMRI Pension Fund in accordance with RBA Act and with the assistance of consultants. The Fund was a defined benefits. The KEMRI Pension Fund was formed and appointed Genesis Kenya Investment Management Limited and the Barclays Bank of Kenya Limited as the Fund Manager and Custodian respectively. The Fund also appointed Actuarial and Benefit Consultants Ltd and Anduuru & Co., CPA, as Actuarial Service Providers and Auditors respectively.
2001–2004	Payment of terminal benefits to the leavers (those officers on permanent and pensionable service leaving the service of the Institute for whatever reason) continued and pension contributions to the Custodian began as per the arrangement reached between the Fund Manager and the Board of Trustees. Audit of the Fund shifted from Controller & Auditor General to the appointed external auditors. The signed audit reports are available at RBA and copies are in the relevant files. Extracts of the relevant portions of the audit reports are attached.

2004	Actuarial Report detailing individual member contributions as well as the net assets of the Fund is presented to the Board of Trustees. Actuarial Report put the net assets of the Fund as of 30 June 2004 at KES 321 million. Out of this, KES 173 million was owed to the Fund by KNAC, and KES 131 million is owed by the Employer (KEMRI) due to under-contributions, while the balance of KES 17 million is held in a reserve account at the bank or invested with the Custodian. It is important to note that during the same year, a total of about KES 124 million was paid out as overdue benefit claims to leavers. A new Board of Trustees was put in place following the changes in the membership of the KEMRI Board of Management. Agreement was reached whereby the KEMRI Pension Fund (as a defined benefits scheme) was converted to KEMRI Retirement Benefits Scheme (as a defined contribution scheme). The new Scheme was registered with the RBA in 2005. The consultants advised of this change because the defined contribution scheme is predictable, but less burdensome to the employer and easy to manage.
2004–2007	Process of actual conversion from the Fund to the Scheme takes place. As of July 2007, the external audits for the years 2001/2002 to 2004/2005 had been completed by the external auditors and reports submitted to the relevant authorities.

3. On the basis of the foregoing, it is irresponsible to make claims of mismanagement of the scheme. The information given to the Inspection Team and which was later forwarded to KACC officials and which formed the charges against me, was incomplete, selective and deliberate in order to depict my person as an incompetent secretary to the Board of Trustees or to cause aspersions to the contributors. If the intention was genuine, then my contribution to the report would have been sought so that I could make any clarification as deemed necessary.
4. There is also the begging question: How come the auditors and actuarial service providers were not consulted by the Inspection Team? It is clear that they were avoiding the truth. Instead, the said Inspection Team went ahead to investigate transactions of accounts totally unrelated to the scheme.
5. I hold the belief that all along, the report which was relied upon by KACC investigators has been suspect and ill-intentioned. Procedures have been violated right from the beginning. If one looks at the selection of the Inspection Team as well as all other players in this matter, one cannot avoid drawing a conclusion on a conspiracy among the players.

This is the response from the Attorney General to Koech's letter. He notes that the response came exactly two years and four days after he sent this letter.

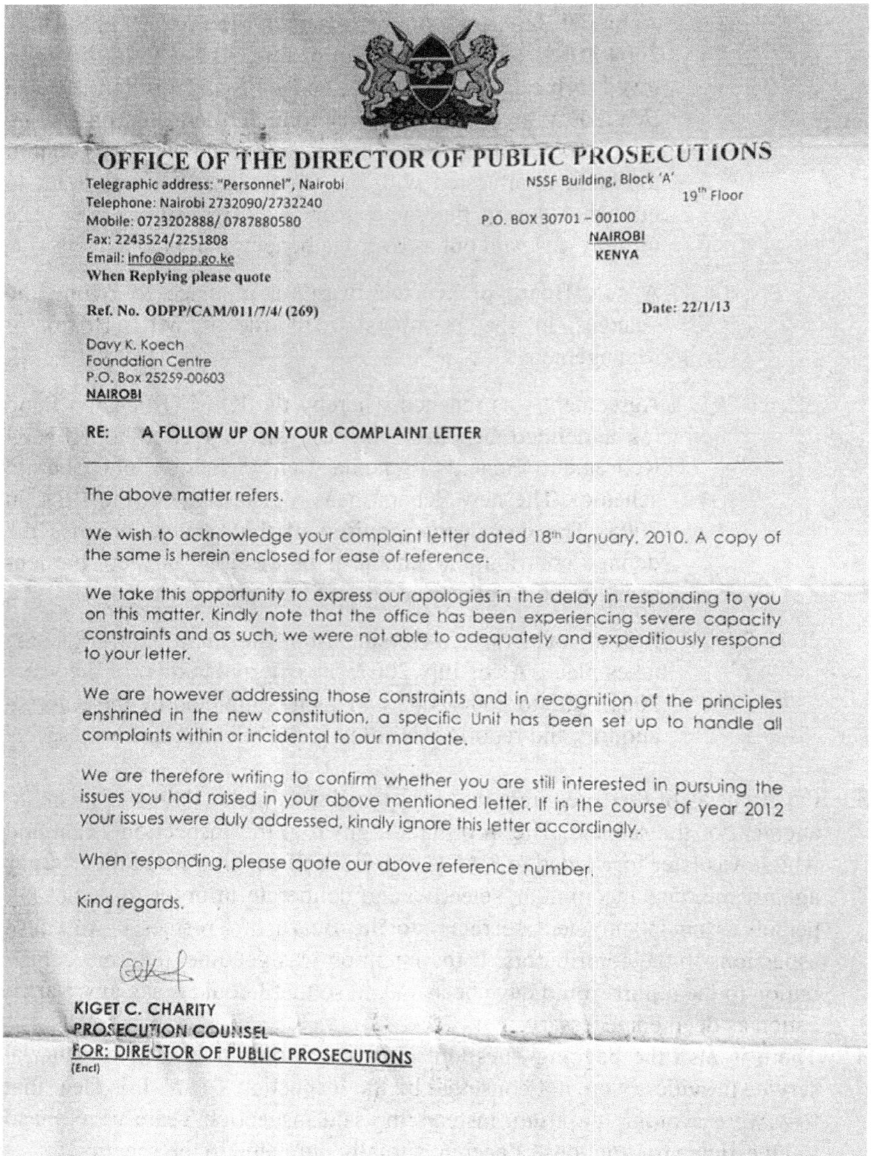

OFFICE OF THE DIRECTOR OF PUBLIC PROSECUTIONS

Telegraphic address: "Personnel", Nairobi
Telephone: Nairobi 2732090/2732240
Mobile: 0723202888/ 0787880580
Fax: 2243524/2251808
Email: info@odpp.go.ke
When Replying please quote

NSSF Building, Block 'A'
19th Floor
P.O. BOX 30701 – 00100
NAIROBI
KENYA

Ref. No. ODPP/CAM/011/7/4/ (269)

Date: 22/1/13

Davy K. Koech
Foundation Centre
P.O. Box 25259-00603
NAIROBI

RE: A FOLLOW UP ON YOUR COMPLAINT LETTER

The above matter refers.

We wish to acknowledge your complaint letter dated 18th January, 2010. A copy of the same is herein enclosed for ease of reference.

We take this opportunity to express our apologies in the delay in responding to you on this matter. Kindly note that the office has been experiencing severe capacity constraints and as such, we were not able to adequately and expeditiously respond to your letter.

We are however addressing those constraints and in recognition of the principles enshrined in the new constitution, a specific Unit has been set up to handle all complaints within or incidental to our mandate.

We are therefore writing to confirm whether you are still interested in pursuing the issues you had raised in your above mentioned letter. If in the course of year 2012 your issues were duly addressed, kindly ignore this letter accordingly.

When responding, please quote our above reference number.

Kind regards.

KIGET C. CHARITY
PROSECUTION COUNSEL
FOR: DIRECTOR OF PUBLIC PROSECUTIONS
(Encl)

Figure 26.1 Attorney General's letter of response.

Notes

1 Davy Koech adds December 2017: As of now, this is where money and political patronage, rather than ethics speak, and where politicians massacre each other. This is also an office where the "chosen" senior public officials spend the rest of their retirement period.

2 Between 2007 and when this goes to press (2018), Koech had received no income or salary from KEMRI.

27 The arrest

When they were arresting me they had told me, "You can come and collect your computer." This was 14th July, six months after they had seized my computer in my home. So when I went to their offices to collect my laptop they kept on tossing me around, yes, tossing me around at their offices. I don't know whether you know Panafric Hotel? In downtown Nairobi there is Kenyatta Avenue and there is a road, Valley Road, as you climb towards Hurlingham. They are just there, Integrity Centre. They are still there until this day. Yes. So when I went there to collect the computer they were purposely delaying in returning to me.

You see they were delaying and so I asked, "What is this? Why is there a delay?" Because they called me to come in the morning so I was there at around 8 or 8:30 am. Then at around 11 o'clock I said, "What is going on?" They said, "We are detaining you. We are putting you under arrest so that you will go to court tomorrow." I looked at my watch. It was around 11 o'clock. I told them, "Is this what you called me for? If you are actually putting me under arrest can you please take me to court now, not to a police station," because they said we are taking you to Kilimani Police Station. I said, "If you want to take me to court why don't you take me now? Why haven't you arranged with the court that you take me to court now and charge me?" So they said no. So that's the time I also called my lawyer. Then when we were leaving the building to go to the police station, you see, there were both local and international press waiting outside the Integrity Centre. Initially, I thought somebody very big like the President was visiting some of the offices. They were there the moment I exited the revolving doors – cameramen everywhere! Oh my God! They were looking at me so in obedience to the law I entered the vehicle, and though the press were trying to talk to me, I kept quiet.

The EACC had issued a statement earlier on saying why they were charging me. They had to do it openly, to make a show of it, to prove to the public that they are doing something about corruption. You see because people were saying that the agency was a toothless bulldog, not doing anything, not arresting anyone. I said okay if that is what they want, let them proceed but some of my rights were actually violated in the process. Yes, some of my very basic rights which is why I took them to court later the following year.

They did not handcuff me. I walked out with my laptop. They claimed later that they had arrested me at home. That did not make any sense at all. I was put into an unmarked car. It was a small car. One of the weirdest things that occurred … I was not armed and it is not like they arrested me running away so why put me in the middle of a vehicle between two officers in this small car, plus more officers in the front, treating me like I am some dangerous criminal? I saw it as a comedy. I told them, if you request that I come to court, I would come. These antics are not necessary. You see. Even if you want me to go to prison, because I am obedient to the law, I will come. Yes. So that is the time I was taken to Kilimani Police Station.

They fingerprinted me and took the photographs in the EACC office when they told me they were arresting me. So they had processed me. I was just being taken to the jail to be locked in. At the police station they said, "Take care of this criminal until further notice. If we don't come to collect him, continue keeping him." At the police station they recognized me and so at the front desk they were trying to figure out where to place me. Inside is a cell for all the ladies and there are cells for men. But just behind the corner they had another space, a large space, where there was a certain young boy who was found loitering in the streets. They don't even know the identity of this boy, some unknown kid who I think was about six or seven years old. So I was told to share the space with this boy. I can laugh about it now but actually it was very bad.

That same evening my family came to see me; they brought me some food. When you want to go to the bathroom, you are taken to a room, and when you are peeing the person is still waiting for you, watching. I said to him, "There is nowhere I am going." I was telling the fellow, "You know, there is nowhere in this place for me to go so why even bother to come and watch me like this?" So the fellow said to me, "When people are after you, they can even kill you in here." So a family member came with a truck and put it outside the police station directly. Yes, he parked it at the station, left with the keys, and walked away. Yes, then he returned at night to sleep in the vehicle in the event I was taken away at night. At least he would be a witness and could testify that he saw me being taken away because at times people have been taken away and then they disappear. It was during a very bad period in Kenya.

When I was at Kilimani Police Station I told these police officers,

> Since you have already prepared a charge sheet and this is a bailable offence, it is not murder, you should have made arrangements for me to be in court so I can make an arrangement for bail to get out. You should have arranged that from here you take me directly to court. Yes. I have done nothing. Why subject me to this? I can't understand.

The officers said, "Those are the orders." At the police station when I was booked in I was told there was nowhere even to sit, there was no chair, there was *nini* [/this thing/] so I had to sit down on the floor. I would stand until I was tired then I would have to sit down on the floor. Then my officers from KEMRI came to see me, yes about 100 of them came when they heard I was at the police station. They were queuing to see me until they allowed me to address them. Yes. My lawyer was also there and so in the evening I ate something. I didn't even sleep. I was just seated now on the edge of this very tiny three-foot blanket that was reserved for this little kid because he could not go to an actual police cell. They could not take me in into the darkroom either. It is so dark that you don't even know whether you are with somebody else inside. It is just a totally dark room so you know you don't know who is there.

Even when I try to look back until today, I ask myself – what is it that I really did to deserve what I have gone through? Even murderers have not been subjected to these situations. Even real thieves have been treated more humanely. In the morning I was finally taken to court where I was formally charged and then I denied the charges. They accused me of taking government property into my own personal use.

So usually people who have been charged with similar offences are required to give about 50,000 KES for bail. Maybe 40,000 KES, but no more than 100,000 KES. The maximum amount of money a person had been required to pay as bail in this country was 400,000 KES, which was given to one of the wealthiest Kenyans, Chris Kirubi. You may have heard of him? Yes, he has a coffee estate towards Thika. In fact, it has a lake within it called Lake Kirubi. He is a flamboyant person and he had been taken to court because they said he misused funds from Uchumu Supermarkets. He was Chairman and then the markets ended up being closed down because of mismanagement and some things of fraudulent nature. He had been accused for some irregularity bordering on corruption. He was only required to pay 400,000 KES bail, and which case was eventually dismissed. For me? One million KES! I said, "Do they want me to stay here forever?" And they know by this time that I am not getting a salary and I have nothing to sell because they have seized my assets. You see. Then, in the following case that appeared the following year they asked for two million KES as bail. Where do they think I am going to get this money? I think the plan was to keep me locked in jail because they knew that I would have difficulties finding this money!

So I spent one night in the holding cell. One night and then when I went to court they said if I failed to pay one million KES bail I would not go back to the police station because from there I became the property of the state so they would take me to an actual prison, which I think was somewhere in the industrial area. Yes. We got the million KES, paid, and then I was out at around three o'clock in the afternoon. Yes. So I came home and we celebrated. Yes. That is it.

This was in 2009 and then in January 2010 I was charged again, but this time, it was with some of my former senior colleagues. That time I told the investigators, "I am not coming for you to take me in, I am sorry. Let us meet in court." Yes. I said let's meet in court. On that day I slept away at someone else's house. I dismantled my phones because they could track me through the GPS on the phone and I went to sleep in my friend's place. I would not go through that again. Yes and then I said, "Farouk, do you know you will not get me even if you try to, you will not get me." Yes. I took my battery out of my mobile. I dismantled my phones so whenever I needed to make a call, I used a friend's phone.

I am being punished by not receiving my salary. I am being punished in court. So a friend who trained in the US, he is a human rights lawyer, stated that whatever had been done to me was just totally immoral and unconstitutional. It was out of the ordinary. Just totally inhumane. You cannot take a person to court, hold everything of his, and then decide to ease him out of his employment! So as a result, I am taking KEMRI to court. But I didn't want to take any action against the Institute because of the love I had for it. How can you go and destroy the baby that you really tried to bring up? So I really tried to be patient and allow the justice system to do its work. Until today my things are still there in the KEMRI office. No one wants to touch it. And I have still not handed over some of the critical things. Yes. Ten years down the line, it is coming to 11 years now, and I have not handed over the office officially.

Yes. I even took some people to court and then a warrant of arrest was issued against the investigating officers. Yes, it is messy. There is a constitutional petition application that I made to the court and then there is another case where I took KEMRI to court. You see, with that one at the court the judge said, "Koech has got a case so he may proceed to make his claims on the Institute." I have been going to court. Even for mention. You see we have what is called mention and hearing. For mention you must appear so they can see that you are around. And then your bond is extended. You are still under the court's jurisdiction. Sometimes you do not know when you will be called. You may not even have time to make official travel plans, say if you want to attend a conference, it is the timing that is difficult to negotiate. They never prevented me from leaving the country; they did not take my passport, no, they did not do that.

You see the matter is no longer with the commission. It is directly under the Director of Public Prosecutions. The investigating authority was the commission with the assistance of the police. That is the standard procedure and then from there, when they have gathered all their documentation and they think they have a sufficient case that can be sustained, they turn it over to the Director of Public Prosecutions. Yes. This is totally different body whose mandate is only to prosecute criminal cases. Before it used to fall under the Attorney General but with the new constitution those powers have been separated. The Attorney General becomes the legal advisor to the state and is no longer involved in prosecution cases. Yes, matters of law, matters of the interpretation of law, formulation of laws, and then the interpretation of those when parliament has passed them and when the President had given assent. But as it is now, the Director of Public Prosecutions is a separate, independent body. They are presented with the charges and he would evaluate the evidence before deciding whether or not the matter can be sustained in court.

It so happened that at the particular time when my matter was being taken forward, such consideration did not occur. It was really bad. Yes. So if it had been up to the Director of Public Prosecutions to examine it, he would have refused to proceed because at times he has said the evidence is not sustainable. Yes, there is not a strong enough case. But when they started this, they were in a rush. There was a reason for that: they were concerned for the security of the jobs at the anti-corruption commission. They had not taken any prominent person to court and I was an opportunity for them. The anti-corruption was about to be disbanded. Yes. I think they were stepping on too many toes so in fact the commissioners were sent home. They left. They were trying to look for a big fish to charge on corruption but they found a very small one in the process.

You cannot go looking for politicians to assist you in these situations because it involves a lot of travelling. If I included a lot of politics into it, one, it was going to be expensive. Yes. It involves a lot of money but, two, these politicians also lie to you. I know this because I have dealt with them. I know exactly who can be good and who can be bad. So I said, why should I have to spend the resources that I don't have? But they have dragged me through the mud all the way through. I have asked them, "What is it that you need? Do you require some money and then I give you what you need then I go my way?" I don't want to waste the rest of my useful life trying to prove my innocence in court. You see? Yes. I feel the situation might be requiring money so that this can go away but I have refused. When I left the office Moi was very angry. He even called Kibaki (then President) himself to ask him, "Where is Koech?" Kibaki then called me and he told me why don't you go back to work? Yes.

It is a total betrayal. Is it that I did something that is totally, totally wrong? And I was telling somebody, if really they wanted to jail me, I would have done my time by now and been released from jail. I would have done my term because they wouldn't jail me for more than three years. If they had just jailed me, I would be free by now. Why keep us in suspense for ten years now?

Intermission

The Ethics and Anti-Corruption Commission released this press release the day they arrested Koech.

KENYA ANTI-CORRUPTION COMMISSION

KENYA ANTI-CORRUPTION COMMISSION
INTEGRITY CENTRE
(Valley Rd./Milimani Rd. Junction)
P.O. Box 61130
00200 - NAIROBI, Kenya

When replying please quote:

Tel.: 254 (020) 2717318/310722
Fax: 254 (020) 2719757
Email: kacc@integrity.go.ke
Website: www.kacc.go.ke

PRESS RELEASE

KACC ARRESTS DAVID KOECH FORMER DIRECTOR OF KEMRI TO FACE CORRUPTION RELATED CHARGES.

CHIEF NEWS EDITOR

Former Director of Kenya Medical Research Institute (KEMRI) Mr. David Kiprotich KOECH was this morning arrested by the Kenya Anti-Corruption Commission investigation Officer and will be taken to the Anti-Corruption court at the **Nairobi High Court at 9am on Wednesday 15th July 2009** to face charges of abuse of office contrary to Section 45(1) as read with Section 48 of the Anti-Corruption and Economic Crimes Act, 2003 and also Fraudulent acquisition of public property contrary to Section 45(1)(a) as Read with Section 48 of the Anti-Corruption and Economic Crimes Act, 2003.

Please find attached the charge sheets for ease of reference.

The Commission would appreciate if you can publicize this press release and highlight the court proceedings tomorrow at the Nairobi law courts.

Your continued support in publishing and broadcasting these cases is highly appreciated and goes a long way in the prevention of corruption.

The Commission does not prosecute criminal cases only the Attorney General does.

Thank you,

Nicholas M. Simani
PRINCIPAL PUBLIC RELATIONS AND PROTOCOL OFFICER

14th July 2009

Figure 27.1 KACC/EACC press release: Koech arrested.

They have also posted the official charge sheet (shared here).

THE KENYA POLICE
CHARGE SHEET

POLICE CASE NO. ……………

DATE TO COURT…………………
O.B.NO………
COURT FILE NO: …………………

Christian names in full or names	Surname or Fathers Name	Identity	Sex	Nationality	Age	Address
1. DAVY KIPROTICH	KOECH		M	KENYAN	ADULT	PO BOX 25259 00603 NAIROBI

CHARGE COUNT I	FRAUDULENT ACQUISITION OF PUBLIC PROPERTY CONTRARY TO SECTION 45(1)(a) AS READ WITH SECTION 48 OF THE ANTI-CORRUPTION AND ECONOMIC CRIMES ACT NO. 3 OF 2003				
PARTICULARS OF OFFENCE (See Second Schedule of CPC.)	DAVY KIPROTICH KOECH On 17th day of August 2006 at Nairobi within Nairobi Area Province, fraudulently acquired public property, to wit, the sum of Kshs 800,000 belonging to the Kenya Medical Research Institute (KEMRI). (FOR OTHER COUNTS, SEE ATTACHED SHEET)				
If Accused Arrested	Date of Arrest	Without/With Warrant	Date App. to Court.	Bond or Bail And Amount	Is Application for Summons to issue
Remanded or Adjourned					
Complainant and Address	Republic of Kenya through Kenya Anti Corruption Commission				
Witnesses	1. Dr. Hezron Nyangito and 10 others				
Sentence Court and date	…………………………………………………… CHIEF MAGISTRATE'S COURT NAIROBI…………If fine paid…………				

………………………………………………………

For *Officer in charge Kilimani Police Station*

1

Figure 27.2 Charge Sheet for Koech.

POLICE 5

INVESTIGATORS ACTION	Date	Time	Initials of recording Officer
Accused informed of Charge,			
Fingerprints Taken by			
Fingerprints to Bureau			
Fingerprints from Bureau			
Completed certificate of previous convictions to Bureau			
First Information and progress Report to Director KACA			
Final report to Director KACA			
Charge Register Completed and case closed			
.. ..			
.. ..			
.. ..			
.. ..			
.. ..			
.. ..			

2. ANTECEDENTS OF ACCUSED (As known to Investigating Officer)

3. BRIEF CIRCUMSTANCES OF CASE (Evidence of Arrest, etc.)

2

Figure 27.2 Continued.

ALTERNATIVE TO COUNT ONE

ABUSE OF OFFICE CONTRARY TO SECTION 46 AS READ WITH SECTION 48 OF THE ANTI-CORRUPTION AND ECONOMIC CRIMES ACT, NO. 3 OF 2003

PARTICULARS OF OFFENCE

DAVY KIPROTICH KOECH: On 16th day of August 2006 at Nairobi within Nairobi Area Province, being the Director of Kenya Medical Research Institute (KEMRI), used his office to improperly confer a benefit upon himself by transferring a sum of Kshs 800,000 belonging to the said KEMRI, from account number 01020-985421-00 held at Standard Chartered Bank (K) Ltd, Kisumu Branch in the name of KEMRI Centre for Vector Biology and Control Research (CVBCR) to account number 01020-690826-00 held at Standard Chartered Bank (K) Ltd, Yaya Centre Branch in the name of African Medical Services Trust (AMSET) that was controlled and operated by himself.

COUNT TWO

FRAUDULENT ACQUISITION OF PUBLIC PROPERTY CONTRARY TO SECTION 45(1)(a) AS READ WITH SECTION 48 OF THE ANTI-CORRUPTION AND ECONOMIC CRIMES ACT NO. 3 OF 2003

PARTICULARS OF OFFENCE

DAVY KIPROTICH KOECH: On 5th day of December 2006 at Nairobi within Nairobi Area Province, fraudulently acquired public property, to wit, the sum of Kshs 6,000,000 belonging to the Kenya Medical Research Institute (KEMRI).

ALTERNATIVE TO COUNT TWO

ABUSE OF OFFICE CONTRARY TO SECTION 46 AS READ WITH SECTION 48 OF THE ANTI-CORRUPTION AND ECONOMIC CRIMES ACT, NO. 3 OF 2003

PARTICULARS OF OFFENCE

DAVY KIPROTICH KOECH: On or about 4th day of December 2006 at Nairobi within Nairobi Area Province, being the Director of Kenya Medical Research Institute (KEMRI), used his office to improperly confer a benefit upon himself by transferring a sum of Kshs 6,000,000 belonging to the said KEMRI, from account number 01020-985421-00 held at Standard Chartered Bank (K) Ltd, Kisumu Branch in the name of KEMRI Centre for Vector Biology and Control Research

P.T.O

Figure 27.2 Continued.

(CVBCR) to account number 01020-690826-00 held at Standard Chartered Bank (K) Ltd, Yaya Centre Branch in the name of African Medical Services Trust (AMSET) that was controlled and operated by himself.

COUNT THREE

FRAUDULENT ACQUISITION OF PUBLIC PROPERTY CONTRARY TO SECTION 45(1)(a) AS READ WITH SECTION 48 OF THE ANTI-CORRUPTION AND ECONOMIC CRIMES ACT NO. 3 OF 2003

PARTICULARS OF OFFENCE
DAVY KIPROTICH KOECH: On 13th day of December 2006 at Nairobi within Nairobi Area Province, fraudulently acquired public property, to wit, the sum of Kshs 12,500,000 belonging to the Kenya Medical Research Institute (KEMRI).

ALTERNATIVE TO COUNT THREE

ABUSE OF OFFICE CONTRARY TO SECTION 46 AS READ WITH SECTION 48 OF THE ANTI-CORRUPTION AND ECONOMIC CRIMES ACT, NO. 3 OF 2003

PARTICULARS OF OFFENCE
DAVY KIPROTICH KOECH: On 13th day of December 2006 at Nairobi within Nairobi Area Province, being the Director of Kenya Medical Research Institute (KEMRI), used his office to improperly confer a benefit upon himself by transferring a sum of Kshs 12,500,000 belonging to the said KEMRI, from account number 01020-985421-00 held at Standard Chartered Bank (K) Ltd, Kisumu Branch in the name of KEMRI Centre for Vector Biology and Control Research (CVBCR) to account number 01020-690826-00 held at Standard Chartered Bank (K) Ltd, Yaya Centre Branch in the name of African Medical Services Trust (AMSET) that was controlled and operated by himself.

....

Officer in charge Kilimani Police Station

4

Figure 27.2 Continued.

28 Corporate executive

When I was younger I was a little bit fidgety. You see I was restless. At times, I would reflect that I had finished my research. I cannot go on drinking endlessly in the evening and expect to be alert in the morning. I can't do that. I can't go to some entertainment spots daily. I had to do something rewarding. My life in Nairobi after school started in Dandora, that is where I lived. Then I moved to Kariobangi and Huruma, all in the Eastern part of Nairobi, called Eastlands, where many Nairobians live. The area also houses a major dumpsite. A lot of birds congregate around the trash. Dandora is also close to where our sewage disposal is, with the big oxidation ponds, and so it smells bad all the time. Then from there I moved over to Kariobangi which was a nice place, a better area, and then from Kariobangi I moved to a place called Huruma Estate. Then from Huruma Estate I crossed over the Atlantic! I used to jokingly call the Uhuru Highway the Atlantic. So I crossed the Atlantic around 1974 or 1975, and since then I started living on this side. I spent probably two years on the other side of the city, hopping from one living unit to another one because I felt uncomfortable.

So I moved this way and eventually ten years down the line I was in Lavington. Yes. So when I was there in Eastlands I recognized something. I saw the disposal of raw sewage. First it is gathered into big collecting tanks, like these big oil tanks. Those big tanks have to be detoxified first through boiling so they have to heat the tank until a certain temperature and then they release the sludge into the oxidation pond. There the sludge is exposed to the atmosphere and so on. Then I realized one day, sometime around 1983, when I was with one the city engineers and he said, "You know to burn this, it takes a lot of time and money." It was approximately 700,000 KES of diesel every month to burn the raw sewage sludge and then after burning it is released into the oxidation pond. I thought about the chemistry of it and I realized the amount of methane that was being released. I asked this guy if it wasn't possible to use the naturally produced methane gas being released to burn the sewage? If they did this, they would save the money on diesel. He said, "I think you are right, but how can we do it?" I suggested he put out a tender for this sort of work. So surprisingly he put up a tender. I made a proposal and I said this is what is going to happen. I approached another friend of mine with whom I was working and suggested we work on this project together. So we tendered for that project. We did the chemistry very well, we did the energy transformation, and conversion of energy, and so on and it made a lot of sense. The raw sludge just like here, it bubbles up and you tap the methane. You tap the gas into the cylinders, the cylinders now will come and burn the sewage, and you don't need to use the diesel. The only thing left to do was find out how to empty the very big drums. The sludge had turned almost cement like. We had to have people actually remove the sediment which was very, very hard inside the tanks so it took us quite a while to get it set up. And we succeeded and I made some money and so I made a small amount of profit that I put down as a deposit for my first house in Lavington. Yes.

I formed a new company to do that kind of work and I am not alone, but I worked with a friend. It worked very well and then we looked for other opportunities. In fact, that system is still working. So I was involved in so many activities that were not routine. Yes. Another business of mine, with a different partner and in a different setting, was in the Port of Mombasa. One of the largest cruise ships then, and I think even now, is Queen Elizabeth II. It used to come to Mombasa but the Likoni channel was full of silt so it could not even sail through to the harbour. Big boats had to go to pick people up and transfer them to the mainland because of the silt. So there was a company that had been doing the dredging of the channel and we knew it was coming up for sale. We bought up the company for nothing. We bought the company cheaply. So that company has cleared the whole of the Port of Mombasa. Yes. It is now a lot deeper so that the big ships can come in. Yes. So this is why one of my businesses was dredging. Then in the process I was given a contract for these ferries, which you must have used, from the mainland to Mombasa Island to the South Coast. These ferries were getting old so now I think we supplied two of them. Yes, after the dredging of the channel they saw that we were an efficient company so they asked us to supply ferries. I had two very good technical people that worked with me.

These are very big businesses. Yes. But then eventually one of these businesses ended up burning my fingers! Which was because of my association with another partner, who was a friend but also a semi-politician. We were going to put up a whole estate with a purchaser finance arrangement with some of the government institutions like the National Social Security Fund. He became a full-time politician eventually. In the process he was involved with YK' 92, which was the youth movement we have discussed. So this flamboyant friend of mine was involved as the Chairman and I was the one laying down strategy, because I was a public servant and I was not supposed to be actively involved in politics. So he and I got involved in a project that is on your way to the airport, in South B. Yes. We had a house financing scheme for our National Social Security Fund staff and it was a very nice project. It was a very nice estate with more than 600 units. It included around 200 maisonettes, another 200 two-bedroomed flats, another 200 three-bedroomed flats, plus a clinic or small hospital; and a school. Yes.

It was all comprehensive and it was going on very well but one weekend after the elections were over I told my friend, "Listen, can you stop politicking and do some business?" But he couldn't listen. He said, "Me and Moi, we are one." You have delivered him back to power so you think he is going to need you after this. So we started arguing with him one weekend. I think there was a meeting so some politicians were making a declaration. So he went against Moi and the others. He made a statement that counteracted those politicians and then it was caught up in the news. Then when I was in State House on a Monday morning they said this fellow Jirongo is finished. They went in and ganged up on this fellow so when I was there I told him, "You are now done." I suggested that he make a statement saying that he was quoted out of context by the press. He said, "How can I do that?" And I said, "With such stupidity you cannot be a politician!" You need to learn very fast but he should have denied it. I further told him to threaten to sue the newspapers for misquoting him. He learned from this but we were already burnt and our business ventures suffered.

This group of powerful politicians from the Rift Valley had gone to see the President and said this person is very bad. They reported to Moi that he had even wired some money to some South African Bank, and that he wanted to overthrow Moi's government. What a lie! They knew that he was powerful and then Moi called me. Yes, because Moi knew I was in business with this fellow. Moi was the one who assisted us. He sort of helped us, and of course he benefited. There is a token of appreciation for this sort of thing. So he called me one evening when I was taking dinner at Yaya Centre. He said, "I am now finishing your friend." I asked him, "But why?" He said, "You know he has done this but I am only telling you so you can *ng'abal*." This is in our local language. *Ng'abal*, in Kiswahili it says *kaa kando* [/evade/], but in English it just means step aside so that you make sure the blood does not spill on you when we are hitting him. I said, "You know that I am a co-director with this guy so why can't you give us some time and let us finish this project?" He said, "We have found out where to hit him. This is the only public project he is involved in so we must terminate this project." And sure enough they terminated the project and then they made us suffer when they took us to court. They stopped the project and then I had even put in some money from my two properties in Lavington, hoping that I was going to make some money but I lost it in the process. I told him but you are finishing me! So eventually they made up recommendations for him to be disciplined and my friend was told to keep quiet.

29 Faith

My mother converted to Christianity when I was very young. She became a church elder and she was the one who helped bring Christianity to our village and helped establish a church under a tree. So at that time we were being told that to become Christian, you must get a name that is also "Christian", basically a foreign name. So she called herself Hellen, and then the wife of arap Mitei, that is my father. So you must have a name to be baptized with.

Our first interactions in the village with Christianity were through the mobile clinics; they would come on certain particular days of the month. These were missionaries from a missionary hospital. They used to come every so often in a month. On particular days … if one of us had a cough, we would go there. We would line up and then we are given some *dawa* [/medicine/]. We just go. Then there was no proper clinic or dispensary … besides, of course, the government hospital in Kericho but that was too far for us to travel to. No, it was basically missionaries who provided medical care. That was why we adopted a particular line of faith. Yes, we adopted the ways of the African Gospel Church.

When I was in school I loved religion. I loved to pray. When I was in secondary school, at Kericho High School, I was a leader of the Christian Union and then I realized that the role of leader of a Christian Union was not totally my role. I recognized that there are "dos and don'ts" if you are a religious leader. You must live in certain ways, very upright. I realized that this path is slippery. I saw it ahead of time that it is a slippery path for me to follow. So I identified a friend of mine and I told him,

> I have seen that you are capable of carrying on the mantle from me so from now on I want to pray and I want to give you this mantle because I have seen the route which I am likely to take is going to embarrass me. And I can see that you are more faithful, more upright and so I now charge you with the responsibility of leading the student Christian Union and beyond.

True enough that person eventually became the Bishop, the head of the Deliverance Church in Kenya, and retired recently. Yes, Bishop William Tuimising. And he is not afraid to also tell this story. A few years ago when we were celebrating 40 years of our secondary school in Kericho, I was invited as the chief guest and Bishop Tuimising was the preacher for the day. We had to remind the meeting about the tree under which I gave my mantle of this Christian leadership to him in 1967, yes. So I gave it to him and sure enough he took it up without any hesitation until now. Yes.

Even at my house we have opened to persons who have come to pray while they are preparing to establish their own individual Christian ministries. We have raised a lot of ministries. We have not denied anyone. There was a room which we had set aside in case you want to come and pray in the house. That is why you see in the photographs mama (his wife) in the church praying, even until today. She is a writer. Yes, she's written quite a number of things related to religion and the Christian ministry. So that is what she does.

As an individual I have been through that but over time I have recognized that there is the presence of a being that is greater than us, or a power beyond our selves, that is greater than our own powers. We can attribute events to this power because I have witnessed it myself on various occasions. It so happens that in most of the faiths if something happens which you cannot explain, you can say this could be witchcraft. Another one it is this, another one it is that but to me I recognize the presence of a force greater than our own individual force. I tend to be a little more spiritual rather than religious because being spiritual and being religious are two different things. There is a force greater than our own. But religion is not binding me, so in as much as I can profess being a Christian, I tend to recognize the spiritual role in myself rather than that, which is demanded by the Christian faith. I have realized that various faiths, various denominations within the Christian faith, have their own way of doing things and they have a lot of fights among themselves. At the end of it there is only one Supreme Being. Being a religious person you must belong to a particular religion that has got rules, the dos and the don'ts. Catholics have one way of doing it, the Protestant churches another, and then there are so many splits within the Christian faith. There are so many orders and so on. I ask myself, why try to follow this so long as you recognize that there is one Supreme Being? Call it whatever you like, but there is no religion without a god. You see. How you practice or pray to that god is up to you.

We tend to, for the purposes of association, say, I go to this particular church. Yes. I go to this particular church to hear the message. I used to be a frequent goer to one of our churches in Nairobi until one day, I think it was about 2009 when I was having my own problems with work. I think it was 2009 when my matters in court were at its height. At that time I remember on a Saturday in the local press a story was carried, because I think I had been in court on the Friday or something like that. I think it was on a Friday but the story came out either on Saturday or on Friday afternoon, one of the days. So when I was in church on that Sunday the senior pastor, who is actually the administrative head or the religious head of the church, was away and one of the lay elders of the church was asked to lead the services. And during the prayers, he said, "Let us pray" and in his prayer he asked God to punish all corrupt people, and so on, and he continues on and on about corrupt people and then, "Amen". I said I am not going to say amen! I am sorry. You see I came here to church with the belief and hope that I am going to be prayed for. I am going to receive some strength. You see, in order to fight my battles I needed strength from my faith. You see, some people have been hanged for the sins they never committed so that is why people pray to God, to this Supreme Being, to intervene so that justice can be done.

But this lay preacher was not interested in justice. So long as you have been mentioned in the news, you should be taken out from society! Yet there is a place where even sinners are welcomed, to be prayed for and they get delivered into the light. So after the service, I walked out and I have never returned. Yes, I have never gone back. I went recently but only for a funeral service for a friend of mine because he used to worship also in that church. I met with senior pastor some time ago and he asked me what had happened. I met him and the pastor said I have not seen you? I said yes, I do come but I need to talk to you later. Yes. That experience made me less religious but more spiritual. Yes, in terms of faith that is where I am, unlike the great scientists, especially physicists and so on, who say in all of these things they have not seen the presence of God in the universe. As if God is somewhere and you must go and look for this guy called God. I think it is a misconception of the idea of God the way I see it. I have read the Bible and I have studied it, not extremely thoroughly but I know it. At some point, in 1966, I did a correspondence course in theology. I got a diploma in theology even before I completed my secondary education.

I noticed that there was a problem with the translation of the Bible from the original tongues into the King James version. It had to be done in a manner that was going to please the authority, King James. It had to be authorized by King James. Yes. So what I believe is there are some chapters or sections which were omitted in the translation and those chapters talked about the human race and then there were some people even praising the dark-skinned race and some person singing very beautiful songs. However, it so happened that this material was not included into the King James version because it was praising other races, other than whites, and King James who was the authority did not want to be shown that there are people who were greater than him. You know King James was a leader of the entire British Empire and its other colonies. If you see, there was a letter that was written by these Christian scholars. I have a copy of that somewhere; it is in the office. It is included in the older versions and actually appears to be a letter of transmission. So there are certain aspects of the Bible that were left behind, that were omitted, and during that particular period they were saying, "We did not include this because we were not divinely inspired", so they had to create some excuses for excluding certain literature from the Bible. That is why I have a quarrel with the King James version, so if you see there is now an African Bible, yes, which now contains all of those previously omitted materials. A sect of the Catholic Church has created it. Yes, an African Bible and it even names communities from Africa: there are Luos, there are Kikuyus spelled in the Bible, or similar ethnic groups, and other communities in the whole of Africa.

Yes, I am a spiritual man but not religious. I used to hear these international preachers say that the only thing that we need to take care of is our relationship with God. We know that there is a God that has a power greater than our own. If you do not listen to him, you see, God is justice....

Epilogue

Davy Kiprotich Koech

This book is a brief account of my life's journey in colonial and independent Kenya. It also reflects experiences, which the persons of my generation went through in rural Kenya, where we had a common birth. This is a unique book. I have a story to tell through Denielle Elliott, a person who makes the argument out of it, and communicates the same to the greater public. I am sure she has made a great deal of effort to achieve this. I am yet to seek my inner soul to find out whether or not my co-author has given a fair and honest critique of my storytelling. I am not a student of history or of anthropology or of ethnography. Denielle Elliott is not a student of science either; but we allowed our shadows to merge into one so that our various competences would produce a solid product. As a scholar, I would not refuse another scholar, in the person of Denielle, in finding academic comfort in my stories. But there have been occasions when the red lines had to be drawn.

I must apologize to Denielle for the long period she spent tracing me, yet I was only a phone call away. Our meeting at Meriada Gardens in the suburbs of Lavington in Nairobi was relaxing and homely, thanks to my social friends who entertained us when we were tired. Charles Nyabera and his siblings made us comfortable as we went ahead with our interviews. Their maternal uncle, Mzee Edmund Oyuga, was my secondary school teacher at Kericho High School 1965/66 and I had the opportunity of meeting with him again in 2016 after 50 years! I appreciate the professionalism in Denielle and especially the way she critiqued my stories. She had the courage to put down some of the negative comments made by others about me, and as I accepted those criticisms, I had the opportunity to tell my story. And if there is anyone who knows me best, it is me. I do, however, have my own strengths and weaknesses. Denielle has been a worthy co-author, and I am indeed indebted to her.

During my youth, my world was within the boundaries of my village, aiming to be a better hunter and a honey gatherer; but this was interrupted by my father who convinced me to go to school so that I could be able to purchase some clothes for myself and be able to read like him. I had no serious ambition, probably because I was too young to critique my surrounding. But making the first step of going to school brought in new challenges and promises for opportunities that I could hardly comprehend. I slowly came to realize that there was a world there beyond my village; a world with unique possibilities and opportunities, and these are summarized in this book, however inexhaustible they may be.

Because of the nature of my background, every step on the way was full of challenges to the point of feeling frustrated and planning to give up. Walking 4 km to school every day at the age of five years, and walking 20 km one way for another four years to attend intermediate school were not only challenging but torturous, let alone breaking my leg and facing the danger of it being amputated as a result of negligence by the hospital staff. The alternative opportunities were limited; and when they availed themselves, new challenges came to play. As I set my journey to distant lands where I also matured, I encountered one obstacle after another, but I was determined to overcome them; and every hurdle overcome was a triumph which came with a crown. Secondary and university education were no better, but I was more prepared to face any challenge.

These challenges have been described in brief in this book; from choosing and changing my degree courses, graduate studies and employment. In the midst of these challenges, there are some initiatives which I participated in and which formed the greater part of my joy and satisfaction. These were the introduction of the credit/unit system in our public universities in the 1970s; the amendment of the Science & Technology Act of 1979 that facilitated the establishment of research institutes in Kenya, including the Kenya Medical Research Institute (KEMRI). KEMRI is an institution where I was privileged to be Director and Chief Executive for a record 22 years, and where I became the longest-serving Chief Executive of a public organization in the history of Kenya; the introduction of tissue-typing technique and later DNA technology for use in donor-related tissue transplants in Kenya (1985); and the enactment of Universities Act (Cap 210B of 1985) that led to the establishment of the Commission for Higher Education (now renamed Commission for University Education, under Universities Act, No. 42 of 2012). Whenever I visit or see learners, including my own children, streaming to private universities in Kenya, I feel very happy, proud and satisfied. It is the consequence partly of my 20 years of participation in serving the Commission, initially as chair of the Technical Committee, for five years, which set out standards of private university infrastructural facilities, a further five years as the Vice-Chairman and another ten years as the Chairman of the Commission.

I came to realize that it is difficult to change the policy in a bureaucratic system especially if the change does not favour or benefit the political elites. If there was no authority ready to listen and agree to make changes, no amount of persuasion would make those changes. My luck was that somebody was ready to listen. The amendment of the Science & Technology Act took place at that time because President Moi was ready to listen, and Attorney General Charles Njonjo agreed to Moi's request. The Commission for Higher Education was established at that time because the Minister for Higher Education, Prof. Jonathan Ng'eno, had the patience to listen and to agree to act. I learned that one has to have the art of negotiating with, and convincing government officials and political leadership to agree to, and to act on anything.

My friendship with President Moi is cited a couple of times in this book. These are the fruits of this friendship. I never used the friendship either to enrich myself or to undermine other Kenyans. I used it for the benefit Kenya and Kenyans; and, as part of collateral benefits of our friendship, I accepted to be part of any team that was chosen to push the government's idea and agenda forward.

Like those in public service in most governments of the world, I came to notice that some self-serving agents of the State no longer valued my services. I was simply being tolerated, frustrated and vilified. So, I realized that it was time for me to move on and to have a new start elsewhere and where I am celebrated. I felt saddened to be forced to leave KEMRI, an institution I helped to establish, to nurture and to grow, and where I spent my prime active life. That aside, my happiness was that I spent 36 years in the public service with utmost dedication. I undertook every assignment I was given with dedication and the seriousness it deserved and I never disappointed any appointing authority. My reward did not come from my employers, but from the satisfied public; and it is in the interest of the same public that I have derived extra strength in order to continue to serve them. Additionally, as I reflect on my humble contribution to humanity, interrupted by the myriad of challenges, I have come to believe that the energy, tolerance, patience and focus have been granted to me by the grace of one who is way above my mortal self.

If I have made any modest contribution in education, health, science and scholarship, it is because I have always believed in being the custodian of my own conscience. If my conscience fires my soul to venture into any untested grounds, I have never hesitated to do so, no matter the risks that abound with such ventures. I believe that by doing so, I cannot cause for others and myself any unknown harm, but I could, at the very least, pioneer a thought, an idea or a technique that may alter or better the lives of others. Similarly, I have never worried myself if I could be a success in life, nor expected any reward or credit for what I am doing, but rather, if I could be of value in my service to humanity.

The penultimate story is yet to be written.

Bibliography

Abraham, Tara. 2016 *Rebel Genius: Warren S. McCulloch's Transdisciplinary Life in Science*. Cambridge: The MIT Press.

Abu-Lughod, Lila. 2008 *Writing Women's Worlds: Bedouin Stories*. Berkeley: University of California Press.

Adar, Korwa and Isaac Munyae. 2001 Human Rights Abuse in Kenya Under Daniel arap Moi, 1978–2001. *African Studies Quarterly* 5(1): 1–17.

Anderson, David. 2005 *Histories of the Hanged: The Dirty War in Kenya and the End of Empire*. New York: W.W. Norton and Company.

Anderson, David and Øystein Rolandsen. 2014 Violence as Politics in Eastern Africa, 1940–1990: Legacy, Agency, Contingency. *Journal of East African Studies* 8(4): 539–557.

Arendt, Hannah. 1979 *Daguerrotypes and Other Essays*. Chicago: University of Chicago Press.

Atieno-Odhiambo and Elisha Stephen. 2002 Hegemonic Enterprises and Instrumentalities of Survival: Ethnicity and Democracy in Kenya. *African Studies* 61(2): 222–249.

Bangstad, Sindre. 2017 Doing Fieldwork among People We Don't (Necessarily) Like. *Anthropology News* website, 28 August. doi: 10.1111/AN.584.

Behar, Ruth. 2014 *Translated Woman: Crossing the Border with Esperanza's Story*. Boston: Beacon Press.

Blum, Allan. 2001 Scenes. *Public* 22/23: 7–35.

Bonneuil, Christophe. 2000 Science and State Building in Late Colonial and Postcolonial Africa, 1930–1970. In Nature and Empire: Science and the Colonial Enterprise, *Osiris* 15: 258–281.

Booth, Karen. 2004 *Local Women, Global Science: Fighting AIDS in Kenya*. Bloomington: Indiana University Press.

Branch, Daniel. 2011 *Kenya: Between Hope and Despair, 1963–2011*. New Haven: Yale University Press.

Branch, Daniel, Nic Cheeseman and Leigh Gardner, eds. 2010 *Our Turn to Eat: Politics in Kenya Since 1950*. Berlin: Lit Verlag.

Brown, Stephen. 2001 Authoritarian Leaders and Multiparty Elections in Africa: How Foreign Donors Help to Keep Kenya's Daniel arap Moi in Power. *Third World Quarterly* 22(5): 725–739.

Burke, Jason. 2017 Kenyan Election Official "Tortured and Murdered" as Fears of Violence Grow. *Guardian*, 31 July, www.theguardian.com/world/2017/jul/31/kenyan-election-official-christopher-msando-dead-before-national-vote, accessed 16 January 2018.

Burton, Timothy, dir. 2003 *Big Fish*. Culver City: Sony Pictures. Motion Picture.

Carney, Judith. 1996 Landscapes of Technology Transfer: Rice Cultivation and African Continuities. *Technology and Culture* 37(1): 5–35.

Cavarero, Adriana. 1997 *Relating Narratives: Storytelling and Selfhood*. London: Routledge.

Chernoff, John. 2003 *Hustling is Not Stealing: Stories of an African Bar Girl*. Chicago: University of Chicago Press.

Citizens for Justice. 2003 *We Lived to Tell: The Nyayo House Story*. Nairobi: Friedrich Ebert Stiftung.

Clifford, James. 1986 Introduction: Partial Truths. In *Writing Culture: The Poetics and Politics of Ethnography*, edited by James Clifford and George Marcus, 1–26. Berkeley: University of California Press.

Cohen, David William and E. S. Atieno-Odhiambo. 2004 *The Risks of Knowledge: Investigations into the Death of the Hon. Minister John Robert Ouko in Kenya, 1990*. Athens: Ohio University Press.

Comaroff, Jean and John L. Comaroff, eds. 2008 *Law and Disorder in the Postcolony*. Chicago: University of Chicago Press.

Crapanzano, Vincent. 1986 *Waiting: The Whites of South Africa*. New York: Vintage.

Crozier, Anna. 2007 *Practising Colonial Medicine: The Colonial Medical Service in British East Africa*. New York: I.B.Tauris.

Cruikshank, Julie. 1991 *Life Lived Like a Story: Life Stories of Three Yukon Native Elders*. Lincoln: University of Nebraska Press.

Cummins, Joseph and Jerzy Georgiades. 1993 How It Began. *Archivum Immunologiae et Therapiae Experimentalis* 41: 169–172.

De Boeck, Filip. 2012 Infrastructure: Commentary from Filip De Boeck. Curated Collections, *Cultural Anthropology* website, 26 November, https://culanth.org/curated_collections/11-infrastructure/discussions/7-infrastructure-commentary-from-filip-de-boeck.

De Laet, Marianne and A. Annemarie Mol. 2000 The Zimbabwe Bush Pump: Mechanics of a Fluid Technology. *Social Studies of Science* 30(2): 225–263.

Disch, Lisa J. 1993 More Truth Than Fact: Storytelling as Critical Understanding in the Writing of Hannah Arendt. *Political Theory* 21(4): 665–694.

Dodd, Rebecca. 1996 Patients Sue "AIDS-cure" Kenyan Scientist. *Lancet* 347(9016): 1688.

Droney, Damien. 2014 Ironies of Laboratory Work during Ghana's Second Age of Optimism. *Cultural Anthropology* 29(2): 363–384. https://doi.org/10.14506/ca29.2.10.

Edwards, Paul. 2003 Infrastructure and Modernity: Force, Time, and Social Organization in the History of Socio-Technical Systems. In *Modernity and Technology*, edited by Arie Rip, Philip Brey and Andrew Feenberg, 185–225. Cambridge: MIT Press.

Elkin, Caroline. 2005 *Imperial Reckoning: The Untold Story of Britain's Gulag in Kenya*. New York: Henry Holt and Company.

Elliott, Denielle. 2014 The Protected Lab: Securitization and Spaces of Exclusion in Global Medicine. *Medical Anthropology Theory* 1(1): 81–113.

Elliott, Denielle. 2016 The Problem with the Truth: Political Alliances, Science, and Storytelling in Nairobi. *Critical African Studies* 8(3): 306–318.

Elliott, Denielle. 2017 Transnational Scientific Projects and Racial Politics: The KEMRI Six Case Against the KEMRI-Wellcome Trust Research Programme in Contemporary Kenya, *MEDIZINETHNOLOGIE*, www.medizinethnologie.net/the-kemri-six-case/.

Fassin, Didier. 2007 *When Bodies Remember: Experience and Politics of AIDS in South Africa*. Berkeley: University of California Press.

Fassin, Didier. 2008 Life & Times of Magda A: Telling a Story of Violence in South Africa. *Current Anthropology* 49(2): 225–246.

Foeken, Dick and Ton Dietz. 2000 Of Ethnicity, Manipulation and Observation: The 1992 and 1997 Elections in Kenya. In *Election Observation and Democratization in Africa*, edited by Jon Abbink and Gerti Hesseling, 122–149. London: Palgrave Macmillan.

Foreign Broadcast Information Service. 1990 Moi Launches Anti-AIDS Drug. *JPRS Report: Epidemiology*, AIDS, August 1990.

Fortun, Kim. 2001 *Advocacy After Bhopal: Environmentalism, Disaster, New Global Orders*. Chicago: University of Chicago Press.

Fox Keller, Evelyn. 1983 *A Feeling for the Organism*. San Francisco: W. H. Freeman and Company.

Fullwiley, Duana. 2011 *The Enculturated Gene: Sickle Cell Health Politics and Biological Difference in West Africa*. Princeton: Princeton University Press.

Gathii, James Thuo. 2009 Defining the Relationship Between Human Rights and Corruption. *University of Pennsylvania Journal of International Law* 31(1): 125–202.

Gathii, James Thuo. 2011 Kenya's Long Anti-Corruption Agenda–1952–2010: Prospects and Challenges of the Ethics and Anti-Corruption Commission under the 2010 Constitution. *The Law and Development Review* 4(3): 184–237.

Geissler, Wenzel. 2011 Parasite Lost: Remembering Modern Times with Kenyan Government Medical Scientists. In *Evidence, Ethos and Experiment: The Anthropology and History of Medical Research in Africa*, edited by Wenzel Geissler and Sassy Molyneux, 297–232. Oxford: Berghahn.

Geissler, Wenzel and Noémi Tousignant. 2016 Capacity as History and Horizon: Infrastructure, Autonomy and Infrastructure in African Health Sciences and Care. *Canadian Journal of African Studies* 50(3): 349–359.

Gibb, Camilla. 2006 Telling Tales out of School, a Research in Society Lecture Delivered at the 2007 Congress of the Humanities and Social Sciences. *ESC* 32(2/3): 39–54.

Gordimer, Nadine. 1989 *The Essential Gesture: Writing, Politics and Places*. London, UK: Penguin Books.

Graboyes, Melissa. 2015 *The Experiment Must Continue: Medical Research and Ethics in East Africa, 1940–2014*. Athens: Ohio University Press.

Green, Mott. 2007 Writing Scientific Biography. *Journal of the History of Biology* 40: 727–759.

Gupta, Akhil. 1995 Blurred Boundaries: The Discourse of Corruption, the Culture of Politics, and the Imagined State. *American Ethnologist* 22(2): 375–402.

Gupta, Akhil. 2012 *Red Tape: Bureaucracy, Structural Violence, and Poverty in India*. Durham: Duke University Press.

Hamilton, Carolyn. 2011 Biography, and the Life of the James Stuart Archive. *History of Africa* 38: 319–341.

Hasty, Jennifer. 2005 The Pleasures of Corruption: Desire and Discipline in Ghanaian Political Culture. *Cultural Anthropology* 20(2): 271–301.

Hecht, Gabrielle. 2012 *Being Nuclear: Africans and Global Uranium Trade*. Cambridge: The MIT Press.

Hecht, Tobias. 2007 A Case for Ethnographic Fiction. *Anthropology News* 48(2): 17–18.

Hempstone, Smith. 1997 *Rogue Ambassador: An African Memoir*. Sewanee: University of South Press.

Hinton, Alexander Laban. 2004 *Why Did They Kill? Cambodia in the Shadow of Genocide*. Berkeley: University of California Press.

Hinton, Alexander Laban. 2016 *Man or Monster? The Trial of a Khmer Rouge Torturer*. Durham: Duke University Press.

Hornsby, Charles. 2012 *Kenya: A History Since Independence*. London: I.B. Tauris.

Hsien-Yu, Chin. 1989 Colonial Medical Police and Postcolonial Medical Surveillance Systems in Taiwan, 1895–1950s. *Osiris* 13: 326–338.

Hull, Matthew. 2012 Documents and Bureaucracy. *Annual Review of Anthropology* 41: 251–267.

Human Rights Watch. 2002 *Kenya's Unfinished Democracy: A Human Rights Agenda for the New Government*. New York: Human Rights Watch. Available online, www.hrw.org/report/2002/12/12/kenyas-unfinished-democracy/human-rights-agenda-new-government.

Hunt, Nancy Rose. 2008 An Acoustic Register, Tenacious Images, and Congolese Scenes of Rape and Repetition. *Cultural Anthropology* 23(2): 220–253.

Hunt, Nancy Rose. 2013 *Suturing New Medical Histories of Africa*. Berlin: Lit Verlag.

Hunt, Nancy Rose. 2016 *A Nervous State: Violence, Remedies and Reverie in Colonial Congo*. Durham: Duke University Press.

Hutchinson, Lauren. 2017 Planning National Malaria Research in Kenya 1977–2010: Space and Place in Global Biomedicine. PhD thesis, London School of Hygiene and Tropical Medicine. DOI: 10.17037/PUBS.04645399.

Ireri, Elijah Njagi. 2016 Assessment of Problems Facing State Owned Enterprises in Kenya. *International Journal of Business, Humanities, and Technology* 6(4): 40–45.

Jackson, Michael. 2004 *In Sierra Leone*. Durham: Duke University Press.

Jackson, Michael. 2013a *The Wherewithal of Life: Ethics, Migration, and the Question of Well-Being*. Berkeley: University of California Press.

Jackson, Michael. 2013b *The Politics of Storytelling: Variations on a theme by Hannah Arendt*. Chicago: University of Chicago Press.

Jacobs, Nancy. 2006 The Intimate Politics of Ornithology in Colonial Africa. *Comparative Studies in Society and History* 48(3): 564–603.

Jordan, Wilbert. 1994 Three Open-Label Studies of Oral Interferon Alpha in the Treatment of HIV Disease. *Journal of the National Medical Association* 86(4): 257–262.

Josephson, Paul. 1997 *New Atlantis Revisited: Akademgorodok, the Siberian City of Science*. Princeton: Princeton University Press.

Kagwanja, Peter Mwangi. 2003 Facing Mount Kenya or Facing Mecca? The Mungiki, Ethnic Violence, and the Politics of the Moi Succession in Kenya, 1987–2002. *African Affairs* 102: 25–49.

Kagwanja, Peter Mwangi. 2005 "Power to Uhuru": Youth Identity and Generational Politics in Kenya's 2002 Elections. *African Affairs* 105(418): 51–75.

Kanyinga, Karuti, and John Murimi Njoka. 2002 The Role of Youth in Politics: The Social Praxis of Party Politics Among the Urban Lumpen in Kenya. *African Journal of sociology* 4(2): 89–111.

Kareithi, Amos. 2013 Math Guru, Magician and Man of Steel. *Standard Digital*, 12 May, 2013, www.standardmedia.co.ke/lifestyle/article/2000083434/math-guru-magician-and-man-of-steel, accessed 14 January 2018.

Kariuki, James. 1996 "Paramoia": Anatomy of a Dictatorship in Kenya. *Journal of Contemporary African Studies* 14(1): 69–86.

Khapoya, Vincent and Baffour Agyeman-Duah. 1985 The Cold War and Regional Politics in East Africa. *Journal of Conflict Studies* 5(2): 18–32.

Koech, Davy. 1999 Totally Integrated Quality Education and Training (TIQET): Report of Commission of Inquiry into the Education System of Kenya. Nairobi.

Koech, Davy. 2009 *I Remember: Eye-witness Account of the Historical Development of the Kenya Medical Research Institute (KEMRI)*. Unpublished manuscript.

Koech, Davy and Arthur Obel. 1990 Efficacy of Kemron (Low Dose Oral Natural Human Interferon Alpha) in the Management of HIV-1 Infection and Acquired Immune Deficiency Syndrome (AIDS). *East African Medical Journal* 67: ss67–70.

Krotz, Larry. 2012 *Piecing the Puzzle: The Genesis of AIDS Research in Africa.* Winnipeg: University of Manitoba Press.

Kuhn, Annette. 2002 *Family Secrets: Acts of Memory and Imagination.* London: Verso Books.

Lachenal, Guillaume. 2017 *The Lomidine Files: The Untold Story of a Medical Disaster in Colonial Africa*, translated by Noémi Tousignant. Baltimore: John Hopkins University Press.

Lampland, Martha, and Susan Leigh Star, eds. 2009 *Standards and Their Stories: How Quantifying, Classifying, and Formalizing Practices Shape Everyday Life.* Ithaca: Cornell University Press.

Larkin, Brian. 2008 *Signal and Noise: Media, Infrastructure, and Urban Culture in Nigeria.* Durham: Duke University Press.

Larkin, Brian. 2013 The Politics and Poetics of Infrastructure. *Annual Review of Anthropology* 42 (2013): 327–343.

Latour, Bruno and Steve Woolgar. 1979 *Laboratory Life: The Construction of Scientific Facts.* Princeton: Princeton University Press.

Lucas, Sarah. 2017 The Primacy of Narrative Agency: Re-Reading Seyla Benhabib on Narrativity. *Feminist Theory* 18, DOI: 10.1177/1464700117723591.

Lynch, Gabrielle. 2008 Moi: The Making of an African 'Big-Man'. *Journal of Eastern African Studies* 2(1): 18–43.

Lynch, Gabrielle. 2011 *I Say to You: Ethnic Politics and the Kalenjin in Kenya.* Chicago: University of Chicago Press.

Lynch, Gabrielle. 2015 The International Criminal Court and the Making of a Kenyan President. *Current History* 114(772): 183–188.

Mains, Daniel. 2012 Blackouts and Progress: Privatization, Infrastructure, and a Developmentalist State in Jimma, Ethiopia. *Cultural Anthropology* 27(1): 3–27.

Mavhunga, Clapperton Chakanetsa, ed. 2017 *What Do Science, Technology and Innovation Mean from Africa?* Cambridge: The MIT Press.

Menchú, Rigoberta. 2010 *I, Rigoberta Menchú: An Indian Woman in Guatemala.* London: Verso Books.

Mialet, Hélène. 2012 *Hawking Incorporated: Stephen Hawking and the Anthropology of the Knowing Subject.* Chicago: University of Chicago Press.

Mohanty, Chandra Talpade. 1991 Introduction: Cartographies of Struggle, Third World Women and the Politics of Feminism. In *Third World Women and the Politics of Feminism*, edited by Chandra Talpade Mohanty, Anne Russo and Lourdes Torres, 1–47. Bloomington: Indiana University Press.

Moore, Sally Falk. 1998 Systematic Judicial and Extra-Judicial Injustice: Preparations for Future Accountability. In *Memory and the Postcolony*, edited by Richard Werbner, 126–151. London: Zed Books.

Morton, Andrew. 1998 *Moi: The Making of an African Statesman.* London: Michael O'Mara Books Limited.

Muhammad, Askia. 2002 Farrakhan Vows to Fight AIDS in Zimbabwe. *The Final Call*, 23 July 2002.

Murunga, Godwin. 2004 The State, its Reform and the Question of Legitimacy in Kenya. *Identity, Culture and Politics* 5(1/2): 179–206.

Murunga, Godwin. 2007 Governance and the Politics of Structural Adjustment Programs in Kenya. In *Kenya: The Struggle for Democracy*, edited by Godwin Murunga and Shadrack Nasong'o, 263–301. London: Zed Books.

Murunga, Godwin and Shadrack Nasong'o. 2007 *Kenya: The Struggle for Democracy*. London: Zed Books.

Musila, Grace. 2015 *A Death Retold in Truth and Rumour: Kenya, Britain and the Julie Ward Murder*. Suffolk: James Currey.

Musyoka, Stephen Kalonzo with Caleb Atemi. 2016 *Against All Odds*. Hong Kong: Peace Books.

Mutongi, Kenda. 2017 *Matatu: A History of Popular Transportation in Nairobi*. Chicago: University of Chicago Press.

National Institute of Allergy and Medicine. 1992 *Executive Summary: AIDS Research Advisory Committee*. Washington, DC: National Institute of Allergy and Infectious Diseases, available on line at https://aidsinfo.nih.gov/news/44/executive-summary-aids-research-advisory-committee-national-institute-of-allergy-and-infectious-diseases.

Nattrass, Nicoli. 2013 *The AIDS Conspiracy: Science Fights Back*. New York: Columbia University Press.

Neill, Deb. 2009 Paul Ehrlich's Colonial Connections: Scientific Networks and Sleeping Sickness Drug Therapy Research, 1900–1914. *Social History of Medicine* 22(1): 61–77.

Neill, Deb. 2012 *Networks in Tropical Medicine: Internationalism, Colonialism, and the Rise of a Medical Specialty, 1890–1930*. Stanford: Stanford University Press.

Ninetto, Amy. 2001 "Civilization" and its Insecurities: Traveling Scientists, Global Science, and National Progress in the Novosibirsk Akademgorodok. *Kroeber Anthropological Society Papers* (86): 181–202.

Nye, Mary Jo. 2006 Scientific Biography: History of Science by Another Means? *Isis* 97(2): 322–329.

Ogot, Bethwell. 1963 British Administration in the Central Nyanza District of Kenya, 1900–60. *The Journal of African History* 4(2): 249–273.

Okuro, Samwel Ong'wen. 2009 Daniel arap Moi and the Politics of HIV and AIDS in Kenya, 1983–2002. *African Journal of AIDS Research* 8(3): 275–283.

Oliech, Joseph. 1990 Editorial: The AIDS Situation and its Containment. *East African Medical Journal* 67(7): 1–9.

Olingo, Allan. 2015 KEMRI under Investigation over Cash Scandal. *The East African*, 28 March, 2015, www.theeastafrican.co.ke/news/Kemri-under-investigation-over-cash-scandal/2558-2668296-4yxk0v/index.html, accessed 16 January 2018.

Osseo-Assare and Abena Dove. 2008 Bioprospecting and Resistance: Transforming Poisoned Arrows into Strophantin Pills in Colonial Gold Coast, 1885–1922. *Social History of Medicine* 21(2): 269–290.

Pandian, Anand and M. P. Mariappan. 2014 *Ayya's Accounts: A Ledger of Hope in Modern India*. Bloomington: Indiana University Press.

Parr, Joy. 2010 "Don't Speak For Me": Practicing Oral History amidst the Legacies of Conflict. *Journal of the Canadian Historical Association* 211: 1–11. DOI: 10.7202/1003040ar.

Peters, Rebecca and Claire Wendland. 2016 Up the Africanist: The Possibilities and Problems of "Studying Up" in Africa. *Critical African Studies* 8(3): 239–254.

Peterson, Kris. 2014 *Speculative Markets: Drug Circuits and Derivative Life in Nigeria*. Durham: Duke University Press.

Piot, Peter. 2012 *No Time to Lose: A Life in Pursuit of Deadly Viruses*. New York: W. W. Norton.

Poissonnier, A. 1990 African Mobilization against AIDS: After the Kinshasa Conference. *Jeune Afrique* 1556: 30–31.

Pollock, Anne. 2014 Places of Pharmaceutical Knowledge-Making: Global Health, Post-Colonial Science, and Hope in South African Drug Discovery. *Social Study of Science* 44(6): 848–873.

Portelli, Alexandro. 2005 A Dialogical Relationship: An Approach to Oral History. In *Expressions Annual*, edited by Manish Jain, available at www.swaraj.org/shikshantar/expressions_portelli.pdf.

Porter, Theodore. 2006 Is the Life of a Scientist a Scientific Unit? *Isis* 97: 314–321.

Psirmoi, Daniel. 2016 How KEMRI Staff Formed NGO to Get Donor Cash. *Standard Digital*, 10 February, www.standardmedia.co.ke/article/2000191156/how-kemri-staff-formed-ngo-to-get-donor-cash, accessed 16 January 2018.

Redfield, Peter. 2002 The Half-Life of Empire in Outer Space. *Social Studies of Science* 32(6): 791–825.

Richards, Joan. 2006 Introduction: Fragmented Lives. *Isis* 97: 302–305.

Robertson, Leslie and Dara Culhane, eds. 2005 *In Plain Sight: Reflections on Life in Downtown Eastside Vancouver*. Vancouver: Talonbooks.

Robertson, Leslie and the Kwagu'l Gixsam Clan. 2012 *Standing Up with Ga'axsta'las: Jane Constance Cook and the Politics of Memory, Church, and Custom*. Vancouver: UBC Press.

Royles, Dan. 2012 "We've Been Doing This for a Few Thousand Years": The Nation of Islam's African AIDS Cure. Paper presented at the James A. Barnes Graduate History Conference, Philadelphia, 17 March 2012.

Schacter, Daniel. 2013 Memory: Sins and Virtues. *Annals of the New York Academy of Sciences* 1303: 56–60.

Schnitzler, Antina. 2013 Traveling Technologies: Infrastructure, Ethical Regimes, and the Materiality of Politics in South Africa. *Cultural Anthropology* 28(4): 670–693.

Shilaho, Westen K. 2017 *Political Power and Tribalism in Kenya*. Johannesburg: Springer.

Shostak, Marjorie. 2014 *Nisa: The Life and Words of a !Kung Woman*. London: Routledge.

Simone, AbdouMaliq. 2012 Infrastructure: Introductory Commentary by AbdouMaliq Simone." Curated Collections, *Cultural Anthropology* website, 26 November, https://culanth.org/curated_collections/11-infrastructure/discussions/12-infrastructure-introductory-commentary-by-abdoumaliq-simon.

Sium, Aman and Eric Ritskes. 2013 Speaking Truth to Power: Indigenous Storytelling as an Act of Living Resistance. *Decolonization: Indigeneity, Education & Society* 2(1): I–X.

Smith, Daniel Jordan. 2007 *A Culture of Corruption: Everyday Deception and Popular Discontent in Nigeria*. Princeton: Princeton University Press.

Song, Priscilla. 2017 *Biomedical Odysseys: Fetal Cell Experiments from Cyberspace to China*. Princeton: Princeton University Press.

Star, Susan Leigh. 1999 The Ethnography of Infrastructure. *American Behavioral Scientist* 43(3): 377–391.

Stoler, Ann. 2002 Colonial Archives and the Arts of Governance. *Archival Science* 2: 87–102.

Straw, Will. 2001 Scenes and Sensibilities. *Public* 22/23: 245–257.

Straw, Will. 2015 Some Things a Scene Might be. *Cultural Studies* 29(3): 476–485.

Taussig, Michael. 1999 *Defacement: Public Secrecy and the Labor of the Negative*. Stanford: Stanford University Press.

Tilley, Helen. 2011 *Africa as a Living Laboratory: Empire, Development, and the Problem of Scientific Knowledge, 1870–1950*. Chicago: University of Chicago Press.

Tomaselli, Keyan. 2003 Stories to Tell, Stories to Sell: Resisting Textualization. *Cultural Studies* 17(6): 856–875.

Tousignant, Noémi. 2013 Broken Tempos: Of Means and Memory in a Senegalese University Laboratory. *Social Studies of Science* 43(5): 729–753.

Transparency International. 2015 People and Corruption: Africa Survey 2015. Available at www.transparency.org/whatwedo/publication/people_and_corruption_africa_survey_2015.

Umlauf, René and Sung-Joon Park. 2017 Stock-Outs! Improvisations and Processes of Infrastructuring in Uganda's HIV/AIDS and Malaria Programmes. *Global Public Health* 1692 (December): 1–14.

Vaughan, Megan. 1991 *Curing their Ills: Colonial Power and African Illness*. Stanford: Stanford University Press.

Verran, Helen. 2001 *Science and an African Logic*. Chicago: University of Chicago Press.

wa Thiong'o, Ngũgĩ. 2011 (1981) *Detained: A Writer's Prison Diary*. Nairobi: Sitima Printers.

Waldram, James. 2012 *Hound Pound Narrative: Sexual Offender Habilitation and the Anthropology of Therapeutic Intervention*. Berkeley: University of California Press.

Waris, Attiya. 2007 Taxation without Principles: A Historical Analysis of the Kenyan Taxation System. *Kenya Law Review* 1: 272–304.

Wendland, Claire. 2008 Research, Therapy, and Bioethical Hegemony: The Controversy over Perinatal AZT Trials in Africa. *African Studies Review* 51(3): 1–23.

Wendland, Claire. 2010 *A Heart for the Work: Journeys through an African Medical School*. Chicago: University of Chicago Press.

Wesangula, Daniel. 2015 KEMRI Develops First Malaria Vaccine, *The Standard*, 2 August, www.standardmedia.co.ke/health/article/2000171275/kemri-develops-first-malaria-vaccine, accessed 15 January 2018.

White, Luise. 2000 *Speaking with Vampires: Rumor and History in Colonial Africa*. Berkeley: University of California Press.

Woo, Rennie and Poyntz. 2015 Scene Thinking: Introduction. *Cultural Studies* 29(3): 285–297.

Wright, Stephen E., David P. Hutcheson and Joseph M. Cummins. 1998 Low Dose Oral Interferon Alpha 2a in HIV-1 Seropositive Patients: A Double-blind, Placebo-controlled Trial. *Biotherapy* 11(4): 229–234.

Wrong, Michela. 2009 *It's Our Turn to Eat: The Story of a Kenyan Whistle Blower*. London: Fourth Estate.

Wrong, Michela. 2014 "Everyone is Corrupt in Kenya, Even Grandmothers": Is East Africa's Economic Powerhouse Becoming the Continent's Newest Lootocracy? *Foreign Policy*, 6 May, available at http://foreignpolicy.com/2014/05/06/everyone-is-corrupt-in-kenya-even-grandmothers/.

Yoshimizu, Ayaka. 2015 Bodies that Remember: Gleaning Scenic Fragments of a Brothel District in Yokohama. *Cultural Studies* 29(3): 450–475.

Index